CORRUPTION IN INDIA

Origin, Causes and Solutions

Edited by

R.K. GUPTA
H.D. BIST

Foreword

C.P. BARTHWAL

ANAMIKA PUBLISHERS & DISTRIBUTORS (P) LTD.
4697/3, 21A, Ansari Road, Daryaganj
New Delhi 110 002
Phone: 23281655, 65827616

First Published 2007

ISBN 81-7975-164-3

PRINTED IN INDIA

Published by Anamika Publishers & Distributors (P) Ltd.,
4697/3, 21A, Ansari Road, Daryaganj, New Delhi 110 002.
Typeset by Phoenix Computer Centre, New Delhi and
Printed at Nagri Printers, Delhi.

CORRUPTION IN INDIA
Origin, Causes and Solutions

FOREWORD

I am pleased to see that the proceedings of the National Seminar on "Corruption in India: Origin, Causes and Solutions" which was organized by Department of Political Science., Govt. P.G. College, Haldwani (Kumaun University, Nainital), jointly with Dev Sanskrit University, Haridwar, under the auspices of Indian Political Science Association, are being published now in an organized fashion in the form of a book. I had also a privilege of serving as one of the organizers of this seminar as the General Secretary of the Indian Political Science Association.

One of the prominent requirements for a meaningful progress in solving any problem in any specific field is to identify the root causes behind the menace. The next task is to chalk out directions and strategies for next decade and onwards for tackling the problems. For this, it is essential that competent persons should critically review the recent trends that are cropping up in the society. They should choose small areas, evaluate the current situation, and suggest fruitful avenues for future changes in the era of liberalization and globalization. It is extremely important that the system advances with time, continuously adapting itself with the ever changing scenario of fast developments in different fields. The Seminar was sponsored by the UGC and ICSSR. Several distinguished scholars in the field had presented papers, participated in discussions and evinced keen interest in the proceedings.

I have gone through the impressive list of papers which are being included in the book. I have been able to read few of them in greater detail. I am happy to say that subject experts have critically reviewed the problem in our country form different angles. A total of 37 articles have been grouped into four sections, for convenience of readers. The book highlights the extent of corruption that has crept in various fields of public life, especially in this fiver year old state of Uttaranchal.

However, the problem is extremely menacing and omnipresent in the global context. The political will and the honesty of the persons at the top in the government and administration are very essential to tackle the problem. It is becoming increasingly evident that the corrupt practices are producing dissatisfied youth in the country. With the continuous population explosion and the inherent desire in the modern man to be rich by quick-fix methods, the menace of corruption has spread throughout the world. It has been institutionalized throughout the country in all aspects of life. The strategies of eradicating it have acquired utmost importance. Efforts need to be made to control the menace.

The relevance of the themes dealt in various chapters of the book in the four sections is of very high significance to the general problem of eradication of corruption form the public life. I am very happy to note that this book would be useful to students, educationists, academicians, politicians, bureaucrats and the general public. The book will provide them a very valuable document in their pursuit of understanding and rooting out corruption.

I take this opportunity to appreciate the efforts of the organizers and the editors to bring out this valuable and useful volume which would be a wonderful addition to the world of literature on the subject.

(Prof. C.P. Barthwal)
V.C., Kumaon University,
Nainital (UA)

Dated: 25.08.2006
Nainital

PREFACE

In recent years, the Govt. P.G. College, Haldwani has taken a lead in organizing several major Seminars and Symposia on the contemporary topics of provincial, national and international importance. For example, a two day National Seminar on Quality of Higher Education in General and Uttaranchal in Particular was held under the auspices of Directorate of Higher Education Uttaranchal, jointly with Dev-Sanskrit University, at Dev-Sanskrit University Shanti Kunj, Haridwar on July 28-29, 2003 to remove the malady in the system of Higher Education, producing unemployed and unemployable youth, in the state and the country. The Proceedings of this Seminar were first published in March 2005 in the form of a book titled *Higher Education: Challenges for the Future* (ed. R.K. Gupta and H.D. Bist). In an identical fashion, another National Seminar on "Corruption in India: Origin, Causes and Solutions" was organized by the Department of Political Science, Govt. P.G. College, Haldwani (Kumaon University, Nainital, UA), jointly with Dev–Sanskrit University. The seminar was sponsored by UGC and ICSSR India and was held at Dev–Sanskrit University, Haridwar on October 1-2, 2004. The reviewed, selected papers from the seminar are being published in the form of this book titled "Corruption in India: Origin, Causes and Solutions".

One of the main aims of any such Seminar is to highlight the presentations and preserve them in the form of a book to keep the contemporary thinking for the future reference. The competitive persons in the field should critically review the problems and outline the recent progress and problems in the field. We have chosen 37 articles for this book, to demonstrate a state–of–the–art narration of the problem by the experts in the field. The salient features and observations of corruption in general and India in particular, from various angles, of the authors, have been brought out. The genesis, consequences and remedies of the general problems have to be sorted out through the Parliament by Legislative (Political) means, in the Executive arm by the Bureaucracy through honest implementations of the law-makers' intentions, by the Judiciary by interpreting the law in an efficient manner and by the Societal and the Journalistic means by bring an awareness in the masses. These themes have been highlighted in various chapters. The whole book is divided into four sections to depict the main themes of the various topics in a group of chapters included in it : (i) Corruption and its Various Manifestations, (ii) Corruption in Contemporary India, (iii) Corruption in Politics and Public life, and (iv) Culture, Ethics, Religion and Yoga Aspects. It is, of course, only an artificial division to club together the topics of similar nature, and it should be appreciated that there could not be any hard and fast division of the chapters into a particular section. We hope the authors and the readers will realize the difficulty in making sections in this manner and pardon us to take liberty for such a division.

The first section has 12 papers. In the very begining R.K. Gupta and Shankar Birdi have nicely elaborated the factors that cause corruption and resultant consequences emanating from them. They have also suggested different methods to prevent the corruption. Pushpa Devi in her paper discussed 'what', 'how' and steps needed to improve our understanding of corruption and enhance government's effectiveness in combating it. R.C. Dikshit, former DGP in UP has summarized the all pervasive, dishonesty for private advantage by public servants, NGO's etc in a variety of criminal acts in all walks of social and cultural life. 'No paper moves in most government offices unless chased from office to office and from seat to seat by the applicants with the help of "speed money" is quite frank and revealing! The apathy of the government and tolerance of the public has made us believe that 'the government has become an instrument for the enrichment of politically dominant group.' He has described the situation in ancient and present day India, and other South Asian and African countries through various periods in history. He has nicely elaborated on the factors that cause corruption and resultant consequences emanating from them. He believes that corruption could be cured and eventually totally stamped out by a firm determination on the part of the political leadership by increasing efficiency, bringing transparency and accountability in the system of governance. The illicit enrichment of individuals should be checked and deterred. Further, a system of honest-incentives and corruption- disincentives should be introduced in the public and private individual life. Whereever possible, International cooperation should be taken to eradicate corruption. At the end of his paper he has quoted from the "Action plan for an effective and responsive government from IIPA journal of 1998 to eliminate corruption in public services. Various forms of corruptions have been discussed by R. Dwivedi. Political, Educational, Police, Business, Medical Departmental, White collar, Social, Defence, Religion, Games and Entertainment fields have caught her eyes. K.Srivastava has described the mother of all corruptions—the Political corruption. In the fourth chapter "Corruption—Is It An Issue" S.C. Arora points to the way the widespread Nazarana tradition is, during Diwali, Birthdays etc. The only way to improve the present situation is to inculcate through education, proper age-old Indian traditional social value system in younger generations. N. Swaminathan from Annamalai University has presented a conceptual framework to comprehend corruption. G.P. Singh ex-VC has pointed out the four C's—Casteism, Communalism, Criminalization—of Politics and Crimes Politicization as the main pillars of Corruption, which have become widespread in both the political and social fields in India. However, he agrees that first and foremost form of corruption is Political. The other causes contributing to widespread of corruption in India are Economic (lust for wealth by every citizen in system where unequal sharing of riches exists traditionally); Social (where parents, wife, children etc, aspire with internal ethos for income above the fixed salary); and Moral-degradation of the society as a whole. I.C. Diwedi, from CBI New Delhi has described some formidable constraints in the fight against corruption. S. Parthasarathy from Dev Sanskrit Viswavidyalaya, Haridwar, has also enumerated the origin, causes and solutions to the problem of corruption. He concludes that only Vedantic Philosophy can give the permanent solution for the menace of corruption. S.U. Rahman, elaborates that the poor are less corrupt than the richer people. Hence it is the aspiration of limitless wealth, not the economic needs driving the corruption in our country, the top rank is of Politics in the corruption field. It could be reduced through, religious and cultural emphasis by education. Choices of politicians who are not corrupt, efficient administration and a sound grievance redressing machinery have been suggested by him. Likewise C.S.

Misra emphasizes that the corruption started with the origin of the man and has become a global phenomenon and is being considered a "low-risk, high-profit business" today by the corrupt persons. He elaborates the definitions of corruption and gives 12 reasons for corruption. He maintains that corruption could be minimized by right education and e-governance.

The next 8 chapters have been grouped into 'The Corruption in Contemporary India' section as all of them have 'India' as one of the words on the topic of each chapter. In the first chapter in this section J.L. Rao from Osmania University has remarked that it is difficult to identify corruption; as it thrives in darkness and invisibility. He argues that it is rooted in human nature and is a part of human vices, such as greed and lust for power and wealth, that have made corruption habitualized, and institutionalized both in private and public life. The projections of the political corruption fall in all fields of societal activity. He then quotes Gerald Caiden to enumerate 14 commonly recognized forms of corruptions where unethical transactions are carried out by an individual either in public or in private life. The human nature, the economic scarcity, lack of transparency in administration, complicated legal procedures along with the globalized and developed technology have all contributed to make corruption as a profitable business for those who indulge in it. He has described the details of some of the stories in the Fodder Scam. He has given several instances where the career of a person starts with corruption, e.g. election of MLA or MP with fales declaration of election expenses are the starting point of the career. In the 2nd chapter A. Sharan elaborates on the genesis, cause and cure of corruption and in Indian perspective. In the next chapter A. Saxena discusses corruption and emphasizes that corruption is living in Indian society because of corrupt people, corrupt practices and existence of corrupt system. He mentions Police, Health and Education, Telephones, Power, Land and Building, Administration, Judiciary and Politician, in this connection. He describes the Indian stories of corrupt practices in various fields. Finally he suggests methods to curb and eliminate corruption. In the 4th chapter, A.K. Singh defines the types and causes of corruption, and gives examples of it during various periods of history in different societies and countries. In the 5th chapter, J.K. Das describes the magnitude of corruption by citing various examples in pre- and post-independent India and suggests 28 measures to facilitate a near corruption-free democratic society and its governance. In the 6th chapter, B. Singh and V.S. Shekhawat enunciate few examples of misrule by administrators; and public rising against them. They point out that the corruption has been facilitated by the erosion of law, extension in the range of reservations, unholy alliance between politicians and Bureaucrats, Tyranny of power brokers, the tussle of power (say, between the PM, the President and the Judiciary), and the Politics of the Vote Bank; to name a few. He concludes that the people of India will make a sound decision and will win eventually to root out corruption. S.S. Tiwana in the 7th chapter gives a few examples of corruption cases taken up by CBI between 1990 and 1996. He gives few remedial measures and an action plan to eradicate corruption from India. And 8th chapter by R. Singh deals in the sociological appraisal of corruption in India.

In the third section there are 11 chapters dealing with Corruption in Indian Politics, Administrative and Public Life. H.D. Bist in his paper discussed corruption in society mentioned typical cases, changing scenario, political constraints. He suggested profession education also along with other measures to check corruption. J.S. Narwal and R.S. Gulia have a re-look on this corruption which started at the time of Pt. Nehru. Scanning through various PMs and Ministers, till George Fernandes, and Chief Ministers in various states, he points out to the influence of corruption in the economic and social fields. The role of Election Commission, President, Governors, the Lokpal and Lokayukta Bills, CBI and Central Vigilance Commission has been pointed out to curb the Pollution created by corruption Industry in politics. Finally they point that peoples participation through education is essential to root out the disease, for which a committed leadership is essential. M. Dixit, quotes Gandhi Ji saying in May 1939 "I would go to the length of giving the whole Congress a decent burial, rather than put up with the corruption that is rampant". The author goes historically through some of the prominent cases of political corruption and its criminalization, where a network of mafia runs a parallel govt. In the next chapters the advantages of public participation in administration have been discussed. A critical review has been made by S.S. Chahar and R. Kundu, to the proposed. Lokpal Bill, 2001, in the 4th chapter. V. Gupta exposes some other salient features of corruption in society and increasing social needs. One of the main deterrent for corruption could be to empower people with the knowledge of their rights and claim them! In the next chapter R. Kundu and S. Lata, have slated various strategies and measures to curb corruption. They have also described the advantages of Public interest Litigation (PIL) and suggested few anti-corruption measures for a holistic analysis consisting of the socio- cultural, economic, political, administrative legal, judicial, and even technological aspects of reforms in the governance system. The next chapter written by S. Kumari emphasizes the significance of social values, joint family system, and Hindu Philosophy to root out the corruption from Govt., political and public life, under new globalized society. The next chapter by M.K. Misra, is on Corruption in Public life. In the next chapter M.V.S.K. Rao and B.P.C. Bose highlight the corruption in the field of Power Sector in Andhra Pradesh. They have quoted the CAG's observations on some Power Plants in the state, and conclude that there are avenues to improve the power in the state if corruption could be controlled. In the last chapter, A. Ravishankar laments that prevalence of "speed money" in India's public life has become a matter of grave concern. He concludes that corruption in India can be controlled by a multi-pronged attack; reforms in political process, restructuring and reorienting the public administration, empowering the people and creating sustained public pressure on speed money.

The fourth section titled "Corruption: Culture, Ethics, Religion and Yoga" has 6 chapters. The first chapter deals with Corruption–Culture and Corporate Governance. In this chapter B. Jayanti from Institute of Labor Studies, Chennai outlines the nexus between public, big business houses, and the bureaucrats. However, for good corporate governance it is essential to have a cherished value system by the management based on a sound moral framework (with transparency and integrity in business operations); keeping in view the legal and administrative framework created by the govt. along with other external factors, affecting the business. The individual and social sense of values accepted by the business and industry, and the system encouraging the corporate governance is needed for flourishing the business in a society in this era of globalization. The author has suggested basic elements of corporate culture with a view to improve corporate governance with transparency, fairness and accountability. The second chapter by G. Sinha illustrates the episodes of the fall of bureaucratic morality and ethical values in administrative culture. He concludes that short and long term measures should be initiated concurrently to combat the menace of corruption, by emphasizing a work culture in all offices. The efficient help from judiciary may also be helpful in this direction. In the 3rd chapter, T. Barthwal and A. Pandey take up the topic of corruption and ethics; and divide it into Money / facility related and human resource development related corruptions. The emphasis on selection of capable human resource is very significant for top positions in any field. The authors have enumerated the five fundamental principles of Ethical management in any company as : (i) Purpose, (ii) Pride, (iii) Patience, (iv) Persistence and (v) Perspective. They have also suggested means to reduce corruption in public dealings. In the 5th chapter D.N. Mishra, A. Misra and S.R. Tripathy suggest methods to fight bureaucratic corruption through moral education to change the mind-set of these officials and to inculcate in them high sense of morality through a series of seminars, workshops and written codes of ethical conduct and positive role models who work as whistle blowers to uncover dubious practices. In the 6th chapter K. Kumar from Hardwar, suggests that Yoga deals the level of consciousness and can change the behavior and whole personality of an individual. Hence Yoga may prove a better solution to the all pervading problems of corruption. The last chapter on "corruption in the name of God", R. Madan feels that the economic dimension of corruption has entered even in religious sphere. The various charity and trusts, in the name of God and Goddesses, are built up and often misused as are some places where temples are made! Likewise it is known that corruption (monetary power or other spheres) is rampant amongst church leaders! The corruption in educational institutions under religious control and the bane of casteism, ethnicity and communalism are often instigated in the name of God. The authors conclude with the hope that a great leader will appear at appropriate time to change the current conditions in India through ethical and religious approaches for solution of the problem of corruption. Finally he suggests that instead of waiting for such an eventuality, we should act now to eradicate the corruption from public life.

R.K. Gupta
H.D. Bist

CONTENTS

CONTRIBUTORS

1. Dr. A. Ravishankar, Reader, Department of Political Science, Presidency College, Chennai, TN.
2. Mr. Abhay Saxena, Lecturer, Department of Computer Science, Dev Sanskrit Vishwavidyalaya, Haridwar, UA.
3. Mr. Amit Pandey, Assistant Professor, Lal Bahadur Shastri Institute of Management and Development Studies, Lucknow.
4. Mr. Arabindbandhu Misra, Reader, Police Training College, Angul- 759122.
5. Dr. Ashok Kumar Singh, Lecturer, Department of Political Science, Y.N. College Chapra, Dighwara, Saran, Bihar.
6. Mr. Ashootosh Sharan, Lecturer, Department of History, Government P.G. College, Uttarkashi, UA.
7. Dr. B. Jayanthi, Assistant Professor, Tamilnadu Institute of Labour Studies, Chennai, T. N.
8. Dr. B.P. Bose, Professor, Department of Political Science and Public Administration, Acharya Nagarjun University, Nagarjun Nagar, Guntur, Andhra Pradesh.
9. Ms. Bibhuti Gupta, Research Scholar, Department of Public Administration, Lucknow University, Lucknow.
10. Dr. C.S. Misra, Department of Computer Science, Bankey Bihari College of Technology, Agra (UP).
11. Mr. Durga Nandan Misra, Sr. Lecturer, PG Department of Psychology, G.M. College, Sambalpur – 768004.
12. Mr. Gaurav Sinha, Department of Public Administration, Lucknow University, Lucknow.
13. Dr. Gopal Prasad Singh, Ex-Pro-Vice Chancellor, (LNMU), Sanhouli, Khagaria, Bihar.

14. Dr. H.D. Bist, Ex-Professor and Emeritus Scientist (CSIR) IIT Kanpur, [14/35, G B Pant Marg, Haldwani, Uttaranchal.]
15. Mr. I.C. Diwedi, IPS, Retired CBI, New Delhi.
16. Mr. J. Laxminarasimha Rao, Associate Professor, Osmania University Hyderabad.
17. Mr. Jagbir S. Narwal, Lecturer, Department of Public Administration, MD University, Rohtak.
18. Mr. Jogendra Kr. Das, DK College, Mirza, Kamrup, Assam.
19. Mr. Kamakhya Kumar, Department of Yoga, Dev Sanskrit University, Hardwar, UA.
20. Kamal Srivastava, Department of Public Administration, University of Lucknow, Lucknow.
21. Dr. M.V.S. Koteswara Rao, Reader, Department of Political Science and Public Administration, Acharya Nagarjun University, Nagarjun Nagar, Guntur, Andhra Pradesh.
22. Mr. Manoj Dixit, Reader, Department of Public Administration, Lucknow University, Lucknow.
23. Dr. Mritunjay K. Misra, Head of Department, Political Science, Government P. G. College, Lohaghat.
24. Dr. N. Swaminathan, Professor and Head, Department of Political Science, Annamalai University, Tamil Nadu.
25. Professor Bhawani Singh, Ex-Professor and Head, Department of Political Science, University of Rajasthan, Jaipur.
26. Professor Raj Singh, Department of Sociology, CCS Haryana Agricultural University, Hisar, Haryana.
27. Dr. (Mrs) Pushpa Devi, Sr. Lecturer in Sociology, MBGPG College, Haldwani, Uttaranchal.
28. R.C. Dikshit, I PS, Former DGP, UP Police.
29. Dr. R.K. Gupta, Reader, Political Science, MBGPG College, Haldwani, Uttaranchal.
30. Dr. Rajesh Kundu, Lecturer, Department of Public Administration, M D University, Rohtak, Haryana.
31. Dr. Ramesh Madan, Assistant Director, ICSSR, New Delhi.
32. Mr. Ranbir S. Gulia, Lecturer, Department of Political Science, MD University, Rohtak.

33. Richa Dwivedi, Department of Computer Science, SRK College, Firozabad, UP.
34. Dr. S. Balamurugan, Lecturer, Political Science and Public Administration, DDE, Annamalai University, Annamalai, TN.
35. Mrs. S. Suchitra Verma, Project Associate, Political Science and Public Administration, DDE, Annamalai University, Annamalai, TN.
36. Dr. S.S. Chahar, Professor and Head, Department of Public Administration, M D University, Rohtak, Haryana.
37. S.S. Tiwana, Professor and Head, Department of Public Administration, Panjabi University, Patiala, Punjab.
38. Sahnawaz ul Rahman, Junior Research Fellow, Department of Public Administration, University of Lucknow, Lucknow.
39. Ms. Sanjukta Rani Tripathi, Reader, Department of Home Science, Govt. Women's College, Sambalpur- 768001.
40. Shankar Birdi, J.R.F., Political Science, MBGPG College, Haldwani, Uttaranchal.
41. Subhash C. Arora, Professor and Head, Department of Public Administration, MD University, Rohtak, Haryana.
42. Ms. Sudha Kumari, Reader, Department of Education, Aligarh Muslim University, Aligarh, U P.
43. Ms. Suman Lata, Lecturer, Department of Public Administration, M D University, Rohtak, Haryana.
44. Dr. Swami Parthasarathy, Research Scholar, Dev Sanskrit Viswa Vidyalaya, Haridwar, UA.
45. Dr. Tripti Barthwal, Associate Professor, Lal Bahadur Shastri Institute of Management and Development Studies, Lucknow.
46. Dr. Vibhuti Singh Shekhawat, Head, Department of Humanities and Social Science, Malviya National Institute of Technology, Jaipur, Rajasthan.

Part - 1

CORRUPTION AND ITS VARIOUS MANIFESTATIONS

1

Corruption: Causes, Consequences & Prevention

R.K. GUPTA
Reader Pol. Sc.
M.B.Govt. P.G. College,
Haldwani
SHANKAR BIRDI
J.R.F. Dept. of Pol. Sc.
M.B. Govt. P.G. College,
Haldwani

The dictionary defines integrity as "soundness of moral principles, the character of uncorrupted virtue; uprightness, honesty; sincerity." Integrity is, indeed, the most essential attribute of a welfare state. The First Five Year Plan rightly emphasized: "Integrity in public affairs and administration is essential and there must, therefore, be an insistence on it in every branch of public activity. The influence of corruption is insidious. It not only inflicts wrongs which are difficult to redress, but it undermines the structure of administration and the confidence of the public in the administration. There must, therefore, be a continuous war against every species of corruption within the administration..."

Corruption is the use of public office for private gain, Section 161 of the Indian Penal Code defines 'corruption' in legal terms, as under:

"Whoever being or expecting to be public servant accepts, or obtains, or agrees to accept, or attempts to obtain from any person for himself or for any other person any gratification whatever other than legal remuneration as a motive or reward for doing or forbearing to do any official act, or for showing, or to show, in the exercise of his official function, favours or disfavour to any person, or for rendering or attempting to render any service or disservice to any person, with the Central or any State Government or Parliament or Legislature of any State or with any public servant as such, shall be punished with imprisonment of either description for a term which may extend to three years, or with fine, or with both."

Another species of corruption not generally recognized as corruption is extravagant expenditure of public money. The Prevention of Corruption 1947 calls it criminal misconduct and defines it as follows:

(a) If he habitually accepts or obtains or agrees to accept or attempts to obtain from any person for himself or for any other person, any gratification (other than legal remuneration) as a motive or reward such as is mentioned in Section 161 of the Indian Penal Code, or

(b) If he habitually accepts or obtains or agrees to accept or attempts to obtain for himself or for any other person, any valuable thing without consideration or for consideration which he knows to be inadequate, from any person, whom he knows to have been or to be, or to be likely to be concerned in any proceeding or business transacted or about to be transacted by him, or having any connection with the official functions of himself or of any public servant to whom he is subordinate, or from any person whom he knows to be interested in or related to the person so concerned; or

(c) If he dishonestly or fraudulently misappropriates or otherwise converts for his own use any property entrusted to him or under his control as a public servant or allows any other persons so to do: or

(d) If he, by corrupt or illegal means or by otherwise abusing his position as public servant, obtains for himself or for any other person any valuable thing or pacuniary advantages: or

(e) If he or any person on his behalf is in possession or has at any time, during the period of his office, been in possession, for which the public servant cannot satisfactorily account of pecuniary resources or property disproportionate to his known source of income.

(f) Any public servant who commits criminal misconduct shall be punishable with imprisonment for a term which shall not be less than one year but which may extend to seven years and is liable to fine.

Provided that the court may, for any special reasons recorded in writing, impose a sentence of imprisonment of less than one year.

MAJOR SCANDALS

Year	*Description*
1949	Rs. 216 crore Jeep scandal case involving Krishna Menon who was India's Ambassador in United Kingdom.
1956	Serajuddin Affair, K.D. Malviya, Minister of Mines and Fuels in Nehru's Cabinet, charged with major involvement.
1958	Feroz Gandhi exposed the Life Insurance Corporation Affairs involving sale of bogus shares to the LIC. T.T. Krishnamachari, Minister in Nehru's Cabinet, had to resign.
1964	S.R. Das Commission of Inquiry appointed against Punjab's Chief Minister Pratap Singh Kairon. Kairon had to quit on charges of amassing wealth for his family while in office.
1971	Rustom Sohrab Nagarwala episode; fraud the State Bank of India (SBI) of Rs. 60 lakhs. In 1971, the chief cashier of SBI received a telephone call from Prime Minister's office asking him to make available Rs. 60 lakhs from the Bank. Nagarwala took the box containing the money and fled. Later, Nagarwala was sentenced to four years rigorous imprisonment.
1981	HDW sub-marine deal, a kick back of Rs. 100 crore paid to certain middlemen.
1982	A.R. Antulay allegedly charged fees for granting lincensed cement and industrial alcohol and exhorted crores of rupees for the trusts founded by him. He resigned following an adverse court verdict.
1983	Churhat Lotteries Scandal allegedly implicating Congress minister Arjun Singh.
1987	Fairfax affair where an inquiry was ordered into the arrangements made with Fairfax Group to probe into

	FERA violations and former finance minister, V.P. Singh, was falsely involved.
1988	Bofors gun deal. Rajiv Gandhi government was alleged to have received bribes to secure the Rs. 1,600 crore contract.
1991	Purchase of the out-dated Westland helicopters.
1992	Multi-crore securities scam exposed with Harshad Mehta at the helm. Highly placed politicians and civil servants were involved in the deal. (Rs. 5000 crore)
1992	Karnataka Chief Minister S.B. Bangarappa forced to resign after being accused of involvement in classic computer deal.
1994	Sugar Muddle – Kalpanath Rai forced to resign on the basis of Gian Prakash Committee report which alleged the lack of timely imports as the main reason for escalation of sugar price (Rs. 650 crore).
1994	Telecom Scam – Sukhram faced opposition from M.Ps over the lack of transparency in the bidding of the telecom tenders on charges of favouritism. CBI raid in 1996. Huge amount of money found.
1995	Rs. 950 crore (Bihar) Fodder Scam – on the basis of Accountant General's report large scale discrepancies found between the amounts withdrawn budgetary grant I and the amount in the Annual Husbandry department top level officials suspended, suspected involvement. Lallu Prasad Yadav, Bihar's Chief Minister, allegedly involved.
1995	Hawala Scam – Large scale involvement of political bodies and several Bureaucrats in the illegal transaction and receipt of money through Hawala agents S.K. Jain and J.K. Jain under the supervision of the Supreme Court, CBI enquiry going on indicating a large number of top politicians and bureaucrats.
1995	Housing Scam – out of turn allotments made by the then minister Sheila Kaul and P.K. Tungon, Sheila Kaul did not resign on Supreme Court's insistance but on that of the President (Rs. 17.4 crores).
1995	JMM Bribery Scandal – Four MPs of Jharkhand Mukti Morcha (JMM) Suraj Mandal, Shailendra Mahto, Shibu

Soren and Simon Marandi had allegedly received huge amount of money to vote against the no confidence motion of the Narsimha Rao Government. CBI enquiry on (Rs. 3 crore).

1996 Urea Scandal – Advance payment of Rs. 133 crore to a little known Turkish firm, Korsan Ltd. for import of urea which was never delivered. This fraudulent deal shows how senior politicians and bureaucrats squander public funds.

1996 Mumbai Port Trust Scandal – The Chairman and Deputy Chairman of the Port Trust allegedly flouted government instructions and guidelines in the allotment of prime commercial and to its counsel, Kiran Chaudhary at a throw-away price, causing the Port Trust huge losses.

2001 (March) The tehelka scam in which video cameras were used to photograph politicians and public servants accepting bribes while negotiating defence deals.

N. Vittal warns: "if we still hesitate to take action against the corrupt people at all levels, it only means that democracy is sustained in India only by a heavy dose of hypocrisy. There is a Tamil proverb which says that a person who is sleeping can be woken up but you cannot wake up a person who is pretending to be sleeping. All those who claim that they are against corruption will have to prove whether they are really sleeping or pretending to be sleeping when it comes to the issue of fighting corruption."

CAUSES OF CORRUPTION

Corruption is a complex phenomenon which naturally has complex causes. A curious mixture of historical, social, political and economic factors cause the phenomenon of corruption. We describe below some of these causes:

(I) Historical Causes

(a) The colonial Government paid his own senior officers handsomely. The local officers, working mainly at lower levels, were paid very poor salaries. This definitely affected their integrity.

(b) During World War II, there was scarcity of goods, even articles of common consumption like food, clothing etc. were available on ration cards. All these controls provided opportunities for corruption.

(c) The climate for corruption created by wartime controls and scarcity was further aggravated by the post-war flush of money and inflation. The salaries of the employees did not keep pace with inflation. The increasing economic activity with excessive Government controls created the climate for corruption on a large scale.

(II) Post-independence Problems

The administrative machinery of the independent India was considerably weakened by

(a) War time neglect;

(b) Sudden departure of a large number of British and Muslim Officers. A large number of promotions of people of unproved merit had to be done. A large scale recruitment also brought down the quality of the staff recruited. All this resulted in a great turmoil in the administrative system. The stability and the continuance of traditions received a jolt.

(III) Environmental Causes

A very important cause of corruption is the vast urbanization and industrialization. This created an environment in which material possession and economic power determines the status and prestige of a person in the society. Since the salaries of the Government servants were not enough to afford this ostentatious living, it caused a lot of strain on the Integrity of the administrative officers.

(IV) Economic Causes

Inadequate compensation to the Government servants in the form of low salaries and benefits is by far the most important cause of corruption in the society. The increasing prices have brought down the real income of the Government employees, specially those in a higher position whose salaries have not at all been protected against inflation. When the salaries are not enough to meet even the basic needs of the employees, they naturally succumb to the temptations of illegal money.

(V) Lack of Strong Public Opinion against Corruption

The corrupt officials, even when they are known to be corrupt are often not looked down upon in the society. In fact they are often more respected than their honest counterparts because of their ability to help and entertain their friends and relatives. Sometimes the corrupt politicians are re-ejected to high offices by the people as a way of life and they do not complain against it.

(VI) Corrupting influence of big industrial magnates

A number of big businessmen try to oblige the Government servant in many ways to obtain some favours in future. They take it as an investment for the future. This acts as a initiation to the Government servants.

(VII) Complicated and cumbersome procedure

The procedure of the Government even in respect of simple things like getting a ration card or diesel permit etc., have unnecessarily been complicated. This provides the Government employees an opportunity to extort money from the clients. The situation probably can be remedied by simplifying procedures and reducing the discretion of the lower staff.

(VIII) Existence of influence peddlers

The cumbersome procedures of the Government and all pervasiveness of Government controls have created a tribe of influence peddlers. These people maintain liaison in the Government offices. They get the work of the clients done through their contacts in the Government. They operate at all levels. In fact, they are the Middlemen of the corruption between the Government employees and their clients.

(IX) Inadequate provisions and enforcement of the Law

The India Penal Code and Prevention of Corruption Act do not provide adequate framework for punishing the guilty officers. Moreover the administration of these laws leaves much to be desired. Not many prosecutions are launched. Out of the prosecutions launched not many are pursued vigorously. This encourages the dishonest employees in continuing their corrupt practices.

(X) Undue protection given to the Government Employees

The Constitution of our country as well as the disciplinary procedures etc., makes it almost impossible to take action against corrupt employees. Naturally, there is nothing to deter them from following their corrupt practices with a vengeance if they are so inclined.

CONSEQUENCES OF CORRUPTION

Corruption in high places affects the very fabric of the social system, it has many direct and indirect harmful effects. Some of the important ones are described below:

(i) Corruption in high places reduces the faith of the people in the Government. The people expect high standards of morality from their rulers. When these standards are not met, it may result in the alienation of people from the Government.

(ii) Corruption increases the effective cost of administration. The people who are in any case paying to the Government for its services in the form of taxes are unofficially required to pay more to its officers.

(iii) The widespread corruption in the bureaucracy causes cynicism and social disunity. This may reduce the willingness of the people to make sacrifices for the economic development of the society.

(iv) Corruption comes in the way of making decision on merits. When the decisions are made on the basis of pecuniary benefits to be obtained from the transactions, the merit naturally gets the second place. There is even a possibility of sacrificing the national interest for the sake of these benefits. This may, for example, happen in case of purchase of substandard arms, which may not be effective during a war.

(v) Corruption has very adverse effect on the morale of the honest officers. In fact, it militates against the very basis of the principles of a pure bureaucracy. When the evaluation of work, placement and promotion are dependent on considerations other than merit, the whole system may be vulgarized and demoralized.

(vi) Corruption has often resulted in a tremendous waste of national resources. For example, purchased goods not used for years result in the depreciation of goods as well as increase in inventory cost.

LIST OF ACTS TO CHECK CORRUPTION

Existing legal and institutional framework to check corruption and redress citizen's grievances in India list of the following:

- Public Servants (Enquiries) Act, 1850
- Indian Penal Code, 1860
- Special Police Establishment, 1941
- Delhi Police Establishment Act, 1946
- Prevention of Corruption Act, 1947
- Commissions of Inquiry Act, 1952 (against political leaders and eminent public men).
- All India Services (Conduct) Rules, 1954
- CentralCivil Services (Conduct) Rules, 1955
- Railway Services (Conduct) Rules, 1956
- Vigilance organizations in ministries/departments, attached and subordinate offices and public Undertakings
- Central Bureau of Investigation, 1963
- Central Vigilance Commission, 1964
- State Vigilance Commissions, 1964
- Anti-corruption bureaus in States
- Lokayukta (Ombudsman) in States
- Divisional Vigilance Board
- DistrictVigilance Officer
- National Consumer Disputes Redressal Commission
- Commission for SCs and STs
- Supreme Court and High Courts in States
- Administrative Tribunals (quasi-judicial bodies)
- Directorate of Public Grievances in the Cabinet Secretariat, 1988
- Parliament and its Committees
- 'File to Field' programme in some states like Kerala. In this innovative scheme, the administrator owes to the village/area and hears public grievances and takes immediate action wherever possible.

COMBATING CORRUPTION

Various methods suggested for Combating Corruption are as follows:

1. Focus should be on law, administration and procedure Law should not be too harsh, complicated and ambiguous. Too much scope should not be given to discretion.
2. Administrative factors include structural and functional aspects. Structure of the Organization should be well defined leaving no scope for lacunae.
3. No lapses should be permitted in procedures and functioning.
4. Artificial shortages/scarcities which promote illegal gratifications should be controlled.
5. Vigilance should be increased.
6. Liberalization policy should be introduced slowly and with caution.
7. General awareness should be created among the people. Corruption can be fought only with collective effort. While many intellectual, educated, articulate and well informed citizens are worried about this monstrous problem of corruption, they fail to channelise their unhappiness into strong public opinion. A collective and concerted effort by the youth will drive this monster away.

   Funding of elections by business houses has a great impact on the corruption. This should be put to an end too. The Election Commission in recent times has fixed certain norms on spending on electioneering and has effectively controlled such expenditure. This practice should be encouraged. Further state funding of elections will eliminate vested interests and will draw persons of integrity into the legislative wings.

   Appointing Lok Pals and Lok Ayukts will help to keep watch on the highest power positions. They should have independent investigative machinery at disposal.

   So long as corruption fails to attract legal, moral and social censure, it will go on increasing. Corruption is like a disease and every citizen of India should fight it at every level. People should not tolerate corruption. They should stop viewing corruption as a 'necessary evil' to continue to live. Then there is hope for the country to come out of the dubious destination of being in the top ten most corrupt countries.
8. To design defensive system one has to strike at the roots of corruption. One such root is the lack of transparency. The Official Secrets Act in India is replaced by the Freedom of

Information Act (which is in the offing), will help in accessing information. A part of bureaucracy's powe r over the public stems from its access to information. Simultaneously, there should also be a general effort at educating the public about their rights. Every citizen should know what type of service he can get from each government body and when and how.

9. Red-tapism results in corruption. If the entire system is made transparent and simple, much of the red-tapism can be avoided. Hence, efforts should be made by the Government to simplify the system. In addition, industries, trade associations, voluntary agencies etc. should also contribute to a simplified system in their spheres of operation.
10. Scarcity of basic products is another factor leading to corruption. Scarcity of products rises not only from shortfall of production but also due to improper management and distribution. Therefore, efforts to increase production should be made along with adoption of proper distribution and management policy to avoid this situation.
11. Laws should be made responsive to the changing conditions and needs, as archaic laws sometimes lead to corruption. Obsolete laws should be reviewed or deleted from statute books. The Jain Committee appointed by the Government to study absolete laws has found that out of 2,500 administrative laws, 1,300 are outdated and obsolete.

The other measures as had been prepared by the former Central Vigilance Commissioner, Mr. N. Vittal are also effective in fighting/ combating corruption.

1. A Corruption Perception Index should be prepared for all Government organizations, public sector enterprises and banks. Each year, it should be published so that one can see which department is more corrupt and also note if any improvement has been made in that office.
2. Departmental action should be aimed at trapping and taking speedy disciplinary action against the corrupt. Legal action through judicial process may take long but departmental action should be completed within six months.
3. Like all Government servants, Members of Parliament and Ministers should file annual property returns. This would help in setting up a healthy tradition to check corruption in public life.

4. There should be a Corrupt Public Servants (Forfeiture of Property) Act. The Benami Transactions (Prohibition) Act, 1988 should be implemented.
5. Youth should be mobilized to fight corruption. Like the National Cadet Corps, there should be a National Vigilance Corps to take up anti-corruption cases. The entire education system should be energized. Finally, it can be said that, fighting corruption is not the responsibility of Government only. It is the responsibility of each individual/person, hence he should contribute in making the 'system' corruption-free as he is also a part of this system. A careful analysis shows that, not a single measure is comprehensive/complete in itself. Every measure (be it a law or organization) lacks in some aspect or other. For example, Prevention of Corruption Act has the authority to punish the corrupt but is unable to keep a strict vigil over corruption at various levels of Government. CVC though empowered to keep a watch on corruption, lacks judicial authority to enforce any punitive action against it. The Freedom of Information bill still retains the power to hide information with the government officials. There is no provision in it for an independent administrative body to review refusals of information. There has not been any attempt by the government either to plug in these loopholes or to change the obsolete laws to deal with corruption. These loopholes, it seems, are allowed to stay for some vested interests.

REFERENCES

1. Kaushik Basu, *Economic Graffiti*, (Bombay: Oxford University Press, 1991), p. 57.
2. Atul Kohli, *Democracy and Discontent: India's Growing crisis of Governability* (New York: Cambridge University Press, 1991), p. 3.
3. U.C. Agarwal, "Galloping Corruption: Need for Effective Vigilance", in *Fifty Years of Indian Administrative: Retrospect and Prospect*, Ed. by T.N. Chaturvedi, New Delhi, 1998, p. 178.
4. Sunil Sondhi, *Corruption: The Asian Experience* New Delhi, Sanjay Prakashan, 2002, p. 10.
5. T.N. Seshan with Sanjay Hazarika, 'The Degeneration of India' New Delhi, Viking, Penguin Books, 1995, p. 13.
6. Bala, K. Dey, "Ethics in Public Administration: Maladies and Remedies", in *Ethics in Public Life* Ed. by T.N. Chaturvedi, New Delhi, IIPA, 1996.

2

COMBATING CORRUPTION: CAUSES, CONSEQUENCES AND POLICY FRAMEWORK

PUSHPA DEVI
Department of Sociology, M.B.G.P.G. College, Haldwani

Over the last few years, the issue of corruption—the abuse of public office for private gain-has attracted renewed interest, both among academics and policymakers. There are a number of reasons why this topic has come under fresh scrutiny. Corruption scandals have toppled governments in both major industrial countries and developing countries. In the transition countries, the shift from command economies to free market economies has created massive opportunities for the appropriation of rents (that is, excessive profits) and has often been accompanied by a change from a well-organized system of corruption to a more chaotic and deleterious one. With the end of the cold war, donor countries have placed less emphasis on political considerations in allocating foreign aid among developing countries and have paid more attention to cases in which aid funds have been misused and have not reached the poor. And slow economic growth has persisted in many countries with malfunctioning institutions. This renewed interest has led to a new flurry of empirical research on the causes and consequences of corruption.

We know quite a bit about the causes and consequences of corruption. An important body of knowledge was acquired through theoretical research done in the 1970s by Jagdish Bhagwati, Anne Krueger, and Susan Rose Ackerman, among others (Mauro, 1996). A key principle is that corruption can occur where rents exist—typically, as a result of government regulation—and public officials have discretion in allocating them. The classic example of a government restriction resulting in rents and rent-seeking behaviour is that of an import quota and the associated licenses that civil servants give to those entrepreneurs willing to pay bribes.

More recently, researchers have begun to test some of these long established theoretical hypotheses using new cross-country data. Indices produced by private rating agencies grade countries on their levels of corruption, typically using the replies to standardized questionnaires by consultants living in those countries. The replies are subjective, but the correlation between indices produced by different rating agencies is very high, suggesting that most observers more or less agree on how corrupt countries seem to be. The high prices paid to the rating agencies by their customers (usually multinational companies and international banks) constitute indirect evidence that the information is valuable. These indices are obviously imperfect owing to their subjective nature, but can yield useful insights.

CAUSES OF CORRUPTION

Since the ultimate source of rent-seeking behaviour is the availability of rents, corruption is likely to occur where restrictions and government intervention lead to the presence of such excessive profits. Examples include trade restrictions (such as tariffs and import quotas), favoritist industrial policies (such as subsidies and tax deductions), price controls, multiple exchange rate practices and foreign exchange allocation schemes, and government-controlled provision of credit. Some rents may arise in the absence of government intervention, as in the case of natural resources, such as oil, whose supply is limited by nature and whose extraction cost is far lower than its market price. Since abnormal profits are available to those who extract oil, officials who allocated extraction rights are likely to be offered bribes. Finally, one would expect that corruption is more likely to take place when civil servants are paid very low wages and often must resort to collecting bribes in order to feed their families.

While all of the hypotheses described above are empirically testable, in the sense that data are available for that purpose, only a few have actually been tested. What empirical studies have been done to support certain hypotheses; namely, that there is less corruption where there are fewer trade restrictions; where governments do not engage in favoritist industrial policies; and perhaps where natural resources are more abundant; and that there is somewhat less corruption where civil servants are paid better, compared with similarly qualified workers in the private sector (Van Rijckeghem and Weder, 1997).

CONSEQUENCES OF CORRUPTION

From economic theory, one would expect corruption to reduce economic growth by lowering incentives to invest (for both domestic and foreign entrepreneurs). In cases where entrepreneurs are asked for bribes before enterprises can be started, or corrupt officials later request shares in the proceeds of their investments, corruption acts as a tax, though one of a particularly pernicious nature, given the need for secrecy and the uncertainty as to whether bribe takers will live up to their part of the bargain. Corruption could also be expected to reduce growth by lowering the quality of public infrastructure and services, decreasing tax revenue, causing talented people to engage in rent-seeking rather than productive activities, and distorting the composition of government expenditure. At the same time, there are some theoretical counterarguments. For example, it has been suggested to exact bribes, might work harder and that corruption might help entrepreneurs get around bureaucratic impediments.

One specific channel through which corruption may harm economic performance is by distorting the composition of government expenditure. Corrupt politicians may be expected to spend more public resources on those items on which it is easier to exact large bribes and keep them secret-for example, items produced in markets where the degree of competition is low and items whose value is difficult to monitor. Corrupt politicians might therefore be more inclined to spend on fighter aircraft and large—scale investment projects than on textbooks and teachers' salaries, even thoug the latter may promote economic growth to a greater extent than the former.

Empirical evidence based on cross-country comparisons does indeed suggest that corruption has large, adverse effects on private investment and economic growth. Regression analysis shows that a country that improves its standing on the corruption index from, say, 6 to 8 (0 being the most corrupt, 10 the least) will experience a 4 percentage point increase in its investment rate and 0.5 percentage point increase in its annual per capita GDP growth rate (Mauro, 1996). These large effects suggest that policies to curb corruption could have significant payoffs. The association between corruption and low economic growth remains broadly unchanged when estimated for a group of countries with extensive red tape. Therefore, there is no support for the claim that corruption might be beneficial in the presence of a slow bureaucracy. The most important channel through which corruption reduces economic growth is by lowering private investment, which accounts for at least one-third of corruptions's overall negative effects. At the same time, the remaining two-thirds of the overall negative effects of corruption on economic growth must be felt through other channels, including those mentioned above. While it is difficult to disentangle those other channels, there is some evidence that one of them—the distortion of government expenditure—plays a significant role.

Based on cross-country comparisons, it seems that corruption alters the composition of government expenditurel; specifically, corrupt governments spend less on education and perhaps health, and probably more on public investment. Regression analysis shows that a country that improves its standing on the corruption index from 6 to 8 will typically raise its spending on education by ½ to 1 per cent GDP, a considerable impact. This result is a matter for concern, because there is increasing evidence that educational attainment fosters economic growth.

Of course, empirical results related to a phenomenon that is, by its very nature, difficult to measure must be treated with a high degree of caution. Two issues that merit special attention in this context are those of causality and the possible role of other forms of institutional inefficiency.

Why do countries judged to be corrupt experience slow economic growth? Is it that corruption harms growth or simply that low growth leads consultants to give bad corruption grades to a country? To deal with this issue, one can take variables (such as a country's colonial history or the extent to which its population is divided along ethnolinguistic lines) that happen to be correlated with corruption but have no effect on economic growth or government spending other than through their impact on the efficiency of institutions, and use them as instrumental variables in the regression analysis. Through this statistical trick, it is possible to get around problems relating to the subjectivity of the corruption indices, and it can be shown that corruption—together with other forms of institutional inefficiency—causes low economic growth.

Corruption is most prevalent where where there are other forms of institutional inefficiency, such as political instabililty, bureaucratic red tape, and weak legislative and judicial systems. This raises the question of whether it can be established that corruption, rather than other factors correlated with it, is the cause of low economic growth. Regression analysis provides some evidence that if one controls for other forms of institutional inefficiency, such as political instability, corruption can still be shown to reduce growth. Nevertheless, it is hard to show conclusively that the cause of the problem is corruption alone, rather than the institutional weaknesses that are closely associated with it. The truth is that probably all of these weaknesses are intrinsically linked, in the sense that they feed upon each other (for example, red tape makes corruption possible, and corrupt bureaucrats may increase the extent of red tape so they can extract additional bribes) and that getting rid of corruption helps a country overcome other institutional weaknesses, just as reducing other institutional weaknesses helps it curb corruption.

POLICY FRAMEWORK FOR COMBATING CORRUPTION

While there is a well established body of theoretical knowledge, as well as some tentative results on the causes and consequences of corruption, several more questions need to be answered to enable governments to design effective policies aimed at curbing corruption. Once a corrupt system is in place, and a majority of people operate within that system, individuals have no incentive to try to change it or to refrain from taking part in it, even if everybody would be better off. Type of the system in which we live plays a big role. For example: You live in a society where everybody steals. Do you choose to steal? The probability that you will be caught is low, because the police are very busy chasing other thieves, and, even if you do get caught, the chances of your being punished severely for a crime that is so common are low. Therefore, you too steal. By contrast, if you live in a society where theft is rare, the chances of your being caught and punished are high, so you choose not to steal.

Another example also explain the same thing such as, You are a new junior civil servant in an administration where everybody, including your superiors, is very corrupt. Somebody offers you a bribe to help him avoid paying taxes. You decline the offer. A few hours later, you receive a telephone call from your boss, who would have liked a cut of your bribe. Your boss suggests that if you treat a friend nicely (by accepting the bribe), you may be promoted, while if you don't, you will be transferred to a remote provincial office. You then take the bribe and share it with your boss and colleagues. If, instead, the administration in which you work is very honest, you are likely to behave honestly to avoid the risk of being fired.

The last example again explains the same, Individuals *A* and *B* are members of the same government. Suppose, on the one hand, that *A* is very corrupt and has established a private bribe-collection system for her own gain. The need to pay substantial bribes reduces entrepreneurs' incentives to invest and imposes a significant burden on economic growth. Citizens realize that economic growth is being harmed by the corrupt government, though they may not know exactly who is soliciting bribes. Therefore, they decide not to reelect the government. This shortens *B*'s horizon, making him more inclined to extract a large proportion of current output and to disregard any ensuing adverse effects on future output. In other words, *B* will seek to obtain a large slice of the cake today since he knows that the government that he participates in will soon be ousted. On the other hand, following a similar line of reasoning, if *A* does not collect bribes, then *B* will also refrain from doing so.

The last example may provide an explanation not only for the persistence of corruption but also for the empirical observation that, on average, countries that are more corrupt tend to be more politically unstable. It also suggests that both corruption and political instability may result from the failure of members of the same government or ruling elite to coordinate their actions. In that sense, corruption and political instability may be two sides of the same coin. This example may fit the cases of countries that are bedeviled by frequent coups whereby corrupt regimes succeed one another. At the same time, it does not explain a number of other relevant cases, such as those of dictators who have remained in power for many years by allowing their supporters to collect large bribes, or those of governments formed by groups of individuals who have been able to agree on bribe levels that are high, but not so high as to cause them to be ousted.

All of the above examples show that once corruption has become ingrained, it is very difficult to get rid of. As a result, corruption tends to persist, together with its adverse consequences. This leads to an important policy conclusion, which is consistent with international experience over the past few decades. Attempts to eliminate corruption tend to succeed when reforms are undertaken in a very sudden and forceful manner and are supported at the highest levels of government. However, an equally relevant question is what characteristics make countries more likely to fall into a high-corruption, low-growth trap.

CO-RELATED FACTORS

1. Poverty
2. Forms of Corruption
3. Existing Practices
4. Miscellaneous

Poverty

One striking empirical finding is that poorer countries are usually considered to be more corrupt. This result mustbe treated with caution, since it may well be driven by the observers' perceptions. However, if one assumes for a moment that this finding reflects a genuine correlation, it may be useful to explore its sources. We have seen that there is evidence that corruption lowers economic growth, thereby breeding poverty over time. At the same time, poverty itself might cause corruption, perhaps because poor countries cannot devote sufficient resources to setting up and enforcing an effective legal framework, or because people in need are more likely to abandon their moral principles. Researchers have begun to analyze the link between civil servants' wages and the extent of corruption. It has been suggested that reasonable wages are a necessary condition for avoiding corruption, though not a sufficient one.

Forms of Corruption

Available indices of corruption are general and do not distinguish between high-level corruption (such as kickbacks paid to a defence minister in exchange for his country's purchase of expensive jet fighter aircraft) and low-level corruption (such as petty bribes paid to a junior civil servant for expediting the issuance of a driver's license). Nor do they distinguish between well-organized corruption and chaotic corruption. (When corruption is well organized, the required amount and appropriate recipient of a bribe are well known, and payment guarantees that the desired favour will be obtained.) Therefore, we still do not know which kinds of corruption are more deleterious and should be tackled first. Country-specific studies and anecdotal evidence suggest that high-level and low-level corruption tend to coexist and reinforce each other. Thus, this distinction may not be relevant. On the other hand, the distinction between well-organized corruption and chaotic corruption may be more relevant, since a fairly convincing theoretical case can be made that the latter has worse effects than the former.

Under a well-organized system of corruption, entrepreneurs know whom they need to bribe and how much to offer them, and are confident that they will obtain the necessary permits for their firms. It has also been argued that well-organized corruption is less harmful because, under such a system, a corrupt bureaucrat will take a clearly defined share of a firm's profits, which gives him an interest in the success of the firm. In contrast, under chaotic corruption, entrepreneurs may need to bribe several officials, with no guarantee either that they will not face further demands for bribes or that the permits they seek will actually be delivered. In addition, if multiple agents request bribes from the same entrepreneur without coordinating bribe levels among themselves, they are likely to make excessive demands, with the result that entrepreneurial activity comes to a halt. While chaotic corruption seems a priori to be more deleterious than well-organized corruption, there is currently little empirical data available to test this hypothesis.

Existing Practices

Many countries and institutions have paid increasing attention to the problem of corruption, and the debate on possible policy options is still ongoing. In deciding how to allocate aid funds, some donor countries have begun to give more importance to recipient countries' actions to curb corruption. Member countries of the Organization for Economic Cooperation and Development have acted to criminalize the bribery of foreign public officials. International institutions, which have always played an important role in reducing the scope for corruption, are now giving more prominence to the issue. For example, the IMF has always encouraged countries to liberalize their economies (for example, by eliminating trade restrictions), terminate off-budget operations, and ensure budget transparency. The guidelines on governance, which were approved by the IMF's Executive Board in August 1997, formalize the IMF staff involvement in such tasks.

Miscellaneous

One of the most difficult policy issues is how to prevent corruption from distorting government expenditure. This important issue goes to the heart of donors' concerns about the possible misuse of aid funds. Donors find it difficult to ensure that aid funds are spent wisely, because resources are fungible. For example, a donor may give aid funds to enable the recipient country to build a school, which the recipient may indeed use for that purpose; however, the availability of aid funds to build the school makes it possible for the recipient to use the resulting savings to buy sophisticated weapons, whose purchase may provide more scope for illegally diverting funds into individuals' pockets than school construction could. How should this problem be addressed? Clearly, donor countries should pay attention to the overall composition of government spending and not focus narrowly on how their own funds have been spent, but many donors may not have sufficient resources to do this. One possible approach that has been suggested is to have an international institution monitor the overall composition of government expenditure, as a service to both the recipient country's citizens and the donor community. This approach would not, however, be easy to implement. Recipient countries would probably resist attempts by the rest of the world to play a role in determining the composition of their public spending. In addition, as a practical matter, it may be difficult to ensure that spending items are not simply relabeled, with no real improvement in the composition of government expenditure.

Conclusion

We have a reasonable theoretical understanding of the causes and consequences of corruption, and have begun to get a sense of the extent of these relationships through empirical research. A consensus is emerging that corruption is a serious problem, and several bodies in the international arena have begun to take policy measures to curb it. At the policy level, although we may still be at the stage of learning by doing, action is being taken. It is important to ensure that ten years from now, we can look back on today's focus on corruption and observe that some concrete results were attained in this domain. To that end, those bodies that are taking action against corruption ought to establish criteria to evaluate their policies. Each entity would need to devise its own evaluation criteria, and it should do that now, so that the effectiveness of its policies can be assessed accurately and fairly over the next decade.

The need to define "concrete results" might appear to be a tall order in an area where quantification is difficult. A place to begin, however, could be the well-established body of knowledge on the causes of corruption. For example, efforts to curb corruption could be assessed on the basis of how effectively they were in bringing about the implementation of policies known to reduce corruption, such as the elimination of government restrictions that create rents.

3

CORRUPTION: CAUSES, CONSEQUENCES AND CURE

R.C. Dikshit
I.P.S. (Retd.)
Former D.G.P. (U.P. Police)

Corruption means 'dishonest or illegal behaviour especially of people in authority" and it includes the 'act or effect of making somebody change from moral to immoral standards of behaviour'. (Oxford–Advanced Learners Dictionary).

Oxford Dictionary defines "Corruption as the perversion or destruction of integrity or fidelity in the discharge of public duties by bribery or favour". Leslie Palmier defines corruption as, "the acquisition of forbidden benefits by the officials or employees, so bringing into question their loyalty to their employers," or it may be regarded, 'as the use of public power for private advantage in ways which transgress some formal rules or laws'.

Ingredients of Corruption: Corruption, as defined above, lays emphasis on 'dishonest, illegal, perverted or deviant behaviour of an employee or official for private advantage'. The private advantage could be 'bribe, price, reward, gift, or favour, bestowed or promised'. (Websters' Third New International Dictionary) or it could be gratification i.e. 'Satisfaction of desire or appetite of body or mind'. The definitions further emphasise that such deviant behaviour ought to be 'illegal' 'forbidden by law' or in 'transgression of law' and they exclude those corrupt acts which don't transgress laws or rules. The corruption, violating ethical laws or moral code may not be illegal therefore not actionable by law enforcement agencies but it seriously determines the public perception regarding corruption.

Not only public servants: In addition to above mentioned ingredients namely dishonest, or illegal behaviour for personal gain or gratification, the element of integrity or fidelity to the employer was also mentioned, which suggests that only public servants are susceptible to corruption. However, in view of new concepts in the field of public administration and governance, the public functions and management of governmental business are increasingly slipping to private sector, i.e. private sector undertakings, corporations, companies, firms, contractors and hordes of other extra governmental organizations (EGO), which means that functionaries working in private sector are discharging function in which public is interested. Therefore they are also susceptible to corruption and come within the purview of our study. Transparency International defines corruption as the "abuse of entrusted power for private profile" to include corrupt practices of the private sector where employees may not be classed as public servants strictly speaking.

The complexities of economic development and commercial imperatives have changed the relationship of public functionaries and beneficiaries therefore initiative in most cases of graft comes from private functionaries or the so-called victims of corruption. In certain cases the bribe giver is the actual beneficiary and the public servant is the minor partner who succumbs to the designs of the manipulator.

Corruption is not an offence in general sense of the term but '*a general classification for a variety of criminal acts*', including, delay in transaction of public functions, accepting bribe in cash or kind, causing undue influence, neglecting lawful duty mutilating changing or corrupting any information and so many other ways to indulge in corruption. As economic complexities increase in our commercial environment, so the new, novel and innovative ways also emerge to consummate the offence of corruption. Some of these have been recognized as criminal acts while others have not been recognized as crime in statute book. Efforts are being made at international level to bring in uniformity in law.

Corruption is all-pervasive: In our country the public perception goes to suggest that all wings of government, all discernible sectors of economy and all walks of social and cultural life are smeared with corruption. Public perception may be exaggerated a bit but not grossly exaggerated. Among the many ills that afflict administration, corruption is the most serious and most damaging to good governance. The general complaint is "that no paper moves in most government offices unless chased from office to office and from seat to seat by the applicants with the help of "speed money". This kind of corruption in public dealing offices and counters has become almost open during the last few years".[1] In the year 1997, some one published "Bribe Index" listing some of the public utility services and also the prevalent rate of bribe or speed money required to be paid for the job. Again the *Sunday Times of India*, New Delhi April 2, 2002, published the prevalent rates for securing admissions in schools/colleges, paper leaks, good jobs and routine payments made to hordes of public servants who inspect an industrial unit. Even the birth and death certificates also have a price. Not only the public servants but also the 'privileged members of the public' have their share of loot. If any body starts construction of a house he has to pay 'bricks and cement' for philanthropic works like construction of a place of worship if he fails then 'protectors of the weaklings' appear on the scene and demand regular money for your protection in their kingdom of crime. For such information, related to crime, enlightened public servants have no time and governments, who suffer chronic paucity of funds; have no grievance redressal system whatsoever. The degree of apathy of the government shown to such complaints and matching tolerance of public helps the corruption to take epidemic form.

In other countries also public perception about corruption in public life is very high specially in Africa and in South and Southeast Asia where people consider that 'government has become an instrument for the enrichment of members of politically dominant group'.[2]

Corruption is a global phenomenon – Our's is not the only country which is suffering from corruption in epidemic form. Other countries also have their share of the scourge. U.S.A. the most prosperous and powerful country of the world today has a very brief history as compared to countries like China, Egypt and India and some of the European countries but history of corruption in that country is quite rich. In 19th century corruption was quite common but it was confined to local levels, until the exposure of Grant Administration followed by Tammany Hal Scandal of New York, which involved political leaders, business interests and political party leaders. The corrupt activity centred around 'kickbacks, extortion and election fraud and bribery which has considered detrimental to political system and economy both. This consensus among the reformers led to Pendleton Act, which created federal civil service system. The prohibition era 1919-

33] also saw rise in corruption and emergence of Mafia as a criminal force on national scene. Besides corruption at cutting edge level, the scandals like Watergate (President Nixon) "Abscam" scandal of 1978-80 (involving FBI and Senators), Wedtech scandal (1986-89) involving representatives and officials and 'Keating Five" (1987) scandals are worth mentioning. Recent scandals with respect to President Clinton are too recent to be forgotten. Scores of other scandals are being investigated by federal agencies.

In U.K. also the scandals spring regularly right from the days of Queen Victoria. The high officials of East India Company were charged and impeached. The scandal against John Profumo and similar other continue to rock the nation. Recent scandal specially after the death of Kelly has shaken Tony Blair, the Prime Minister of U.K.

The countries like Indonesia, Korea, Philippines and scores of African countries have come to news only because of interesting scandals. In Philippines, the regime of Ferdinand Marcos was known as 'Kleptocracy'.

THE INDIAN SCENE

In India people were aware of public official's susceptibility to corruption as early as Mauryan period of our history. Kautilya in his famous classical treatise on statecraft the *Arthashastra* has mentioned that it is as difficult to resist the temptation of utilising state funds for personal use as to resist the temptation of tasting honey or poison kept on one's tongue. He further elaborates how difficult it is to detect corruption of public officials.[3] He not only mentions administrative and punitive measures to deal with such officials but also discusses in detail the procedure of their recruitment and also procedure and mode of character verification.[4] Not only Kautilya but other Acharyas while elaborating duties of King also clearly mention that King has to protect public from the enemies (invaders), thieves or criminals, high officials of the state, kinsmen of the King and also the greed of the King himself. Acharyas apprehended danger to public from above mentioned five quarters.[5] Some of the enlightened groups even led the movements against the kings who transgressed their limits.

During middle ages also, corruption of every type was prevalent and all palace intrigues were financed and executed by those public servants who were close to the ruler. Bribe was considered to be very effective tool in the hands of conspirators. During the time of Jehangir a magistrate was punished by the emperor himself and was ordered to be bitten by a cobra. Emperor took pains to see the execution of the punishment and remained seated till the magistrate died. During British period – during company rule as well as crown rule – corruption was rampant and proceedings of British Parliament bear the testimony of impeachment of high officials and recall of governors on charges of corruption.

When on August 15, 1947 we 'awoke to freedom' every body thought that at least corruption will be controlled as the followers of Gandhi will not indulge in corruption. All those hopes were shattered within very short time and scandal after scandal rocked our national life. Even before the dawn of freedom the symptoms of this dreadful disease, started appearing on the body politic.

When our freedom fighters started misappropriating the public contributions (Thaili Presentations) ignoring public criticism as well as brotherly admonition by the party leaders. In one case of Madras Presidency even Gandhi Ji had to intervene when advice of lesser mortals was ignored. This and other events of similar nature forced Rajaji to mention (1922) that "Elections and their corruption, injustice and the power and tyranny of wealth and inefficiency of administration will make hell of life as soon as freedom is given to us, men will look regretfully back to the old regime of comparative justice and efficient, peaceful more or less honest administration". The scandals, like "Jeep Scandal (1948), Mundhra case (1957), "Kairon Case", Kuo Oil Deal (1980), "Thal Vaishet Fertiliser Case" (1980), "Antulay Files" (1981) then "Bofors", "Fodder Case", "Float Pump" and JMM case throw enough light on standards of our national life. The sensation created by Bhatnagar murder case followed by murder of Madhumita Shukla of Lucknow also gives an idea about our social and moral values. Arrests of High Court Judges, senior administrative service officers, police service officer, officials of public service commission have become almost a routine event and do not evoke any public reaction. This indifference is very dangerous for society because it emboldens the functionaries indulging in corruption as said Claire Safian "The accomplice to the crime of corruption is frequently our own indifference".[6] Nani J. Palkiwala reacted to the current situation in following lines, "*The quality of our public life has reached the Nadir. Politics has become tattered and tainted with crime. The moral standards of our politicians, policemen and criminals are indistinguishable from one another. India to–day is living example of the fact that cynicism corrupts and absolute cynicism corrupts absolutely".* – In our country we are facing a situation wherein people have accepted corruption as part of their lives. A man commands respect and status on the basis of his acquisition and not by merit.[7] The respectability acquired by wealthy though corrupt people, vitiates the social environment and corrupts the social institutions.

CORRUPTION – THE CAUSATIVE FACTORS

"In nature there are neither rewards nor punishments, there are only consequences". Wrote Robert Ingersoll not long ago which simply means that our present day situation with respect to corruption and crumbling moral standards in public life are nothing but the consequences of our doing in the past. If we closely analyse the political, social and economic factors operating in a particular period of history and try to co-relate them with general ethical standards of society and then compare them with similar studies of other periods of history then perhaps such comparison will give an idea about the impact of these factors on the value system of the society, its ethical standards, the extent of corruption and also the peoples perception about corruption. Similarly if we scan geographically the countries, which are very low or very high on corruption scale and co-relate the factors with prevailing standard of corruption, then causes can be discerned to some extent.

The studies made by the sociologists in connection with commission of crime in general suggest that lack of integration with society or faulty upbringing and socialization is to a large extent responsible for deviant behaviour, the group of criminal acts called corruption included. The societies, known for their permissiveness, result into broken homes, inadequate parental contacts, and problems of emotional instability leading to social disturbance or rise in deviant behaviour.

The economists, in their quest for the causes of crime specially those related to corruption, find that economic crime is related to faulty economic policies, and improper development strategy which results into unjust and inequitable distribution of wealth and services. The 'acquisition of such goods and services becomes a matter of privilege and not a normal entitlement as declared in the preamble of our Constitution and also various international declarations of Human Rights. The sense of economic insecurity leads people to acquire wealth for difficult days. Lack of employment opportunities and sources of livelihood are some of the economic causes adduced for spread of corruption at lower level.

Other studies suggest the general consumerism as one of the important causes of corruption. The factors like illiteracy, general decline in social values, social acceptance of corrupt people or their respectability in society and weakness of governmental enforcement system, weak and erratic judiciary, lack of nationalism and acquisition the sole aim of life have also contributed in a big way in making a prosperous but corrupt world.

If we analyse corruption from common man's angle then it would appear that corruption can be the result of following factors:

(a) Desire to have undue personal advantage as public functionary which may be conditioned by the economic needs (real or imaginary) social status value system, sub-culture, degree of social insecurity and the degree of resistance against social sanction. These may be termed as human factors. These human factors may be conditioned by various socio-economic conditions.

(b) Desire or willingness to provide undue advantage to some one for certain cause or the degree of willingness to succumb to pressure. Again this may be the result of human factors.

(c) Opportunity to indulge in corruption may be provided by nature of work, discretionary power, amount of superior supervision, sharing of information without accountability, chances of detection and punishment and other systemic factors such as secrecy, delay, inefficiency, insecurity, instability in administration and lack of objectivity at higher level. Administrative intervention can change these conditions and can definitely influence a large number of 'fence sitters'.

The problem of corruption specially monetary corruption has been studied from various angles but no universal theory explaining its causation could be propounded. Like other acts of crime this cann't be related to or explained by familial maladjustment or lack of social integration. It is a complex problem and in some cases economic factors may be dominant and one can link poverty or lower wages with corruption but bigger corruption prevailing in corporate world on the other hand negates any such linkage. Corruption in high places involving powerful people, and practiced in utter disregard for the welfare of masses, defies all explaining and can be regarded as one of those inexplicable human traits. Further a man may remain honest up to a stage in his life but a single incident may change course of his life. In my opinion most important factor with respect to corruption at high places is the value system one adheres to and other socio-economic factors affect only marginally while the petty corruption is more and more an outcome of enveloping socio-economic environment. Similarly corruption consummated after considerable planning and conspiracies is always a conscious decision and it is never mandated by emergent need but always a result of well-weighed decision taken in consonance with one's cherished value system. In this category we can place cases of Harshad Mehta, Sukh Ram and Sandhu.

CONSEQUENCES

Consequences of corruption are very serious for the community. The monetary corruption at every level leads to a kind of helplessness in the minds of people who find no alternative but to comply with the illegitimate demands of the public dealing officials of government and local bodies for legitimate work. The general perception is that "all occasions and opportunities of public dealing are said to be utilized to harass the people to extort illegal money from them without fear or sense of guilt. This near total break down of any sense of duty and moral values among public servants is indeed a matter of shame and serious concern. Already government has lost its credibility and confidence of the people".[8] The lack of confidence and frustration leads to agitations, attacks on public offices, and officers resulting into damage to government and public property. This type of violence as a result of direct action by the public attracts equally tough reaction from law enforcement agencies leading extra strain on law enforcement machinery and extra cost of governance.

Consequences of rampant corruption are to be suffered by the community everywhere. No part of community life remains untouched. All the institutions—social, political or religious—suffer image loss. The public organizations are not run by codes or rules but by their image in public. In situations where organizations suffer loss of face people run towards the governmental agencies at higher level but if they fail to get redress there also then a sense of helplessness or cynicism takes over which is detrimental for good governance and drastically reduces credibility of the government.[9]

Once corruption becomes wide spread, normal functioning, in public offices, stops as every one tends to keep himself busy in creating opportunities for corruption which increases cost of governance and in a poor country, no amount is left for development as major portion of revenue receipt is spent on public servants and managing public offices. All public servants don't get 'positions' where they can swindle away public money. The 'trusted ones' get the good postings and others are sidetracked or parked on loop lines. If this happens for long the number of honest officers come down or they are also forced to adjust themselves with prevailing culture. Once anybody occupies good position then he earns enough money to retain it or purchase other similar post in future.

When personal gain becomes dominant then it increases cost of a transaction. When computed at national level the figures will be astronomical for a country like India. In 1996 Hong Kong fraud study published by consultants KPMG estimated a total cost (to local respondent) of Hong Kong $ 230 million. In 1995 Australian fraud survey estimated corporate fraud of Australian $ 16 billion, Rajiv Gandhi as P.M also lamented that 85 per cent of the budgeted amount is not spent the way govt. desire. One can very well guess cost of corruption to public with respect to public money. If we include private corruption—corruption in private medical centres, corruption in concealing Sales Tax and Income Tax, extortion by way of donation, capitation fee etc.—then figures will be astronomical. Public burden is increased by non-payment of public dues as road tax, water tax, income tax, sales tax, rail fare etc. A man who makes use of a service available on payment but does not pay for it, means that he is increasing the tax burden on honest tax player. No body wants to be cheated for all time to come therefore even the honest person tries to indulge in corruption for avoiding extra-burden or increasing his income by unfair means, thus setting a vicious circle in motion.[10]

Adverse public perception about corruption is more damaging than the actual corruption. Public perception about corrupt practices gives free play to imagination and new and very innovative methods are found out to swindle away the public money. Public starts believing that "no paper moves in most government offices unless chased from office to office and from seat to seat by the applicants with the help of speed money". This perception helps the dishonest officers and corruption is recognised as 'best practice' and stealthily enters the system then no one has to take any initiative or risk. This paves the way for systemic corruption, which becomes impossible to be uprooted. The systemic corruption, corrupts even in–corruptible as it requires lot more courage and resources to oppose the system to remain honest. The situation prevailing in our country is just like that. Wherein it has become difficult to live 'honestly and simply'.

Corruption destroys relationship as it involves breach of trust. It destroys integrity and fidelity and ultimately questions the very legitimacy of the political system and prepares the ground for the agitations of the type that were witnessed in Eastern Europe and Indonesia,[11] which swept away the rulers in no times. Such situation can sweep away the democratic institutions as well.

Corruption also corrupts the mind and the scientists in love for greener pastures can sell out the defence of the country, and political leaders can mortgage the democratic institutions for private gain. Purchases for fighting forces, leakage of vital information regarding our preparedness can be the target of those who are against us if our personnel are not properly insulated against corruption a fact proved to the hilt by Tehalka recording.

Emergence of organized crime on the global stage is a menace to society and even the world body U.N.O. is anxious to control it. But very few people know that corruption, intimidation and elimination are the potent tools in the hands of organized crime. Once we surrender to corruption, we must know that we are surrendering to Mafia and we are mortgaging our democratic institutions to criminals.

Political corruption has taken control of governments. Even now a sizeable number of die-board criminals have been able to enter the parliament and state legislatures. When our legislatures have a fare sprinkling of corrupt and criminal elements one can very well imagine the plight of those who have to obey them. When temples of learning are full of persons having degrees by corrupt means one can guess the standard of education we are giving to our future generations. When presiding judges of High Courts are arrested for corruption, then what more one required to destroy the faith and confidence of common man in the legitimacy of judicial pronouncements. Everyone knows that material progress is dependent on advancement of science and technology and it requires big money for research and development in these fields. If we continue to syphon away 85-90 per cent resources for private gain then how many decades will we take to come to American or European levels.

Political corruption can take many other forms also. Prime Minister can purchase political support in parliament. Chief Ministers can engineer defection with the help of money at times even muscles. In one case whole of the legislature party defected to save the government. We are again going to witness a similar scene in Arunachal Pradesh if newspapers reports are to be relied. Criminal cases can be withdrawn, instituted and closed on considerations other than merits. The day is not far when high offices like Rashtrapati, Rajyapals can also be auctioned. All this and more can be done with the help of money. If we allow money power to gain in strength further then even the thin line between corruption and honest act will be totally obliterated and 'Corrupt practices' will be included in 'best-practices'.

CURE

Corruption is like a serious disease which has acquired, over the years, the epidemic form. There are many who feel that it has become incurable while others feel that it can be stamped out totally. In my opinion truth ties in the middle of it, i.e. the time has come when we must take a vow to curb corruption, cleanse the public administration and sanitize the governing apparatus so that the government is able to discharge its basic functions efficiently. I am of the firm opinion that corruption cann't be eradicated totally but it can be controlled and brought down to "permissible limits" that our social system can digest or excrete as per need.

Determination to eradicate corruption – Safety mechanism can be installed to take care of residuary part of corruption but the main stream of corruption should be taken head–on with genuine desire and firm determination on the part of political leadership, firm resolve by the government servants and vow by honest and sincere people not to succumb to the pressure of dishonest people and their designs. The 'political will' should be reflected in unanimous acceptance of basic tenets of governance by all political parties and a basic code of conduct to be strictly observed and failure in this respect to be visited by severest possible political punishment such as denial of right to vote or contest election for public offices. Once political determination becomes evident by the actions of political functionaries, the public servant and the public will follow suit.[12] As goes the well known adage that 'in a dead fish, the rot starts from the head', so is the case with corruption. Therefore, if we have to control corruption then cleansing process has to start from the top to prevent rot of body of fish. To summarise corruption cann't be tackled effectively without co-operation of all parties to the problem.[13] This co-operation cannot be sutured by ordinance and resolutions only but something more has to be done and it is the personal leadership, the charishma that can take the masses with him.[14]

Efficiency – One can say that corruption is the by–product of inefficiency. If public functionaries perform their functions efficiently then perhaps no body will like to pay speed money. It is the delay and inefficiency that forces a person to pay bribe to avoid greater loss.[15] If a person is efficient at the ticket counter of railway station, no body will go to travel agents for purchase of tickets. If our public health centres are receptive and efficient, nursing homes and research centres wouldn't make easy money. It is this inefficiency that creates situations where one feels driven to the wall and payment of bribe is the only ray of hope. In order to control corruption, efficiency in public offices has to be ensured and in this respect implementation of recommendations of various reports on administrative reforms should not be delayed even for a day. The efficiency can be brought about not only in government offices but also in factories and other establishments by better time management, accountability, quality control, total-quality management, citizens charter (Clients charter) and then by holding efficiency polls regularly at regular intervals.

Transparency and Accountability – The right to govern is a privilege which a government enjoys in return for its commitment to honour and defend the Constitution. The Constitution is nothing but the collective will of the people. Therefore government should never forget that the legitimacy to govern is derived from people and government is obliged to act in the interest of many over the interest of few.[16] The government is obliged to subject its official conduct to public scrutiny and should consider itself accountable to public, their constituents.

Transparency with respect to decision-making is very important in democracy. If secrecy is maintained even for the transfers and posting of officers, their promotions and also the criteria of promotion then departmental corruption cann't be stopped. If marks obtained by the examinees are published in newspapers and placed on the notice board then perhaps no student will pay speed money to the university assistants working in confidential deptt. I am of the opinion that public should be given free access to all information related to public policies and projects. Such access to relevant information prepares ground on which public can make well informed reasonable judgments that reduces chances of people becoming cynical and losing faith in governing apparatus as happened in eastern Europe. When timely and correct information is easily accessible the false propaganda loses its efficacy and people make reasonable decisions and more often than not, take appropriate action.[17]

Mechanism to deal with illicit enrichment – Public perception about corruption is dependant on certain tangible changes in the economic status of people connected with governance. If a public servant acquires wealth which does not appear to be proportionate to his known sources of income, the natural inference one can draw is illicit enrichment. Ministers, legislators government employees whose acquisition appears to be illicit should be scrutinized and legal action should follow. In this connection strict adherence to code of conduct and faithful disclosure of income, assets and liabilities of persons who are performing public functions is essential. The matter should not stop here. There should be some well established mechanism so that the statements so received should be thoroughly verified and scrutinised. The law should be clear the legal process brief and adjudication prompt to restore confidence in the working government.

Preventive mechanism – Prevention of a disease is any time better than its cure. In case of corruption also it is better to prevent corruption than its detection and prosecution. The aim of preventive mechanism are:

1. To restore confidence of public and public functionaries in the impartial working of the government.
2. To check preventable loss.
3. To discourage the fence sitters.

4. To scrutinize and identify the weak points and to strengthen the system to avoid future loss.
5. Constant review of the process and reaction of the employees to charge.

These preventive monitory mechanism if practiced properly, can reduce corruption considerably.

One can analyse functions of some of the department where corruption pinches most and plug the loopholes with the help of preventive and monitoring mechanisms.[18] Big corruption in a developing country is largely associated with industrial commercial development, infrastructure projects (road, power plants, ports, etc.) or areas where government approval or license is required. Such deptts. be subjected to thorough scrutiny and their corruption risk factor be identified. The experts can device mechanism to plug the loopholes in these areas. By this process we can sanitize some department, whose operational efficiency affects our rate of progress and well being of masses.

Deterrence – To eradicate corruption from public life is very essential, as was felt by our national leaders even before adoption of the Constitution, unfortunately this did not happen. Whenever there was any voice of dissent (immediately after independence) it was considered anti–national. If there were charges of corruption, it was considered to be an attempt to spoil good name of our country. If there were proposals to modernize the society apace with "Time Spirit" it was considered an attack on our civilization and culture. This tendency on the part of elderly national leaders led to a situation when political leaders started thinking that their sacrifices, made during freedom struggle, are license to indulge in corruption and avoid its consequences. The scandals of early years were brushed under the carpet. With the result no political leader was punished even after findings of commissions and committees.

The officials, in higher ranks were also not touched as it was considered demoralizing for the services specially the civil services. All these factors led to a belief that perhaps government lacks will power to punish "vested interests". This situation continued for a long time. Now there is growing realization that deterrence is a must to tackle graft and unabashed corruption in public life.

On international fora also importance of deterrence came up for discussion and it was agreed that a balanced view be taken and both

"Discourse and Force" be tried in our fight against corruption. Force signifies disciplinary action, which deters public officials from resorting to corrupt practices. Deterrence does not mean only the legislation with deterrent punishment prescribed for certain offences. Deterrence means differently to different persons. A man who enjoys very high place in society a clean disclosure of crime may be classed as deterrent punishment but for a hardened criminal the sentence of life imprisonment may be termed as 'bit lenient'. Generally speaking it is not the length of prison sentence or enormity of fine that deters a man but it is certainty of detection, followed by conviction and proper execution of punishment that deters a man. When some scandal comes up people (even enlightened and experienced) start demanding "Death sentence" without realizing that it is difficult to secure conviction in court of law when punishment provided is very stringent.

We must streamline our detecting and prosecuting machinery so that the culprit knows that there is every likelihood that his crime will be detected and conviction is sure to follow. No amount of lobbying and pressurising will be able to stop execution of punishment.

Incentive and disincentives: Just as deterrent punishment can dissuade a person from indulging in corrupt practices the rewards may also achieve similar result. Those who are upright efficient and honest should be given incentives by way of salary increase, accelerated promotion and other honest benefits while those who lack integrity and sincerity can be visited with disincentives. The supervisory levels should also be made accountable.

Public Co-operation: In addition to the measures suggested above it is imperative to have public cooperation in eradication of corruption from public life. In this connection empowerment of public or Extra Government Organizations to access information with respect to policies and implementation of them, execution of projects and also investigation of complaints of public may also be considered as one of the measures to curve corruption. In a democratic system public is the ultimate beneficiary, therefore 'citizens charter' be prepared and all branches of administration should be directed to strive to fulfil the duties mentioned in the charter. Success and failure of the functionary be evaluated on that basis.

International co-operation: International co-operation is very essential these days in the context of e-business and crimes committed in Cyber Space. The difficulties in tracking criminals in other countries is a real problem. Extradition and confiscation of property are other problems which if not resolved quickly defeat the very purpose of investigation. Our law has to be amended to cope with such situation specially the provisions related to procedure and rules of evidence. Uniformity in law of evidence and procedure is essential to avoid prolonged litigation.

NATIONAL RESPONSE

During world war II all methods were adopted to collect money for war preparation. The level of supervision of the officers declined because of peculiar circumstances operating at that time which resulted into defalcation of money and misuse of resources. Govt. took serious note of it and a cell was created in war department. In 1946 Delhi Special Police Estt. Act was passed and a new agency came into being for investigation of such complaints of corruption. As legal backing P.C. Act—1947 was enacted. It may be mentioned that provisions regarding bribe etc. were included even in I.P.C. drafted by Lord Macaulay. Later on a committee headed by J.B Kripalani submitted a report on "Corruption in the Railways" (1951) followed by Santhanam Committee Report on corruption in 1964. After these pioneering works the committees and commissions are submitting their reports on reform in administrative set–up and mechanism to prevent corruption. In 1988 P.C. Act was thoroughly amended and some sections of I.P.C. were deleted to avoid contradiction.

A watchdog organization called Central Vigilance Commission was created in 1963 in the light of interim report submitted by K. Santhanam. C.B.I. was created to be the main investigation agency. In states also anti –corruption agencies ere created to look into the complaints of corruption. States also have their Vigilance Commissions. In addition to these commissions at central and state level the departments and public sector undertakings also appointed their Vigilance Officers and Chief Vigilance Officers for enquiry of the complaints and also to oversee preventive vigilance.

With the opening of gates to IMF and World Bank Indian administration was exposed to critical examination of international experts. Certain difficulties were brought to the notice of government by the functionaries of world bodies. There was concern about growing corruption and criminalization in public life. Government thought that time has come "for a strong message to be conveyed that administration is for the people and not for the public servants themselves". In November 1996 P.M. inaugurated Chief Secretaries Conference to discuss, 'Agenda for an Effective and Responsive Administration'. The Action Plan included inter alia, 'Measures to cleanse and motivate civil services'. In order to cleanse the administration, it was thought that the service needs to address to preventive surveillance and deterrent prosecution and deal ruthlessly with the nexus between criminals and unscrupulous elements. In action plan certain steps were to be taken for proper investigation and prosecution of cases under the head corruption.[19] Corruption all of sudden became so important that almost all political parties included it in their election manifesto. Even after accepting these recommendations and action as per action plan corruption is increasing leaps and bounds.

INTERNATIONAL RESPONSE

With the collapse of prospering economies of South East Asia in 1996-97 onwards world organisation and regional groups were anxious to know the reasons for this collapse. I.M.F., World Bank and other organizations studied the problem in proper context. These studies revealed that this menace should be tackled internationally as it can afflict any prosperous economy and its impact is felt all the world over. "This has been the result of a recognition that corruption weakens democratic institutions and public administration undermines good governance, fairness and social justice, distorts the economy and competition, hinders economic and social development and damages a society's moral fibre. Of growing concern is that corruption is used as a tool by organized crime to achieve its criminal goals".[20]

On March 29, 1996 organization of American States (OAS) adopted first international convention on corruption which came into force on March 6, 1997, with twin purposes.

(i) To strengthen mechanism to prevent, detect, punish and eradicate corruption.

(ii) Promote co-operation for above purpose among the member states.

On December 17, 1997 the member states of organization for "Economic Co-operation and Development (OECD) signed the convention on combating bribery of foreign public officials in international business transaction.

In the year 1994 the Council of Europe established a multidisciplinary group on corruption to make recommendation for drafting a model code and also the international convention for eradication of corruption. In November 1996 a programme of action was adopted by Committee of Ministers of the Council of Europe. On November 6, 1997 Committee of Ministers of Council of Europe adopted 20 guiding principles for fight against corruption. These guiding principles included public awareness, co-ordination at the national and international levels, independence of those fighting corruption, seizure and forfeiture of property earned out of corruption, transparency of administration and other points. On May 5, 1998, Group of States against corruption (Greco) was formed to improve the capacity of states to fight corruption and also to oversee implementation of 20 guiding principles. Later on January 27, 1999 European states signed criminal law convention.

In 1990 U.N. Congress on Prevention of Crime and treatment of offenders adopted a resolution on corruption in Government. In 1995, 9th U.N. Congress held in Cairo a Special session was devoted to corruption. The background paper was prepared which included 'various characteristics of corruption adverse effects on development, measures and international initiatives. In the year 1996 U.N. General Assembly adopted two resolutions on corruption – (i) Action against Corruption – (ii) U.N. Declaration against corruption and bribery in international commercial transactions.

A meeting of experts was held in April 1999, which submitted recommendations to combat corruption. The Centre for International Crime Prevention in Vienna, Austria, has prepared a Global Programme against corruption, which outlined action against corruption in terms of research and technical co-operation and assistance. A database has been created to have information on "best practices, relevant national legislation and regulatory measures of different countries and international instruments against corruption".[21]

In February 1999, first Global Forum on fighting corruption; Safeguarding Integrity among justice and security official was held in Washington in which 189 countries participated. Now the world body is very much concerned to combat corruption and efforts are afoot to have model code on corruption including procedure for extradition, seizure and forfeiture of property connected with crime.

Good governance is the most important function one expects from a government. If the political leaders who formulate policies and select their team of people to implement them, faultier either in framing the policies or in selection of their team, then people have to suffer from ills associated with bad governance. These ills such as inefficiency, delay, lack of integrity, infidelity breach of trust by the public functionaries breed corruption and whole apparatus designed to manage the affairs of the state for the welfare of all is reduced to a system utilised for illicit enrichment of those in power and positions.

This can be likened to a disease quite contagious. If disease remains unchecked for a long time it is likely to take epidemic form. In our country it has already taken an epidemic form but it is not incurable. It can be cured if we have strong will power and unity of purpose. The success can be achieved only when all parties to the problem, e.g. the political leaders, public functionaries including judiciary and people join hands show determination to wipe out corruption.

Corruption has international implication therefore there is growing realization that it should be tackled effectively if all countries co-operate and agree to ensure uniformity in law and procedure to give strength to our fight against corruption.

APPENDIX – "A"

"Action plan for an effective and responsive government" I.I.P.A. Journal, July-September 1998, p. 652.

1. Elimination of corruption in public services should address preventive, surveillance and deterrent punishment, and deal ruthlessly with the nexus of officials with criminal elements and venal political functionaries.
2. Rules and legal provisions should be amended to enable immediate and exemplary prosecution and removal of corrupt officials without recourse to any political protection.
3. There should be no scope in the rules for any interference in prompt prosecution and punishment of corrupt public servants, and permission for such prosecution should be given within a prescribed period to investigating agencies, like the CBI, where prior approval has been stipulated. At the same time clear norms should be laid down to prevent demoralisation of public servants on account of frivolous complaints or inquires.

4. The investigating agencies and vigilance machinery should be strengthened by provision of adequate staff, powers, resources and independence, accompanied by proper accountability for results. The preventive aspect of corruption in government or the public sector depends on an independent and well-staffed vigilance set-up.
5. Amendments should be formulated to the relevant rules on the lines of those proposed in the rules relating to All India and Central services to provide for the premature retirement of officials at a reasonably early stage of employees' careers to weed out elements which are either inefficient or of doubtful integrity. It is further necessary to amend the relevant Service Rules to enable the review of integrity and efficiency of officials at any stage during their career, and to provide for premature retirement of officers of doubtful integrity in public interest.
6. The existing procedures for departmental enquiries and vigilance proceedings for Central and State Government employees should be revamped in order to ensure their completion within a year. The proposed steps in Central government include:
   (a) Prescribing firm time limits for all the stages from preliminary investigation to issue of charge sheet, to actual enquiry and the issue of final orders of exoneration or punishment;
   (b) Ensuring, through training, compliance with all legal requirements of enquiry and opportunity to the defendant so as to avoid procedural infirmities that lead to legal challenge;
   (c) Agreeing with Public Service Commission and Chief Vigilance Commissioner on time limits for consultation and advice;
   (d) Ensuring adequate number of full-time or part-time inquiry officers, and providing them with adequate incentive and training;
   (e) Suspending or transferring to non-sensitive posts those personnel who are being prosecuted or proceeded against departmentally on charges of corruption;
   (f) Providing for summary procedures in cases where charges relate to penalties other than removal, dismissal and reduction in rank;

(g) Dealing with deficiencies pointed out by the Courts of Law; and

(h) Making a careful distinction between petty procedural irregularities and substantive misconduct to eliminate the former from detailed inquiries and close such case after recording adverse remarks in the CR, issue of warning or counselling the officer.

7. Attachment and forfeiture of properties (movable or immovable) acquired by public servants by corrupt or illegal means not only in their own names but also in the names of their relatives and other under their control can be considered, through provision modelled on the Smugglers and Foreign Exchange Manipulators (Forfeiture of Property Act, 1976) and prompt penal action in respect of proven holding of assets disproportionate to known sources of income.

8. Areas of discretion available to various levels of administration should be curtailed to the minimum, along with steps to prevent their arbitrary use. Equally urgent are steps for deregulation, procedural simplification, elimination of unnecessary controls, decentralisation and delegation, monitoring of service delivery through citizen groups, greater transparency in all areas of public interface and corruption prove agencies, and the review of the rules and procedures governing procurements, contracts and extortion, as these would bring down the incidence of speed money on the one hand and extrusions at the decision-making level.

9. Objective and transparent criteria for the transfer and promotion of officials in order to insulate them from political influence in action taken according to law and in public interest.

10. Strengthening role and powers of Audit in the identification of financial and procedural irregularities to be followed by investigation for possible corruption.

11. Close networking of different agencies like Lokpal / Lok Ayukta, CBI/ CVO, Income Tax authorities, Enforcement Directorate and CAG in terms of sharing of information and intelligence and coordinated investigation.

12. Encouraging adoption of code of Ethics not only by civil servants but also all public functionaries, media, professionals, and the

corporate sector based on constitutional principles and moral values.

13. Assuring adequate remuneration, congenial working conditions and access to housing and health care for the employees.
14. Mobilising public opinion against corruption, increasing awareness of avenues of complains and investigation, and supporting efforts of citizen groups, media and NGOs in this respect.
15. Encouraging officials at all levels to bring irregularities or suspected corruption to the notice of the Chief Secretary, and to rewards such officials in case where the fraud reported by them are established.

REFERENCES

1. U.C Agarwal, "Good Governance: Cutting Edge of Administration", *I.I.P.A. Journal*, July–Sep.1998 p. 432
2. John M.M. Mbaka, "Bureaucrat corruption in Africa", *I.I.P.A Journal*, April-June 2000, p. 239
3. Kautilya, 25/9, p. 117

"मत्स्या यथान्तः सलिचे चरन्तो ज्ञातुं न शक्याः सलिलं पिबन्तः।
यूक्तास्तथा कार्यविधौ नियुक्ता ज्ञातुं न शक्या धनमाददानाः।।
अपि शक्या गतिर्ज्ञातुं पततां खे पतत्रिणाम्।
न तु प्रच्छन्नभावनां युक्तानां चरतां गतिः।।"

4. Kautilya, 5/9, pp. 25-26
   1. मन्त्रिपुरोहितसखः .... शोधयत्।
   2. पुरोहितमयाज्ससाजनाध्यापने .... धर्मोपधा।
   3. सेनापतिरसत्प्रतिग्रहणावक्षिप्त .... शुचिरित्यर्थोपधा।
   4. परिव्राजिका .... कामोपधा।
   5. प्रवहणनिमित्तमेकाऽमात्यः .... भयोपधा।
5. आयुक्तेभ्यश्चोरेभ्यः परेभ्यो राजबल्लभात्।
   पृथ्वीपति लोभाच्च प्रजानां यच्चाभयम्।।

{कामन्दक-5/82-83}

6. Claire Safran, *Time of India*, "Win with the times", 22-08-2003, p. 1.
7. "It is surely a bad thing that the greatest offices ... should be bought. The law which permits this abuse makes wealth of more account than ability and whole state becomes avaricious" – Aristotle – Politics'.
8. U.C Agarwal, "Good Governance: Cutting Edge of Administration". *I.I.P.A. Journal*, July-Sep. 1998, p. 432.

9. Sari Mehmad Pasha (1717), "Bribery is the beginning and rot of all illegality and tyranny, the source and foundation of every sort of disturbance and sedition, the most pervasive of evils and greatest of calamities than this there is no more powerful engine of injustice and cruelty, for bribery destroys both faith and state.
10. U.C Agarwal – 'Worldly wisdom prompts them to adopt the policy of "discretion as the better part of valour". They perforce adjust and adapt to the prevailing culture of corruption", *I.I.P.A Journal*, July-September 1998, p. 434.
11. "While seemingly benign on the surface, corruption breeds distrust and may contribute to more violent crimes as the social injustices accumulate and become more obvious", Thomas Chan–Corruption Prevention–The Hong Kong Experience, Resource Material Series No. 56, UNAFEI, December 2000, p. 367.
12. धर्मस्य तत्वं निहितं गुहाया, येन गतः स पन्था।। (गरूड़ पुराण-109/51)
13. The importance of transparency and accountability in economic sustainability, and "Without the support of all sections of society, working as coalition partners to address the issue of confidence building as part of a long -term strategy to develop and strengthen our national integrity systems, the task is an impossible one", Tunku Abdul Aziz' "Strengthening Integrity: Resource Material Series No. 56, UNAFEI, Japan, December 2000, p. 387.
14. Albert Camus: "Do not walk in front of me, I may not follow.
    Do not walk behind me, I may not lead.
    Walk beside me, and be my friend."
15. "It is said that the British invented the red tape and the Indians subsequently improved it by tying it up in knots. The Malays ever resourceful, turned it into a profitable personal revenue service". Tunku Abdul Aziz,—*International Case Study: Stamping out corruption in Malaysia*, Resource Material Series No. 56, Japan, December, 2000, p. 395.
16. Thunku Abdul Aziz "*Strengthening Integrity: The Importance of Transparency and Accountability in Economic Sustainability*", Resource Material Series No. 56, UNAFEI, Japan, December 2000, p. 387.
17. Thunku Abdul Aziz "*Strengthening Integrity: The Importance of Transparency and Accountability in Economic Sustainability*", Resource Material Series No. 56, UNAFEI, Japan, December 2000, p. 391.
18. Susan Rose- Ackerman:
    1. Program elimination (of corrupt programs).
    2. Privatisation (of current government service).
    3. Reform of public programs (revenue collection, regulation, social benefits).
    4. Administrative reform (make administrative competitive).
    5. Deterrent effect of anti-corruption laws (increase deterrence and reward whistleblowers).

6. Procurement systems (improve the efficiency of government purchasing).
7. Reform of civil service (substitute civil service for patronage and ensure that it is apolitical).

19. Given as Appendix "A".
20. Donald K. Pivagoff, General Counsel, Criminal Law Policy Section Deptt. of Justice, Canada, "International Anti-Corruption Initiatives" – Resource Material Series 56, UNAFEI–December, 2000.
21. Donald K. Piragoff, "International Anti-Corruption Initiatives", Resource Material Series No. 56, UNAFEI, Japan, December 2000, p. 341.

4

VARIOUS FORMS OF CORRUPTION

Richa Dwivedi
Lecturer, Dept. of Computer Science
S.R.K College, Firozabad, U.P.

"Corruption is a willful failure to perform a specified duty in order to receive some direct or indirect personal gains". – Elliot and Merrill.

We can easily find corrupts around us. Corruption is the biggest cancer for India. Wherever we go we find corruption in different forms. All departments and officials are highly depending on corruption. From top to bottom public and most of the officials are involved in corruption. A large number indulge in corruption for relatively small sums of money – at every check-post, at every police station or for every railway ticket. There is corruption in every field in some or other form. Corruption arising from transactions of public service providers with citizens is the most pervasive form of corruption. I would like to highlight various forms of corruption.

- **Political Corruption:** Most of the politicians are responsible for the presence of corruption around us. Booth capturing is a very common field where political parties are directly involved. They don't hesitate to kill the common public for their profit. Politicians are also directly involved in post-election settlement to increase the number of supporters for a particular party. List of scams include names of politicians. Whether it is Bofors scam, Enron power scam, Fodder scam or Stamp scam. Political leaders don't hesitate in spreading misunderstanding between persons belonging to two different religion or caste just for few votes. Politicians are indirectly involved in the appointments at various government posts. Also they are involved in transfer and promotion of employees. They accept heavy bribe from businessmen or industrialists to pass their tenders. There is political corruption in allocating petrol pumps and STD-PCO, giving permit of bars, etc. Sometimes the wrong political policies increase corruption. For example, if a policeman killed by the terrorists, his family is packed off with a compensation of Rs, 25,000, while the terrorist who have killed many such policemen are given a lakh each, a Maruti, assured job and permit retain their weapons, if they "surrender".

- **Educational Corruption:** Education teaches us to be an honest, responsible and loyal to our duties. But now as corruption is spreading in educational field also, how we can find a corruption free society. From getting affiliation to educational institute to paper disclosure corruption is all around. MBA entrance test (CAT) papers were in news. After registration of institute a series of illegal admissions starts, and then appointment of examiner, paper disclosure, cheating in exams, position of a particular student in university, etc. starts. Management compels teachers to sign on salary receipt of higher grade. Teachers compel students to take tuitions from them. Students have to give some extra money to get good marks in practical exams. There is high level of corruption in universities. Students can get address of examiner to approach them in order to get high marks. With the help of clerks, one can easily get the marks changed in mark-sheet issued by the university. Government funds are highly misused. Registrations of fraud institutions are common now day in educational field. From primary schools to universities we can find corruption every where. In primary schools one can easily find the names of many teachers in the staff register but rarely on the spot. Those who go to the school, they are not interested in teaching the students. Also the list of holidays is very long in government primary schools. At the higher level, candidate should get appointment after being eligible for the post or after clearing the eligibility test. But there is also corruption from both the sides, to get the job candidate has to give bribe to get the appointment, also candidate can get posted at his choice of place after offering bribe.
- **Police Corruption:** Police department is the department where one can find corrupts easily. From policeman to IG, most of the personals have link with criminals; they are involved in

small scale crime to high scale crime. Policeman can be easily found in taking bribe from truck and taxi drivers at crossings. They also have commission in robbery. Higher officers are involved in filing false cases or not filing the true cases and deaths in custody. Police officers compel culprit to give his statement as they desire using third degree treatment. Most of the policemen don't' take ticket in local bus or auto-rikshaw. In any cultural function policemen entered whole of his family in VIP block. Recent *'Taj' Mahotsava'* is the example, when actual VIPs and invited guests faced problems at entry gate but family of police officers had occupied seats.

- **Business Corruption:** The economy of whole world depends upon the trade. But business is not excluded from corruption. Political corruption leads to business corruption. Businessmen artificially increase the prices of commodities to get more profit. They are also involved in adulteration and duplicate marketing. Few years ago case of adulterated oil made news. Businessmen usually don't give the sale receipt to the customer and indirectly save the tax. Businessmen never made the correct payment of income tax and sale tax. Also they take their goods from one city to another without correct booking. Registration of fraud companies and fraud schemes are also made to get the public investment.
- **Medical Corruption:** Doctors are placed just next to God. But corruption made these Gods to Devils. Medical practitioners sale human organs illegally. In spite of abortion law they make illegal sex identification and abortions. Doctors subscribe those medicines from which they can get more commission. They also charge extra price for operation. Besides being in a government hospital doctors do their private practice also. Doctors sometimes issue illegal certificates. There are so many persons doing medical practice without having a legal medical degree or certificate. Medical shopkeepers sell duplicate medicines. Some cases of sexual harassment of nurses or patients by doctor have also been registered.
- **Departmental Corruption:** All the departments are full with corruption. Whether we talk about income tax department, sales tax department, custom department, electricity department, telephone department, transportation department, social welfare

department or tourism department. Most of income tax officers have their commission from the persons belonging to high income group to prevent them from paying the corresponding high income tax and also they put a safe hand on them to save them from any departmental action against them. The same case as with the sales tax department. Officials of these departments take action either because of any political pressure or because of less commission. The customs and Excise Act provides excellent opportunities for corruption because of the ambiguity and discretion at different levels to decide what should be the applicable rate. Businessman dealing in import-export prefers to give few per cent of tax to custom officers as gift than the actual custom or excise duty on goods. There are corrupts in electrical department also. Government provides sufficient power to department but even then people face electricity problem daily.

This is due to improper utilization of power and less demand of power. Un-recovery of huge electricity bill from industries and factories also lead to electricity problem. One can get his electricity bill with reduced units with the help of links in department. Officers from lineman to engineer most of the persons are corrupt in telephone department. Lineman charges extra money to repair the phone line. High authorities can reduce the phone bill either due to high source or extra personal charges. Any of this cause lead department in loss. Government faces loss in transportation about every year, because of less recovery from the buses. But the question arises if we see heavy rush in the buses then how there is less selling of tickets? The answer is again corruption, money is taken from the passengers but tickets are not given to them, so money doesn't reach to the government. Other government departments such as social welfare department, tourist department or such other departments take a huge amount of money from the government as funds but only 40 per cent of it is utilized. Other goes to corruption.

- **White-Collar Corruption:** This type of corruption is due to industrialists, judges, administrator and other highly reputed persons in society. Industrialists contribute a large amount of money in the development of any country. But to invest money, they try to make and save more and more money in short time period. For this they wish to get more and more tenders, which is possible with the help of money and ministers. Therefore they have a large stock of black money, which is undeclared money. Recently, about 3 crore hard cash is recovered from the house of a CBI head. The Indian intellectuals are paper tigers. Reports show that today about 25 to 30 per cent directly recruit IAS officers are corrupt. Judge is a person who is expected to be most impartial. But some of judges give biased decision, due to either fear of bully persons or due to money taken from one of the party.

- **Social Corruption:** Man is a social animal and is expected to abide by the laws of society. But unlimited desires of money and sex lead man to break all the rules which his ancestors have made. Now about all the social relations are affected by the corruption in human behavior. Demand for dowry, illegal relationship, prostitution, rape, illegal construction in front of house or shop, illegal possession of someone's property, etc., are few examples of fall in human character. Naina Sahani case and recently Dhananjay case are the examples of such type of corruption.
- **Corruption in Defense:** Army of any country is responsible for the security of the country. But due to some corrupt army persons all army become infamous. Kargil war was the result of corruption in army. Sometimes high authorities are also linked in business dealing of arms. Low ranked army persons sell the items of CSD canteen in the civil market.
- **Religion Corruption:** Religion and Priests show the way to God. But now it is also a part of business. Donation in the name of religion is very common way to make the man fool. Many Crores of rupees is collected during festival season, but how much of it is utilized is a question, for example about 5 to 10 crores rupees are collected from Golden Temple on *Prakash Utsava* and 3 to 5 crores is collected during '*Goverdhan Parikrama*'. Popes are found involved in sexual harassment. Priests and astrologers charge a considerable amount in the name of *Grah-Shanti-Pooja*. Some priests are also involved in compelling people to change their original religion.
- **Corruption in Games:** Appointment of incapable players, wrong judgment by referees, match fixing by players, etc. are due to corruption in games. Just one medal in Olympics reflects

unskilled team. Politicians interfere in the appointment committee and recommend their relatives for the team. Sometimes aspirants offer bribe to be selected in the team. Kale is the example.

- **Entertainment Corruption:** The field of entertainment is also affected by corruption. Acting aspirants whether they are male or female, they have to go through the sexual harassment. Madhur Bhandarkar case is known to all. Approach also work to get a new film, or to get awarded by jury. There is cut-neck competition between various channels, so they don't feel any hesitation to use illegal means to get down other one.

The problem of corruption can be resolved by listening to our inner voice and acting according to that conscience.

5

CORRUPTION—POLITICAL

Kamal Srivastava
Dept. of Public Administration
University of Lucknow, Lucknow.

"Corrupt influence is itself the perennial spring of all prodigality, and of all disorder; it leads us more than millions of debt; takes away vigour from our arms, wisdom from our councils and every shadow of authority and credit from the most venerable parts of our constitution.

— Bruke

The corruption has been defined "Perversion or destruction of integrity in the discharge of public duties by bribery or favour; the use of existence of corrupt practice especially in a state, public corporation etc.

In present scenario, corruption has become synonym of livelihood in society. Because people have lost moral values, they imbibe corrupt practices in day- to-day routine work. Thus, it has been phenomenon Mostly varieties of corruptions, are directly related with a minds set. Moral values and morality have become outdated and history.

Every individual is corrupt because of certain limitations it may be in the form of dishonesty, jobbery, breach, betray *etc*. Today it has become infections type of disease, means who so ever comes in touch starts corrupt practices in life. **Instead of Honesty is the best policy; 'cheating is the best policy' ha been set up in frame of mind.** Degree of corruption has been culminated in society. The percolation starts from top level to grass root level. *Important features of corruption is jealousy Competition is good feature for development and progress, but it should be free from any malpractice* *or by foul means which seems no where in society.* This is irony that corrupt practice is visible by naked eye and has a mushroom growth. Gradually society started to recommend these things which turn into a system.

Basically political nexus of politicians with civil servants is basic cause of spreading corruption. Nomenclature has only changed the style of functioning of politicians is equivalent to feudal system, which is a mockery of democracy. **Political corruption is the misuse of public power for private profit.** Not all acts which benefit the office holder at the expense of the people are corrupt, else the term would include all taxation by an absolute monarch to provide accustomed luxuries for his family and court, all fees and dues paid by serfs to their feudal lords , all sacrifices and gifts given to the priestly class in theocracies. Acts illegal in themselves and calculated to benefit the office-holder are obviously corrupt. But neither the question of formal legality nor that of the sufferance of the act by the mass of the people is of the essence of the concept. Where the best opinion and political morality of the time, examining the intent and setting of an act, judge is to represent a sacrifice of pubic for private benefit, it must be held corrupt.

No political group has been entirely free from jobbery, but corruption has not prevailed to equal degree at all times. It has responded to varying opportunities for the misuse of power created by governmental institutions, to psychological milieu to pressures arising under the existing scheme of economic arrangements. Any analysis of its prevalence must therefore regard corruption as a phenomenon of group psychology, conditioned by the entire cultural setting of the group; and no remedial program can be successful if it limits itself atemistically to prosecution of individual offenders or even to administrative reorganization.

Corruption presupposes the existence of public officials with power to choose between two or more courses of action, and the possession by the government of some power or wealth or source of wealth which can be taken or used to private advantage. Public offices are bought for profit, tenure of office is uncertain. Fortunes are amassed by extortion and embezzlement of funds obtained from taxes, cess, and from international development agencies, ostensibly for public improvements. Principal sources of corruption lies in the regulation of public morals. The administration of legislation against corruption offers an opportunity to the politically controlled police to levy tribute upon the so-called underworld. By overlooking the violations of those who pay and by vigorously enforcing the laws against those who do not, corrupt public servants have a weapon for extorting tribute from those engaged in such activities. Let the inferno of the indignation consume the wrong doer and the indolent alike. Rebrindranath Tagore's equi-contempt for the one who committed a wrong and the one who tolerated such wrong was not merely an emotional outburst but a logical deduction holding both as equal guilty.

From time immemorial, there has been no dearth of attempts to tolerance to offences palpably wrong, on philosophical, material or political counts. The apologist while defending inaction has invariably pleaded either helplessness like the blind Dhritarashtra in Mahabharata or compulsion.

According to Transparency International's Corruption Perception Index 2003, India ranks 83rd position in the list of 133 countries in descending order from the least to most corrupt and based in the bottom half of Asian countries. India's rank is likely to go down further, affecting its future economically as also on moral front.

Corruption in India has been spreading like a plague affecting every sphere of life. Divesting India of its spiritual past in the name secularism destroyed the very foundation that propped up national leaders in the freedom movement like Tilak, Gandhi, Bose who did not find any contradiction between secularism and Hindu spirituality as contained in the Upnishads, Vedanta and Gita. This spiritual orientation in character building strongly advocated by Swami Vivekanand was clearly wanting in Pt. Nehru's prescription for Independent India. The demonic lust, greed for power and wealth, and the desire to lord over the poor and the weak, got unleashed and uncontrolled, witnessing concentration of power and wealth in few hands and the vast multitude languishing in poverty. This distortion in Indian economy by cancerous corruption is clearly determined to investment and growth.

Though in the time of fast growing corruption, moral and ethical value has the controlling power to check corrupt practices and corruption syndrome. Recently, a wife of the senior central government officer started to have fast as much against her husband as against the corrupt system. She would continue her agitation till this systemic corruption was dealt with. Thus, the self realization is the more and more effective measure to check and control corruption.

REFERENCES

1. *Encyclopedia of Social Sciences.*
2. *The Pioneer*
3. *Hindustan Times.*

6

CORRUPTION: IS IT AN ISSUE?

Subhash C. Arora
Deptt. of Public Administration.
MDU, Rohtak

Corruption is no more an issue in Indian society rather it has become a way of life. The *Nazarana* tradition has become widespread and acquired new dimensions. Be it Divali or New Year, in general, and birthdays, marriage celebrations and wedding anniversaries in particular, lavish gifts come one's way and accepted willingly. These are no more just a token affair but an advance payment to be reclaimed in future. This, in fact, is the most widely accepted form of using money to get favour and it works. It is pertinent to narrate an episode which appeared in one of the daily newspapers. An officer of a state government who was gifted nearly three dozen suit lengths on Divali eve, asked a leading cloth merchant to sell them and give him the cash. After a few days, the trader gave him a few lakhs of rupees with the remark that none of the pieces had been sold but the money was found in the folds of the suit lengths along with visiting cards.[1]

Today, corruption has steeped into every pore of this country's public life. The common man who comes face to face with the agencies and officials of the government such as Police Station, the Block Development and Panchayat Officer, Municipal Committee Officials, Sales Tax Officials, Tehsil Office, Electricity, Water and Telephone Departments, Courts etc, either has to resort to some kind of recommendations from political quarters or pay his way through. The situation has reached a stage where people no longer even try to get a recommendation; they just try to find an intermediary who could facilitate the exchange of money, or better still an official who does not even need an intermediary.[2]

Though corruption is not a new phenomenon yet in recent years, it has assumed alarming proportions and has become diversified in nature. In the early seventies, corrupts were singled out and now it is the honest. Corruption has lately been institutionalized. From sporadic cases of malpractices, graft has now become part of public business and public life. Ironically, this business is conducted under the portrait of Mahatma Gandhi amidst the high sounding creed of '*Satyameva Jayate*' inscribed below the Ashoka Emblem.[3] These days it has commonly been accepted that honest is one who has not got a chance to be corrupt. In fact, the earlier saying that 'honesty is the best policy' has undergone a sea-change as it is now said that 'it is the second best policy.' Admittedly, the very definition of concepts like honesty, probity, justice, fair-play has lost its age-old meanings so much so that in the eyes of the masters, those subordinates are 'honest' who handover to them all the illegal and unethical collections without any deductions.

Likewise, the value-system has taken a U-turn. Earlier the social and family vigilance served as a deterrent against indulgence in corrupt practices. There used to be fear of losing social prestige particularly when it came to marrying of daughters to some respectable families. Now this very deterrent has become a support factor as the family induces their vulnerable and potential members to become worldly-wise and advise them to learn lesson from others in keeping and protecting the financial interests uppermost in their mind. Surprisingly, if anyone who fails to do so has to face the wrath and sarcastic remarks from his kith and kin. The Gandhian saying 'good means are necessary to achieve a good end' is no more seems to be relevant and has been substituted by 'end justifies the means.' Today a wealthy person carries respect and is held in high esteem in the society irrespective of the fact how he acquired the wealth. Likewise, that officer or manager is efficient or effective in the eyes of the people and management who achieve or exceeds his targets and nobody questions the methods and means adopted by him to achieve the targets. There was a time when corruption was not only deplored but denounced but now there is a resigned and cynical acceptance of corruption at all levels. A feeling of helplessness has permeated the public mind. There is growing feeling that the malady is too far advance to be curable; that the whole system has been contaminated and has gone beyond redemption.[4]

Politically speaking, there is no denying the fact that independent India inherited clean politics from the national movement led by Mahatma Gandhi, who spiritualized politics. However, with the passage of time a steady degeneration started. It is believed that "corruption that began as an echo during Nehru's times acquired the dimensions of a big bang during the subsequent Congress regimes" and at present, 'acquired the shape of volcanic eruption leaving the people dumbfounded.'[5]

Recently, the infamous Tehelka Scam has exposed how corrupt and porous our system has become as it involved people from different professions at various levels such as army officers, bureaucrats, political leaders, party managers and ministerial staff. And see the height of degeneration in politics that affected political parties and tainted politicians had raised the question of ethics for the journalists exposing them and not for themselves.

The story of scams during the last one year reveals that corruption in the country by its sheer size, magnitude and nature has broken all the previous records and affected the national life in many ways. A Chief Minister of a state had to lay down office in the wake of Taj controversy. A Central Minister was allegedly seen on tape accepting currency notes and reportedly swearing by God, "Money is not God, but by God, it is no less than God." Likewise, an ex-Chief Minister of a state was trapped while negotiating a monetary deal in an alleged attempt to engineer defection. Further, the Telgi Scam, potentially the mother of all scams in the country was reflective of the brittleness of the financial and administrative machinery. Officially, the racket involves money to the tune of Rs. 33000 crore. However, it may be multiple of the official sum. It is hard to believe and digest that a scam of this magnitude cropped up overnight. In fact, it must have continued for decades together with the possible patronage of high ranking politicians and officials. Another such shocking incident pertains to the Burail Jail break case as it is beyond one's imagination to think that a long tunnel could be dug out and that too without the knowledge and connivance of the high ups. Surprisingly enough, unlike the scams of earlier years these episodes raised more of public cynicism and less of despair.[6] This feeling is largely reflected as the Lok Pal Bill which aims at curbing the menace of corruption is still hanging in the Parliament for want of sound and healthy public opinion.

One of the reasons responsible for this cynicism could be the multiplicity of scams on the one hand and miserable outcome of the various inquiries and commissions appointed from time to time. As reported in one of the English Dailies "since independence 40 enquiry commissions have been set-up but nothing has come out of any one of them and their reports have gathered dust."[7]

Consequently almost all the seasoned players got scotfree from the clutches of law and law enforcing agencies and majority of cases they emerged as popular heroes in the eyes of the people as we all know that people's memory is too short. This clearly shows that corrupt and tainted people have not only been accepted by the society rather they got a premium over others.

In brief, the corrupt practices in the society, in present times, have picked up such a supersonic speed that the question of making a distinction between 'who is corrupt' and 'who is not' has been relegated to the background. The primary question is 'who is bigger' or rather 'biggest one.'

This reflects the ugly face of corruption as has rightly been depicted by an Indian poet –

देख तेरे संसार की हालत क्या हो गयी भगवान, कितना बदल गया इंसान।
कही पे लूट, कही पर दंगा, नाच रहा नर होकर नंगा ।।

Many reasons have been put forward for indulgence in corrupt practices, however, the most prominent one as has already been pointed out is the change in our value system. In this context, a reference to the story of 'A Thirsty Crow' perhaps would be most appropriate. In our school days, we were taught the story with the moral 'where there is a will is a way.' Now, the same story is being taught to the new generation but with a different moral meaning thereby that the crow was foolish. Had he been clever, he would have gone to the nearby coca-cola stall, picked up the straw and drank the water.

There is no denying the fact that the situation is grim but let us not become too much pessimist and loose all hopes. We know very well that the evil of corruption can never be eliminated altogether, at the most it can be made an issue and if we really want to make corruption an issue the need is to sensitize the masses and inculcate the age-old moral values through education to our coming generations. In this context, family and educational institutions can play a vital role. Further, the academic meets such as seminars, conferences and workshops can go a long way in highlighting the evil of corruption and making it an issue. The present Seminar is a right and appropriate step in this direction.

Undoubtedly, the problem is Levithanian in nature and the task is very tough but we should not loose heart.

है अन्धेरी रात, पर दीपक जलाना क्या मना है।

REFERENCES

1. T.K. Ramasamy, "Politics and Corruption: Then and Now," *The Sunday Tribune*, Chandigarh, March, 18, 2001.
2. Gurnachan Jagat, "Good- Governance at Grass-roots level," *The Tribune*, Chandigarh, December, 18, 2002.
3. Editorial, *The Sunday Tribune*, Chandigarh, August 25, 1996.
4. L. P. Singh, "Morality in Public Affairs," *Indian Journal of Public Administration*, Vol. XII No. 3 Special Number, July-September, 1995, pp. 618-636.
5. D.R. Chaudhry, "Frightening Shadow of Lure and Lucre," *The Tribune*, April, 25, 2001
6. Gaurav Chaudhury, "Corruption in Politics Touched New High," *The Tribune*, New Delhi, December, 27, 2003.
7. D.R. Chaudhry, *op. cit.*

7

UNDERSTANDING CORRUPTION: A CONCEPTUAL FRAMEWORK

N. Swaminathan
Dept. of Political Science,
Annamalai University, Tamil Nadu.

THE PROBLEM

India is ranked among the most corrupt countries in the world. Corruption in India is omnipresent and is playing unprecedented havoc with the country and its future. Everyday brings to light a new scam and we as a nation have degenerated to such an extent in this respect that rank hypocrisy, double talk and deception characterize our approach and attitude to the question.

With so much corruption all around, one should expect social scientists in the country to be so seized of the situation that there is no dearth of research output in the area, providing policy guidelines to combat corruption. Such however, does not seem to be the case. Gunnar Myrdal, for example, in his *Asian Drama* bemoans the lack of research on corruption in South Asia. Renowned economist Kaushik Basu believes the reason for this to be belief among the region's social scientists that since corruption is so evident all around, to write about it would be lacking in originality[1] .

However, understanding corruption is a complex task and requires serious research by social scientists. The purpose of this paper is in part to focus on this point, and further to develop a conceptual framework for understanding the phenomenon of corruption in India by drawing on the writings of some leading social scientists.

CONCEPTUAL FRAMEWORK

The roots of corruption in India go deep into the nature of the country's democratic politics. They are embedded in the growing 'deinstitutionalistion' of politics, in the systematic erosion of the authority of the leading institutions of our polity including the legislature, the executive, the judiciary, the civil and police services, and above all, the political parties. In other words, corruption is a manifestation of the growing 'crisis of governability' afflicting our system. Atul Kohli, the Princeton political scientist, who has made an intensive study of Indian politics in this respect, recently, describes the crisis:

> The evidence of eroding political order is everywhere, personal rule has replaced party rule at all levels—national, state and district. Below the rulers, the entrenched civil and police services have been politicized. Various social groups have pressed new and ever more diverse political demands in demonstrations that often have led to violence. The omnipresent but feeble state, in turn, has vacillated: its responses have varied over a wide range: indifference, sporadic concessions, and repression. Such vacillation has fuelled further opposition. The ineffectiveness of repression, moreover, has highlighted the breakdown of the civil machinery intended to enforce the law and maintain order. In order to protect themselves, citizens in some parts of the country have begun organizing private armies. The growing political violence has periodically brought the armed forces in to India's political arena, whereas the armed forces once were considered apolitical.[2]

The erosion of the institutional authority of our system is closely linked to the emergence of conditions wherein the vast army of men and women working the vital institutions at every level pay lip service to the core values that sustain the modern institutions while in fact practice and actively promote nepotism. The magnitude of the problem is best captured in the following words of B.K. Nehru, one of our eminent civil servants:

"The governmental machinery is now fast becoming an agency not for serving the people, but for extracting money from them and distributing it to all those who exercise any kind of power."[3]

So much so, there are no public goods in India today, only private goods. All pubic goods and services distributed by the central, state and local governments are sold to the public for a consideration–above the price fixed, where it is priced. On top of all this, we have 'big time' corruption on the part of politicians and bureaucrats.

Political corruption has today become virtually a legitimate activity. Mahatma Gandhi stressed that ministers and legislators should be, like Caesar's wife, above suspicion. He advised them to be watchful of their own personal and public conduct, not to make private gains either for themselves, or for their relatives or their friends. Our politicians today take the convenient stand that they must be seen as innocent until proved guilty[4]. Given the tardiness of our judicial system, this is as good as giving a clean chit to the corrupt politician. How has this situation come about? Who or what is responsible for this appalling state of affairs?

The widespread political and bureaucratic corruption in our country is directly traceable to, and reflective of the growing erosion of our institutions as bearers of authority. This institutional erosion has occurred primarily because of the actions of our political class. That is to say, our political leaders, instead of sustaining and promoting the health of the modern institutions created and bequeathed to us in a fairly good condition by the founding fathers, have consciously brought about their erosion. The key institutions of our political system are in shambles today but the disease, which has spread like cancer, originally began with our political parties—the most vital institution of our democratic system.

Our political parties have increasingly lost their vitality as institutions at the hands of their leadership from about the mid-60s, and thereby, inevitably and correspondingly, brought about the decline of other institutions, resulting in the crisis of gevernability. Our political leaders—both at the national and state levels—have consciously brought about this process of large scale deinstitutionalisation of the politics by turning the parties they are heading into more puppets in their hands sans authority and organization. To understand why this has happened, it is necessary to know how power is won and used by politicians in our system.

Atul Kohli has suggested a hypothesis which succinctly describes the Indian situation. According to him, strong parties, i.e. parties with well-developed political identification, programmatic goals and organization, develop mainly as means for gaining power. Conversely leaders who come to power primarily due to their personal appeal have no incentive to build their parties into strong organizations from above; on the contrary, parties as institutions, often constrain the individual discretion and personalistic power of charismatic leaders.[5] Thus strong parties, i.e. strong in the institutional sense, rarely emerge from above rather than from below.

With rare exceptions, the scenario as regards the health of Political parties in India—both national and regional–presents a sad spectacle of weak organizations with no ideology, and specific programmatic goals, and unable to constrain the discretion and personalistic power of their leaders. Many of India's popular leaders, national and regional, have not only failed to build their parties into strong institutions but have in fact sought to destroy the existing institutional constraints.

Deinstitutionalisation of parties results in a situation which leads to lack of effective party organization linking centre and periphery, and extending into localities. This in turn weakens the ability of rulers to implement policies and makes them vulnerable to "wave effects,"[6] when the electorate is swung in directions in successive elections by particular factors having to do with personalities or events. These developments and the resulting volatility of politics have produced a general 'decline of ideology'. Political conflict has come to be less and less about ideological and programmatic differences, and more and more about personalities. At the national and at state levels, political parties generally offer to the electorate one populist package or another, aimed at appearing to voters across the diversity of interests, and without a coherent programme for the fulfillment of the promises which have been made. As a result, elections have become more and more like populist referenda, or plebiscites on the performance of particular leaders. And lacking local organization that reflects the 'real issues' before the electorate, politicians take recourse to 'black money' derived from the informal and illegal economies in order to fund their campaigns during elections. This in turn has contributed to the enormous corruption in and criminalisation of politics. Politics has increasingly become a cynical game in which political capital is turned into private wealth and vice versa.[7]

The roots of corruption, then, lie in the growing 'deinstitutionalisation of politics' brought about primarily by the political class. As such the remedy demands the restoration of the institutional wealth of the polity. But this is not something that can be achieved /done immediately or through legislation. What it requires is the commitment to and practice of modern values of impersonality, professionalism and achievement by us, i.e. all those working/managing our institutions including the legislatures, the executive, the judiciary, the civil and police services and above all, the political parties. In short, what is needed is a revolution (of sorts), and this can happen only over a considerable period of time, as the result of conscious and concerted effort at different levels by a large number of individuals, groups and organizations. This then should be our long term goal, in the realisation of which our research effort should focus on identifying the areas, substance and depth of reforms that need to be carried out in our institutions so that conditions might be created for the spread of the modern values of impersonality, professionalism and achievement by the people at large.

Combating corruption through seeking to arrest the 'deinstitutionalisation of Indian politics' and restoring the authority of institutions is a fairly long-term project. Therefore, there is need to think of short-term measures to control corruption. And here, it is imperative that such measures are based on sound principles rather than adopted mechanically. This is the second point that this paper focusses on.

Kaushik Basu suggests that in devising rules and regulations to control corruption, we should seek to hold corruption down to what he describes as the 'optimum level'. His argument is that it is bad strategy to try to weed out corruption altogether. He argues that this conclusion follows directly from some standard principles of economics [8]. His reasoning is as follows: when economists first began suggesting the notion of optimal amount of pollution, they were criticized. But today it is accepted by most people that though pollution may be an unmitigated evil, it is irrational to try to eliminate it altogether. What this implies is that pollution control is costly, and hence it may be reasonable not to seek to remove all pollution. There may be differences as to where the optimum lies but that clearly does not call into question the validity of the principle.[9]

In the same way, corruption control is also costly. But unlike in the case of pollution and other such areas / issues, the costs of controlling corruption are unusual and diffused.

The direct cost of maintaining a bureaucratic machinery to detect and punish corruption is rather small when compared to indirect costs involved. Rules and regulations framed to curb corruption may end up putting an end to many legitimate activities, when they become too many or too intrusive. Hence, the main cost of controlling corruption through regulation takes the form of loss of production and delivery of public goods and services, i.e. losses of economic activities owing to the fact that excessive regulation induces cessation of certain economic activities. Those losses are, it is true, difficult to trace and calculate but that is no reason for ignoring them.

It is therefore necessary that in framing laws for curbing corruption, "We should stop at a point where the costs associated with the next regulation exceed its benefits".[10] This is where the role of research is called for. Adopting this principle in efforts to control corruption is a difficult project, no doubt. Calculating the costs calls for large amount of data and a large number of man-hours. The calculation of benefits is critically dependent on value judgements. Still, the principle, as argued by Basu, is very important. Every bureaucrat ought to learn it and use it within latitude of his understanding and judgement.

It is necessary to review the elaborate mechanisms for controlling corruption. This cannot be done mechanically and needs to be based on some principles so that we can design an effective system for checking corruption.

REFERENCES

1. Kaushik Basu, *Economic Graffiti* (Bombay: Oxford University press, 1991) p. 57.
2. Atul Kohli, *Democracy and Discontent: India's Growing crisis of Governability* (New York: Cambridge University Press, 1991), p. 3.
3. As quoted by Inderjit in his article "Battling Corruption": Going Beyond Rhetoric and Buzz-worlds", *The Times of India,* 1 October, 1996.
4. Inderjit, *op. cit.*
5. Atul Kohli, *op. cit.*, p. 392.
6. Stuart Corbridge and John Harriss, *Reinventing India Liberlization, Hindu Nationalism and Popular Democracy* (New Delhi: Oxford University Press, 2004). p. 76.
7. *Ibid.*, p. 77.
8. Kaushik Basu, *op. cit.*, p. 58.
9. *Ibid.*, p. 58.
10. *Ibid.*, p. 60.

8

CORRUPTION: DEFYING SOLUTIONS

Gopal Prasad Singh
Ex-Pro Vice Chancellor (LNMU)
Sanhouli, Khagaria – 851205, Bihar

The Indian Political system is besieged with casteism, communalism, corruption and criminalisation of politics and politicization of crimes better known as Four Cs. Here, we are going to deal with corruption 'a global phenomenon'. No doubt it has become 'a way of life' as it is 'widespread. So far as our country is concerned it has already sank deep into this all pervading evil. Really, corruption in public life of India has become 'a fact of life'. It is here, there and everywhere hardly leaving a gap. So, its omnipresence is being felt, horizontally, from top to bottom, i.e. from peon to highly placed bureaucrats, from PRIs functionaries to Chief Ministers, MLAs, MPs, PMs and vertically, from J&K to the Seven Sisters as well as from the North to the South. 'The whole country in every sphere and department of life is plunged in the stagnant ocean of corruption'.[1] The serious national concern is that it is galloping unchecked and unhindered. Undoubtedly, the 'country appeared to be sinking' rather stinking with corruption. The bold and brave pronouncements 'a call to launch a satyagrah' against corruption, such as, to 'wage war' against corruption, 'not to spare any corrupt person, however high' and so on, have repeatedly been made by all top leaders of different political parties in power at the centre and the states.[2] But no effective step has been initiated to stem the rot till the date. When time comes to take action, every body connives by saying that law will take its course. The reality is that law is never allowed to punish the guilty. Hence, the situation is very grave and grim as day by day the scale of corruption is going high and high engulfing the entire society polluting our daily life. Surely, degeneration and decay is going on unabated.

It is difficult to define the word corruption. However, the simple meaning is to abuse the public office for private or personal gain. The public office is called to be abused when an official accepts, solicits or extorts a bribe. It is also abused when private agents actively offer bribes to circumvent public policies and processes for competitive advantage and profit. Public office can also be abused for personal benefit, even if no bribery occurs, through patronage and nepotism.[3] So, bribery, patronage, nepotism, undue favour in curbing the law and rule etc., constitute the corruption. The money involved may be small as well as big running into billion and billion.

No body can deny that corruption remained prevalent in the polity in the ancient times also. Even our religious scriptures testimony it. But what is of grave concern is its ever-rising scale. 'The decline and degeneration of policies and politicians in India is visible, visceral and violent. No more are politicians satisfied with mere loot; they resort to the age-old style of the foreign invader—loot the 'native' and carry of his women folk and children to bondage.[4]

So, the corruption in our country has assumed an ugly form rather it has become like a cancer malignant enough to paralyse the every organ of body social and political. It has taken deep root since the time of Second World War due to the 'License-Quota-Permit Raj' though there were instances of corruption at the time of Congress Ministry in 1937 also. The English people were not quite immune from it. But the righteousness and ethical standard were perceptible clearly in their dealings. That is why some people opine that British Raj was better.

Our religious literature depicts Lord Rama as ideal king. The Emperor Ashoka and Akbar valued right more than might. Even in post-independence era we are proud of Lal Bahadur Shastri. However, the standards of public life have fallen steeply, particularly, since the Congress split 1969. Steadily, corruption has increased to such an extent that people have started losing faith in the integrity of public administration. It has spread even to those levels of administration from which it was conspicuously absent in the past.[5] Presently, it has taken a mega form. From jeep (V.K. Krishna Menon) scandal, the involvement of T. Prakashan, Mr. Kairon, T.T. Krishnamachari to the

Bofors scandal, the Urea Scam, Telecom Scam, The Fodder Scam, Tehelka, Telgi and so many others involving P.Ms., Chief Ministers and the likes are to the point out the scale of growing corruption in India.

Despite the legal efforts, such as, the Delhi Special Police Establishment in 1941 (DSPE Act in 1946), the creation of C.B.I in 1963 and the enactment of 'The Prevention of Corruption Act' 1947, the Foreign Exchange Regulation Act (FERA), The Import-Control Act, The Custom and Excise Act, The Income Tax Act, The Industrial Licensing Act, etc., the Corruption had grown monstrous. They seem to have provided fresh impetus to the corruption.

The Gorwala Report of 1951, the Santhanam Committee Report of 1964 and the Vohra Committee Report are excellent one but they remained more as a piece of papers. They were not implemented and adhered to in the true spirit. The report of different committee was mostly allowed to remain in the dust. Naturally, the corruption remained unhindered.

The first and the foremost cause of corruption is **political**. It is well said that, 'as the king, so the people'. If we have corruption at the top, it must percolate to bottom. It has been observed that if the honey is to pass through on the tip of the tongue of any one person, it is futile to tell him not to taste the same. So, one who deals the Exchequer must taste it. But public man must have the ethos and ideals that the interest of the State is above his personal interest. But these days politicians strive hard to capture power anyhow and then to keep perpetuated with it on all costs. It is here they have to embrace corruption, especially when elections have become costly.

The funding of elections compels them to resort to fair and foul means. The Gandhian prescription of pure means for pure ends becomes irrelevant. Here Marxian prescription 'means justifies end' prevails. So, they accept bribes in form of subscription. Here, we should give serious thought to the State Funding of Election.

Besides, 'power corrupts and absolute power corrupts absolutely'. Generally it has been observed that having legislative majority behind them the influential always escape the punishment. Whole Ministry and party stand on one leg to defend the misdeeds of a Minister on party line making it difficult to take action. It has been suggested that no one, however highly placed is immuned from enquiry if allegations against him are made by responsible parties and a prima facie case exists.[6]

Again, sometimes lack of power also breeds corruption. Leaders in the realm of politics and administration often rely on patronage to secure loyalty in order to have base or hegemony in the constituency. This weakens their grip they need to control the corruption. The result is that contact or relationship gets priority over merit. All these lead to generous distribution of patronage and protection. Further, weak institutional support provides fertile soil for rampant corruption. The very tools for controlling corruption, such as law, police, court, ombudsman, audit, public service commission, media etc. find themselves fragile if they lack support from political actors.

As has already been explained, that Parliament or State Legislatures has to dance on the tune of majority. Even the impartial and objective enquiry reports of various committees or commissions become irrelevant if these are against the member of the party in power. Mr. Gorwala has recommended that there should be arrangement for enquiry for every body even if highly placed by a tribunal. The President in case of Central Government and the Governor in case of State Government acting in consultation with the President should be set up the tribunal. An alternative would be to vest power of appointing such Tribunal in the Supreme Court. All facilities for directing investigation, obtaining evidence, examining document etc. would have to be placed at the disposal of the tribunal. Surely, the purpose of the tribunal should not be to punish but to find out the facts. But sorry to say that we have failed to pass the Lokpal Bill as yet and to allow full autonomy to C.B.I. Certainly, the exemplary punishment to the wrong doers will ensure the lessening of the corruption. Certainly of punishment in case of corruption will be an effective law in itself. Of course, political vendetta should not be allowed to come into the process. Here we should go for legality accompanied by legitimacy. Sometimes, wrongs are committed in the name of legality. Tenders are called and lowest one awarded the work. But free and fair tenders are not given due to the manipulation and manoeuvering of officials and criminal contractors, thus, the work allotted does not acts, hold legitimacy in the eyes of people. Everybody knows that foul has been played. Hence illegal acts should not be allowed to be done under the cloth of legality, only then we can control the corruption.

The second cause of corruption is **economic**. The consumerist culture has produced mad rush for material comforts. Acquisition has become the prime motive. People do not get satisfied with comforts for oneself but think in terms of next generation, not only that they aspired for generation after generation.

This lust for wealth has been described as the real cause of corruption. Corruption is prevalent both in capitalist as well as in socialist systems. Everywhere it is poor and helpless who suffer. The privatization, liberalization and globalisation has similar openings for corruption if it is derived of taking care of the last man in the last row. So, any reform for that matter development must have a human face. What is required is equity and equal share to the deprived and destitute in the benefits of the development.

The industrial houses, business and trading community run after profit. For the same they try to lure bribe the officials to curb the rules in their favour for profits. At times, high officials seek employment after retirement from big business houses. Hence, we find a natural nexus between business houses and officials for well-planned racket. Involvement of politicians have been found in all these.

The **social** factor is the third cause of corruption. In the society everybody even parents and wife aspire for the income above the fixed salary. In this way social ethos provides for fertile ground for the corruption. It is a tragedy that we go for the highest bid for I.A.S. and I.P.S. bridegroom and they accept the dowry with impunity though they are responsible for implementing the Anti-Dowry Act.

Not only that, we as the citizens even vote for the corrupt and unscrupulous thereby providing legitimacy to the wrongs committed by the corrupt. Social sanction or social acceptability encourages corrupt practices. After being involved deep into mega scam and scandal politicians gets clearance at the husting by the voters. They say that they have been exonerated in the court of the people. That is why tainted persons allowed to join Central and State Ministry. Hence, voters should reject the corrupt at the election and, at the same time, society as a whole must boycott the wrong doers in the social function or social relation. Side by side we must frame the rule that tainted person belonging to any party should not get berth in the Ministries or decision making positions in the Government. The Vohra Commission findings that 42 persons with the criminal records had made to the Parliament at that time. The recent survey conducted by Banglore-based Public Affairs Center (PAC) says that 23.2 per cent or almost one in four MPs have a criminal case against them based on the affidavits submitted by them. The obvious fact is that the criminalisation of politics and politicisation of crime has added additicnal booster to the corrupt practices.[7]

The fourth reason for the steep rise in case of corruption is the sharp decline in the *moral values* in our society. The ethical degeneration of individuals, especially of our leaders is responsible for this menace.

'The conduct of ethics has always been associated with adherence to qualities of honesty, integrity, courage, optimism, fairness and impartiality by an individual singly as well as collectively.'[8] So, moral weakness is one of the important cause of corruption. It is relevant here to refer to the role of elites particularly political elites in establishing norms and values providing role model. Here religious leaders should give more stress on character building and setting of moral standard rather politicizing and communalizing the society.

The religious prescriptions of abnegation of wants and an attitude of non-possession advocated by Lord Buddha and Gandhi have to be followed seriously in order to control the corruption.

The last but not the least is the **administrative** factor responsible for the prevalence and preservation of corruption in our public life.

In 1953 Paul Appleby rated the Indian Administration as one of the best among a dozen of then best administered governments of the world. But today we are poorly administered state, having a tag of a 'functional anarchy' or a 'soft state' always lower on the development graph and high on the list of corrupt states.[9]

Gone are the days when the steel frame were known for their honesty and integrity. These days 'speed money' or 'greasing the palm' has become popular. Today 'kickback', pay-off, scamming ethics have become wise technique.[10] Influencing appointments, postings, transfers and promotions of all categories of officials and the kind of money, involved in the process is the greatest source of corruption. The sycophancy and loyalty on the cost of political naturally have played havoc with good governance here. Lack of transparency and accountability has compounded the already deteriorating situation. The single greatest cause of corruption has been earmarked as administrative delay. Dearth of proper democratization of polity and sufficient development of powers has been termed as contributory factor for the corruption. Presently this malaise has assumed an ugly form.

In course of diagnosing the causes of corruption we have gone for remedies also. However, if we seriously and sincerely desire to put our system on rail which has got already derailed due to the corruption we should adhere to all useful recommendations of the Gorwala Report, the Santhanan Committee Report, the ARC Report, the Vohra Commission Report, etc. Besides legal reforms we should support the system with strong institutional innovations, such as Lokpal having the power to enquire even against P.M., the Central and State Vigilance to work effectively, C.B.I. with full autonomy, independent and impartial judiciary free from delay, Neutral bureaucracy, Free media and so on.

For all these our political elites should make a dedicated and determined bid to banish the corruption from the land called India. It is possible only when our political leaders learn to minimize their personal needs; they begin to observe ethical norms in their dealing under strict self-discipline; they stick to treat politics as a service to the people rather a means for power and perk, otherwise corruption – a monster will defy all solutions.

REFERENCES

1. S.P. Sen Verma, The Former Chief Election Commissioner, *The Hindustan Times*, 4th November 1972.
2. U.C. Agrawal, "Galloping corruption: Need for Effective Vigilance." *Fifty Years of Indian Administrative: Retrospect and Prospects*, Ed. by T.N. Chaturvedi, (New Delhi, 11 PA, 1998), p. 178.
3. Sunil Sondhi, *Corruption: The Asian Experience* (New Delhi, Sanjay Prakashan, 2002), p. 10.
4. T.N. Seshan with Sanjay Hazarika, *"The Degeneration of India"* (New Delhi, Viking, Penguin Books, 1995), p. 13.
5. Dr. Haridwar Rai and Dr. S.P. Singh, *Current Ideas and Issues in Indian Administration* (New Delhi, Uppal Publishing House, 1979), p. 198.
6. A.G. Noorani, *"Ministers Misconduct"* (New Delhi, Vikash Publication House, Pvt. Ltd., 1974), pp. 10 -11. He has quoted extensively from Report on Public Administration known as Gorwala Report (Planning Commission, Government of India, 1951, pp. 12-27.
7. *The Times of India*, Patna, 21st September 2004, p. 10.
8. (i) Dr. S.N. Mishra, Anil Mishra and Sweta Mishra, *Public Governance and Decentralization* (New Delhi, Mittal Publication, 2003), p. 22.

   (ii) U.C Agrawal, *"Corruption Hindering Good Governance"* ibid., p. 95.

9. Arun Prosad Mukherjee, "What is Ailing India's Administrative Culture," in *Contemporary Administrative Culture of India*, ed. by T.N. Chaturvedi, (New Delhi, 11 PA, 1996).
10. Bala. K. Dey, "Ethics In Public Administration Maladies and Remedies," in *Ethics In Public Life* ed. by T.N. Chaturvedi, (New Delhi, 11 PA, 1996).

9

SOME FORMIDABLE CONSTRAINTS IN THE FIGHT AGAINST CORRUPTION

I.C. Diwedi
(I.P.S.), CBI
New Delhi

Despite loud declarations of their desire to eliminate corruption made by Governments of the day (at the Centre and in the States) since independence corruption in India has continued to grow. It has gained acceptance amongst the people and now they seem to have reigned to their fate. India is perceived to be quite corrupt by the world community. Transparency International, a reputed N.G.O. engaged in fighting corruption worldwide, published its findings about the perceived level of corruption in various countries. India's raking in the list has risen from 71 in 2001 to 83 in 2003. Only Pakistan, Russia, Indonesia and Bangla Desh are amongst the other (big) countries which are seen to be even more corrupt. That could hardly be any consolation.

Our anti-corruption laws made more stringent by widening their coverage and enhancing the penalties. The enforcement machinery has also apparently been strengthened. All these steps have, however, failed to check the exponential growth of corruption. It has, therefore, become necessary to look for the hidden obstacles which are not allowing our anti-corruption laws to succeed.

I propose to speak about a few such factors, which to my mind, are negating all our efforts to eradicate corruption.

The most important factor which is responsible for the unchecked growth of corruption is the total lack of transparency in our system of governance. Democracy is a participative form of government in which people are expected to play an active role in the process of governance. Effective participation by the people can only be possible if they have prompt and adequate access to official information. Openness is a primary requisite for the good political health of a democratic state. Secrecy in government 'leads to arrogance in governance and defective decision-making'. In a free society it is, therefore, very necessary to strike a balance between people's access to information and preserving confidentiality where disclosure would be against public interest.

In 1975 the Supreme Court of India had declared (State of U.P. Vs Raj Narain) that "The people of this country have a right to know every public act, everything that is done in a public way by their public functionaries. They are entitled to know the particulars of every public transaction in all its bearings." Later, in 1982, the Court ruled that access to government information was an essential part of the fundamental right to freedom of speech and expression and declared that "the concept of an open government is the direct emanation from the right to know which seems implicit in the right of free speech and expression guaranteed under Article 19(1)(a). Therefore, disclosures of information in regard to the functioning of Government must be the rule, and secrecy an exception justified only where the strictest requirement of public interest so demands. The approach of the Court must be to attenuate the area of secrecy as much as possible consistently with the requirement of public interest, bearing in mind all the time that disclosure also serves an important aspect of public interest." (S.P. Gupta v. President of India [1982] AIR (SC) 149, p. 234).

More than half a century after we became independent a deep-rooted mindset of secrecy still pervades all spheres of administration. This may be attributed to the Official Secrets Act, 1923 and the Conduct Rules for government servants which made any unauthorised communication of official information received in the course of official work, an offence, irrespective of the nature of that information. However, but for few cases of espionage endangering the security of the State, the draconian provision of the Official Secrets Act have not resulted in successful prosecution of any public official for unauthorised communication of information. The deterrent provisions have, nonetheless, succeeded in perpetuating the all pervading climate of secrecy (which provides an effective shield to delinquent public officials indulging in corruption and favoritism).

Although all political parties were apparently unanimous about the necessity to urgently bring about transparency in administration concrete steps were not taken well in time. It was only in July 2000 that the Union Government introduced the Freedom of Information Bill, 2000 in the Lok Sabha. Parliament took a long time to enact the legislation (the Rajya Sabha passed it on Dec.18, 2002). But even now the Freedom of Information Act, 2002 continues to be in a limbo as the enabling Rules are yet to be notified. Section 13 of the Act states that as soon as this law comes into force, all the provisions of the Official Secrets Act, 1923, 'shall cease to be operative to the extent to which they are inconsistent with the provisions of this Act'. Since the Rules have not been notified the Official Secrets Act continues to remain in force.

The law, as enacted, is far from adequate. It does not provide for an independent review of refusals to disclose information by authorities. Courts are specifically barred from entertaining any suit (See. 15). Though there is a provision for internal review but in the absence of an independent forum for appeal the ultimate decision whether (or not) to release information rests entirely with the Government. No system for ensuring the right to information can be effective unless it provides for an opportunity for appeal to an authority whose independence is demonstrably guaranteed. Willful tampering with (or destruction) of public records has not been made a specific offence.

Exemptions under Sec. 8(d) and (e) of the proposed Bill (records of deliberations of Ministers/Secretaries and minutes/record of advice etc.,) are not subject to explicit "harm" requirements. Other exemptions too are very broadly defined (being in the nature of class exemptions). None of these exemptions are subject to an over-riding 'public interest' clause to determine whether the harm caused by the disclosure would be greater than the public interest served by it. Public undertakings are not included in the definition of 'public authority'.

There is no protection to 'whistle blowers'. Civil servants and other individuals exposing official wrongdoing need to be protected from being subjected to legal proceedings for disclosing information relating to : - (i) the commission of a criminal offence; (ii) failure to comply with a legal obligation; (iii) a miscarriage of justice; (iv) a serious threat to public health/ safety/environment; and (v) corruption/ dishonesty. The recent Govt. of India Resolution on Public Interest Disclosure and Protection of informer authorizing the Central Vigilance Commissioner as the 'Designated Authority' to receive complaints for disclosure on any allegation of corruption or misuse of office and recommend appropriate action is very inadequate as the CVC can entertain complaints only against Central Govt. employees.

Some of the states had already enacted their Freedom of Information laws before Parliament passed the Freedom of Information Act, 2002. A few of these Acts are indeed better than Central Act as these provide for imposition of penalty for not providing information (or providing it with delay).

An erroneous impression has gone round only the 'middle class' would be benefited from a right to information. It is the poor who need the 'right' more than anyone else for it is they who suffer the most from denial of information. Some NGOs have shown what can be achieved by making Government disclose information about expenditure of public funds. Efforts by 'Mazdoor Kisan Shakti Sangathan' in Rajasthan, 'Parivartan' in Delhi and 'Asha' in U.P. have demonstrated that local people can exercise a very effective check on the proper utilisation of development funds.

We must remember that changes in the mind-sets cannot be brought about merely by enacting laws. People's awareness programs and social movements would be necessary to bring about the desired change at the grass-root level. We should not forget that mere enactment of law has not been able to bring about the intended changes in society (abolition of sati; widow remarriage; abolition of untouchability; stopping atrocities on dalits etc.,) despite enactment of stringent laws many years ago. We have all been a witness to the concerted opposition by all political parties to disclosure of information of criminal antecedents, assets and liabilities and educational qualifications by candidates seeking election to Parliament/State assemblies. As more and more people become aware about their 'right to know' corruption in use of development funds would be substantially reduced.

This brings me to the second major factor hindering effective anti-corruption activity. Over the years people have lost faith in the ability (sometimes even the intention) of government apparatus to eradicate corruption. The public has come to believe that those, who have, or can at a time of need harness, the right kind of resources, can never be brought to book. Consequently they, themselves, are no longer amenable to abide by the law and spend their time and energy in cultivating 'influential' friends. People believe that the higher one is in the official or political hierarchy the lower are his chances of facing the consequences of his misdeeds and corruption is now viewed as a 'low risk high gain' activity.

Politicians in power have not been altogether oblivious of these perceptions. In 1993 the Vohra Committee was set up by the Government of India to look into the activities of crime syndicates / mafia organisations which had developed links with, and were being protected by, government functionaries and political personalities. In its report, the Committee said that 'the network of mafia is virtually running a parallel government pushing the State apparatus into irrelevance." It painted a dismal picture of the existing scenario which 'discloses a powerful nexus between the bureaucracy and politicians with the mafia gangs, smugglers and the under world."

Another Committee constituted by the Government of India in 1997 under the Chairmanship of Shri B.G. Deshmukh, former Cabinet Secretary, observed in its report, "In the past several years, there has been progressive increase in allegations of corruption involving public servants. Understandably, cases of this nature have attracted heightened media and public attention. A general impression appears to have gained ground that the Central investigating agencies concerned are subjected to extraneous pressures and have been indulging in dilatory tactics in not bringing the guilty to book."

In 1969 the Government of India issued a directive to the C.B.I to obtain prior sanction of the designated authority to initiate investigations against senior officers (of the rank of Joint Secretary to Govt. of India and above). These instructions (which came to be known as 'Single Directive') were later amended so as to include officers of equivalent ranks in public undertakings and nationalized banks. Instructions on similar lines were issued by a number of State Governments too.

"The stated objective of the Directive is to protect decision-making level officers from the threat and ignominy of malicious and vexatious inquiries/investigations. It is said that such protection to officers at the decision-making level is essential to protect them and to relieve them to the anxiety from the likelihood of harassment for taking honest decisions. It was also stated that absence of any such protection to them could adversely affect the efficiency and efficacy of these institutions because of the tendency of such officers to avoid taking any decisions which could later lead to harassment by any malicious and vexatious inquiries/investigations. The Directive does not extend to any extraneous or non-official acts of the government functionaries...."

Collection of information about corruption at higher levels of "Government is a very difficult and delicate task in which speed and confidentiality are of great importance. Compliance with these instructions not only hinders the collection of information and its verification as also the registration of cases and their investigation, giving rise to a public perception that senior government functionaries were above the law of the land.

A Division Bench of the Supreme Court of India (presided over by the then Chief Justice of India Hon. Justice J.S. Verma and on which Bench sat the next Chief Justice of India Hon. Justice S.P Bharucha) closely examined all the aspects of the matter relating to Government(s) issuing directions to investigating agencies about initiation and investigation of criminal cases (Vineet Narain and others Vs Union of India, 1998 SCC 226). Defending the right of the Government to issue instructions to the investigating agencies the Attorney General had urged before the Court that the C.B.I. being a special agency created by the Central Government it was required to function according to the mandate of the Central Government which had constituted this special agency for a specified purpose and the ultimate responsibility for the functioning of the agency to Parliament is that of the Minister concerned who has the power to review the working of the agencies which are under his department, to give broad policy direction regarding investigation and prosecution of classes or categories of cases and to call for information regarding progress of cases.

Citing the basic postulate of the concept of equality, "Be you ever so high, the law is above you" Court observed "Everyone against whom there is reasonable suspicion of committing a crime has to be treated equally and similarly under the law and probity in public life is of great significance...."

The Court further observed, "It is sufficient to say that the Minister's general power to review the working of the agency and to give broad policy directions regarding the functioning of the agencies and appraise the quality of the work of the head of the agency and other officers as the executive head is in no way to be diluted. Similarly the Minister's power to call for information generally regarding the cases being handled by the agencies is not to be taken away. However all the powers of the Minister are subject to the condition that none of them would extend to permit the Minister to interfere with the course of investigation and prosecution in any individual case and in that respect the officers concerned are to be governed entirely by the mandate of the law and the statutory duty cast upon them...."

"The agencies concerned must bear in mind, and if needed be reminded of the caution administered by Lord Denning in this behalf in R.V. Metropolitan Police Commr. (1968 All E R., p. 769). Indicating the duty of the Commissioner of Police, Lord Denning stated thus: "I have no hesitation, however, in holding that, like every constable in the land, he should be, and is, independent of the executive. He is not subject to the orders of the Secretary of State.... I hold it to be the duty of the Commissioner of Police, as it is of every Chief Constable, to enforce the law of the land. He must take steps so to post his men that crimes may be detected; and that honest citizens may go about their affairs in peace. He must decide whether or not suspected persons are to be prosecuted; and, if need be bring the prosecution or see that it is brought; but in all these things he is not the servant of anyone, save the law itself. No Minister of the Crown can tell him that he must, or must not, keep observation on this place or that; or that he must, or must not, prosecute this man or that one. Nor can any police authority tell him so. The responsibility for law enforcement lies on him. He is answerable to the law and to the law alone."

Lord Denning further observed as under:

"A question may be raised as to the machinery by which he could be compelled to do his duty. On principle, it seems to me that once a duty exists, there should be a means of enforcing it. This duty can be enforced, I think, either by action at the suit of the Attorney General; or by the prerogative order of mandamus."

The Supreme Court also observed: "There can hardly be any doubt that the obligation of the police in our constitutional scheme is no less.... The Minister's power in these matters has, therefore to be understood as circumscribed by these limitations under the law."

The Police Act, 1861 vests the power of "superintendence" over the State police in the State Government. The Delhi Special Police Establishment Act, 1946 vests in the Central Government the power of "superintendence" over the C.B.I. The Supreme Court examined the scope of the power of "superintendence" and observed:

"The general superintendence over the functioning of the Department and specification of the offences which are to be investigated by the agency is not the same as, and would not include within it, the control of the initiation and the actual process of investigation, i.e., direction. Once the C.B.I is empowered to investigate an offence generally by its specification under Sec. 3, the process of investigation, including its initiation, is to be governed by statutory provisions which provide for the initiation and manner of investigation of the offence. This is not an area which can be included within the meaning of "superintendence" in Section 4(1). The word "superintendence" in Sec. 4(1) cannot be construed in a wider sense to permit supervision of the actual investigation of an offence by the C.B.I. contrary to the manner provided by the statutory provisions. The broad proposition urged on behalf of the Union of India that it can issue any directive to the C.B.I. to curtail or inhibit its jurisdiction to investigate an offence specified in the notification issued under Sec. 3 by a directive under Sec. 4 cannot be accepted."

"...The Single Directive has the effect of restraining recording of FIR and initiation of investigation as in Saldana (State of Bihar v. J.A. Saldanha (1980) 1 SCC. No authority to permit control of statutory powers exercised by the police to investigate an offence within its jurisdiction has been cited before us except K. Veeraswami (K. Veeraswami v. Union of India (1991) 3 SCC 655) which we have already distinguished. The view we take accords not only with reason but also with the very purpose of the law and is in consonance with the basic tenet of the rule of law."

"Once the jurisdiction is conferred on the C.B.I. to investigate an offence by virtue of notification under Section 3 of the Act, the powers of investigation are governed by the statutory provisions and they cannot be stopped or curtailed by any executive instruction issued under Sec. 4(1) thereof... It is settled that statutory jurisdiction cannot be subject to executive control."

There is no similarity between a mere executive order and requiring prior permission or sanction for investigation of the offence and the sanction needed under the statute for prosecution. The requirement of sanction for prosecution being provided in the very statute which enacts the offence, the sanction for prosecution is a prerequisite for the court to take cognizance of the offence. In the absence of any statutory requirement of prior permission or sanction of investigation, it cannot be imposed as a condition precedent for initiation of the investigation.

"The Single Directive has to be examined in this background. The law does not classify offenders differently for treatment thereunder, including investigation of offences and prosecution for offences, according to their status in life. Every person accused of committing the same offence is to be dealt with in the same manner in accordance with law, which is equal in its application to everyone. The Single Directive is applicable only to certain persons above the specified level who are described as "decision-making officers." The question is whether any distinction can be made for them for the purpose of investigation of an offence of which they are accused.

Obviously, where the accusation of corruption is based on direct evidence and it does not require any inference to be drawn dependent on the decision-making process there is no rational basis to classify them differently. In other words, if the accusation be of bribery which is supported by direct evidence of acceptance of illegal gratification by them, including trap cases, it is obvious that no other factor is relevant and the level or status of the offender is irrelevant... It is clear that the accusation of possession of disproportionate assets by a person is also based on direct evidence and no factor pertaining to the expertise of decision-making is involved therein. We have, therefore, no doubt that the Single Directive cannot include within its ambit cases of possession of disproportionate assets by the offender....

The Single Directive cannot, therefore, be upheld as valid on the ground of it being permissible in exercise of the power of superintendence of the Central Government under Sec. 4(1) of the Act...."

Through their clear verdict (noted above) the Supreme Court has unequivocally upheld the principle of 'equality before law'. It, however, did not suit the corrupt politicians in power and the senior officials who colluded with them and shared the spoils. No action was, therefore, taken by the Union Government to withdraw the 'Single Directive' although the then Attorney Generally of India had stated before the Supreme Court in April 2003 that he did not think the Single Directive was appropriate. Later the Union Government chose to circumvent the law and provided a legal (?) cover to the Directive through the CVC Act by amending the Delhi Special Police Establishment Act.

The State Governments have also been unilaterally assuming far greater powers of direction and control than those envisaged under the law (and clearly demarcated by the apex court in the Vineet Narain case) to effectively shackle the police agencies charged with collection of intelligence about corruption and investigation of such cases by specifically preventing these agencies from conducting even secret enquiries without prior permission of the Government. Permission once accorded is many a time withdrawn later without disclosing reasons. A long time is generally taken for according permission for initiating enquiries. At times even the information confidentially conveyed by the enforcement agency to Government somehow reaches the suspect officer enabling him to cover his tracks. All the political parties in power are loath to give up the powers which they have illegally usurped to interfere in the initiation, investigation and prosecution of cases.

The Criminal Procedure Code (Sec. 197) and the Prevention of Corruption Act (Sec. 19) both lay down that prior sanction of the appointing authority has to be obtained before a public servant is prosecuted. This requirement was meant to save public servants from undue harassment and victimization. It has, however, become a major obstacle in the prosecution of corrupt officials. All the evidence available with the investigation agency is placed before the appointing authority to apply his mind before according sanction. In most cases it takes a very long time (at times 2 or 3 years) to get the requisite sanction. The accused thus gets all the opportunity to subvert the evidence against him. Sanction is refused in a number of cases without assigning any reason. Morale of the informant as well as the investigating agency is thus adversely affected and the enforcement agency and the Government both lose credibility.

Investigation and prosecution of corruption cases involving powerful persons usually takes a very long time and some prosecution witnesses and accused before the trial starts. The Bofor case provides a good example. As against this the case against Nick Leeson of the Barings Bank (in Singapore) was detected in 1992. Nick who had fled to Germany was promptly traced and brought to Singapore to stand trial. Within 6 months the trial was over and the accused sentenced. A comparison with the cases against Harshad Mehta would clearly indicate the reasons for our consistent failure to combat corruption.

Active and effective participation of the people in their governance through easy and adequate access to official information is the primary prerequisite of success in anti-corruption work. Functional autonomy of the investigative machinery (as provided in the law) has also to be ensured so as to restore its lost credibility. It must be clarified that the investigating machinery would continue to accountable to law in their work.

All Governments would naturally be reluctant to give up powers which they have usurped. A strong and assertive public opinion and a watchful judiciary would only be of help in our fight against corruption.

10

CORRUPTION: ORIGIN, CAUSE AND SOLUTION

Swami Parthasarathy
Dev Sanskriti Vishwavidyalaya,
Haridwar.

INTRODUCTION

To know the nature and meaning of corruption we are to reach back to root level of ancient and medieval historical periods. The corruption as a practice may have its extension in all vital systems of the tree of modern time. Indeed its root origin lies in times itself. Which cropped up in Buddhist period. It reached to neplusultra level in Muslim rulers time. The English had realistic approach. The development of Science and Technology gave blubber to think for 'self' only. The deep sea you search for self convenience oriented approach the more prone you become for malpractices. Herbert Rizley and Sir Jadu Nath Sarkar spoke very high of unique features of practices prevalent in Modern India. But the artificial touch in the way of manipulation is altering the naturalization of the unique feature, culture, practices, rules, regulation, processes, methods, governance, style, system and that in *toto* is corruption. Therefore, "*corruption is manipulation by artificial touch in normalization and naturalization of a practice.*"

ORIGIN

The Brahmin played diplomacy in Vedic times. Manu classified the society into four divisions—but the major fault are that to inherit this caste system family-wise instead of merit, quality and profession-wise. The breaking of the society by cessation of a part of it from development may find an alternation in natural practices. In Mahabharta enumerated that Aekalvya had to loose thumb being a prey of mal-practices in system. The madunend period was Buddhist. They started to cease the lethality prevailed in Brahmanic times. At last they met end due to aberrations in moral culture by male and female teachers in monastery. By this time the practices had only the seed level, they germinated when Muslim rulers ruled Indian masses. The Muslim men played unethical role and kept women only as a constituent of recreation. The Hindus had no such alteration, but to follow up the ruling system Hindu women started 'Pardah' they perpetuated retrogressive metamorphosis commenced simplification. Other sectors of system had same level. The more you followed up aberrated system the more you had chances of economic development. The British had a straightforward policy of dir. They had long extension of falsification of disystematisation and non-organized management of Indian population; even by the moment leaving the country they produced a scar on the face of governance in the name of Pakistan.

VARIOUS ISMS

Many philosophers wanted to homogenize the social system by their notion in Western and Indian land parts. Our land has Vivekananda, Aurovinda Ghosh, Mahatma Gandhi, Shankaracharya, Mahavir Jain, Guru Nanak Dev, etc. to talk to few for spirited system which function as a control mechanism of naturalization of practices keeping it away from aberrations. The development of Science and Technology and the feeling of self centeredness as supreme with absolute blend of non-belief in our fundamental cultural roots became the prime cause of abundance in mal-systems of naturals system corrupting it. The builders of nations, the teachers became the brokers. The policy-makers are rule breakers. The civil servants are civil rulers, and above all Democracy has a backbone of autocracy. The previous rulers and Jamindars changed the name and ruling the country. The backwards have unsustainable forward movements in mainstream. Because the developments are more economically processes now. The Ambanis have no satisfaction in running business. To give it a shape they want to be policy-maker or a watchdog sitting in institution. The uneducated is the Vice Chancellor of a private university though behind screen.

The industrialists mint money and run away leaving the labourers to commit suicide. The youth is given slow poison by western waves to deplete their vital energy not channelise and unite it to think for naturalization of system. This rat race, this cut throat practices has no limit, till Swami Subash Chandra Bose, Lal Bahadur Shastri, Chandra Shekhar Azad, Bhagat Singh, Raj Guru, Swami Vivekananda are shaped by teachers like Ramakrishna Paramhansa to lead the country. To set the policy by identifying the true aims of Social status to each constituent by relieving from orthodox views and by implementing it with the zeal we forced British to run away. We should have mission to bring revolution for peace, progress and prosperity at every segment of country to yesterday rooted corruption system in our country.

TACKLING CORRUPTION: A STRUCTURAL APPROACH

Why should not we be corrupt? Why should not a country be corrupt? If we look at the way our moral principles have evolved over time, we find that whatever is for the good of society is considered as moral and whatever is against the interest of society is considered as immoral. For instance, if people were free to kill each other there will be no orderly society. If everybody were to become adulterous we cannot have a healthy family life. In developed societies where the divorce rate is high and single parent families are becoming common, there are many sociological problems. The people may be rich but may not be happy. Like this we can look at all the Ten Commandments and find that behind each commandment there is a basic social purpose. Extending the logic therefore, we must hold corruption as bad if it is found to be an anti-social activity.

When it comes to corruption some will justify this as a part of our way of life. The Gita says, '*Swadharme nidhanam shreya, paradharmo bhayavah*'. We should all follow our *dharma*. If you are a businessman and if you have to deal with a corrupt administration, you have to choose between two alternatives. One is not to pay the bribe and thereby lose the contract or permit and thus allowing your company to go to the dogs, make your employees lose their jobs and your shareholders suffer monetary loss. The second is to pay the bribe and go ahead. Get on, get honour, get honest is the policy. There are economists and intellectuals who justify corruption in an economically poor country like India, because it helps to fix priorities when resources are scarce. There are Professors of Plutocracy who explain how in a developing country where resources are limited, corruption decides which project will be cleared and which industrialist will be permitted to flourish. I went to Thailand few years back and I was told that what they had in Thailand was honest corruption whereas in India we had dishonest corruption. What they meant was that in Thailand if a bribe was given the work will be done and if not the bribe will be returned. In India when you pay the work will be done and even if work is not done, money will not be returned.

Then there are businessmen who make a distinction between God-made laws and manmade laws. These businessmen say that they would not disobey God-made laws like the one that prohibits committing murder but they do not mind indulging in *Hawala* or cheating on taxes. After all sometimes the government itself encourages such cheating by asking honest people to pay 40 per cent of the income tax and those who suppress their income could get away only with 30 per cent. I hope in future such open measures, which are encouraging corruption, do not take place. In fact, *I am reminded of Baburao Patil's (of Film India fame) solution to remove corruption from our country : He said with one stroke of the pen we can remove corruption from India. Just call bribes as "Service charges"! It becomes legal.*

There is however another side to the issue of corruption. If stealing or murders are not being in the pubic interest, can corruption also be on the same category? The collapse of the South East Asian nations has brought home the fact that in the era of globalization where investments are taking place across borders, the investors want to be sure not only of good corporate management but also good corporate governance. Good corporate governance that the management will be taken in an ethical manner. Sometimes it may be possible to undertake activities, which are legal but not ethical. Such activities must be avoided in principles of corporate governance. For instance, we had sometime back a company like ITC, which has excellent reputations as a well-run company being accused of indulging in Hawala. We do not know what is the final outcome. Even a company like Barings, which was 400 years old, went down because one of their employees indulged in corrupt practices: Corruption may bring success in the short run but will be ruinous in the long run.

Corruption is not only related to the economic sphere. The Bombay blast case has shown that by giving bribe of Rs. 20 lakh to a customs officials, RDX was smuggled into India and that resulted in the death of 300 people. Corruption is not only bad to business in the long run but it is also dangerous for society. After all, the Hawala case was detected were getting their money and that was the same source from which corrupt bureaucrats and political leaders also apparently got their money. Thanks to the way the investigations were conducted, those who were alleged to be involved in Hawala scam might have escaped. The fact nevertheless remains that Hawala is the common source exploited both by the terrorists and by the corrupt in the country. Terrorism is definitely not good for the country.

On the basis of the above analysis, I hope we now agree that corruption is not good and therefore we should not indulge in corruption. Unfortunately, we are living in a country which is very corrupt. Is there a way out? As I see it, it is possible to try to improve our system and make India a less corrupt country. I will call it a panchsheel approach to corruption. There are five reasons why corruption flourishes in our country. There are four participants in the corruption process. There is a three-point method by which we can tackle corruption. Two of us, the CVC as a statutory authority and every patriotic Indian together can ultimately reach on goal, namely make India a less corrupt country. Let us examine the nutshell concept to fight corruption.

ROOT CAUSES OF CORRUPTION

Transparency International of Germany has listed India as the ninth most corrupt country in the world. Perhaps we are a very corrupt society not by tradition. I would like to quote from Lord McCauley, the author of the British Education in India, submitted his report in the British Parliament on the 2nd Feb., 1835:

"I have traveled across the length and breath of India and I have not seen one person who is a beggar, who is a thief. Such wealth I have seen in this country, such high moral values, people of such high caliber, that I do not think we would ever conquer this country, unless we break the very backbone of this nation, which is her spiritual and cultural heritage, and, therefore, I propose that we replace her old and ancient education system, her culture, for if the Indians think that all that is foreign and English is good and greater than their own, they will loose their self-esteem, their native self-culture and they will become what we want them, a truly dominated nation."

The above reference is the proof of India's high morality and value in the past days, now it is a matter of thought that where we were and presently what we are.

Can we ever have clean organizations in such a society? I would take the stand that we can have clean and non-corrupt organization even in our society. Two examples would show how in spite of social conditions, certain organizations have maintained their ethos. The Indian Army has retained its professionalism while their colleagues in Pakistan and Bangladesh, who shared the same tradition till independence, have become politicized. Calcutta is not a very clean city but every Kolkataiets take pride in the cleanliness of the Calcutta Metro Railway. We should approach the issue of building a less corrupt or corruption free system in our country with a positive attitude.

The level of corruption in a society ultimately depends on the values and morals of that society. However, inculcation of values is something that is only for social reformers or religious leaders to practice. In any population about 10 per cent will be honest by nature and 10 per cent always dishonest. The remaining 80 per cent are those who get influenced by the system and would be corrupt if an opportunity arises. The question is, can we design a system that will check the corrupt tendencies of this 80 per cent?

After the great stock market scam, the explanation given was that it was due to systemic failure. Two simple questions can be asked. Whom do bureaucracy, the political leadership and we design? We are also the system. Explaining away scams by invoking the mystic and mythical systemic failure is just misleading people.

That brings us to the issue of designing corruption-free systems. To stock market scam occurred, among other things, because there was a manual system in the Public Debt Office of the Reserve Bank of India which gave a 15-day float. This was exploited by Harshad Mehta and his friends. Have we since plugged this loophole and changed the system? I do not know.

The Prime Minister of Singapore says that if civil servants are paid only peanuts, we will get only monkeys as civil servants. India, eternally short of resources, can never afford to pay more for the civil servants. Singapore, therefore, has adopted a different strategy, which India cannot adopt.

We have to go to the roots of corruption and design systems that will tackle these root causes. One root of corruption is lack of transparency. If the Official Secrets Act is complemented, if not replaced with a Freedom of Information Act, it will be a welcome step in accessing information. Part of the power of bureaucracy over the public arises from this access to information. In the heyday of the permit-license raj, the liaison men were mainly engaged in finding information.

The word 'transparency' has become a buzzword in the context of liberalization. While we talk the fashionable language of economic liberalization, we also have the Official Secrets Act on the statute book. This Act has been invoked in Rajasthan to prevent the exposure of misdeeds in the implementation of the IRDP program. I understand that Rule 9 of the IAS conduct Rules was invoked to pull up that district magistrates who were bold enough to give the correct facts to the NGOs who were looking into issues of false muster rolls and defalcation of funds in the IRDP.

To introduce transparency, apart from the Freedom of Information Act, there should also be a general effort at educating the public about their rights. Government of India has taken the initiative recently to frame a Citizens Chapter. I do not know how and when this charter will become an operational reality. What is needed is that every citizen should know from each government organization, what types of service he can get, when and how.

The second root of corruption is scarcity. The scandals relating to accommodation or gas connection or telephones relate to scarcity of the product and services. This can be tackled systematically by designing rules and modifying regulations so that scarcity is removed. For example, the National Telecom Policy, 1994, if implemented in the right spirit, should have by now created a telephone-on-demand situation. That it got hijacked into the tender trap is a sad development. Similarly for accommodation, extreme shortage in big cities is the combined effect of the Rent Control Act and the Urban Land Ceiling Act. I understand that about 100,000 facts in Bombay are locked and kept empty because the owners dare not let out the premises. The situation has provided enough incentives for anti-social elements to speculate and generate a lot of black money. We do not see any serious initiative being taken to amend the Urban Land Ceiling Act or the Rent Control Act. If this be done, one major source of generation of black money will disappear and the corruption it breeds. Simultaneously, there will be relief in the availability of accommodation.

The third root of corruption is red tape. In our country, red tape is the greatest incentive for generating corruption. Bribe is treated as speed money. Indian entrepreneurs budget for this in their pre-operative and pre-project expenses. Perhaps this is nothing new compared with some Asian tigers. Much scope for red tape can be eliminated if we do business process re-engineering and combined with transparency, make the system simple.

I have heard businessmen saying that they are prepared to obey God's law but not a man-made law. They say that they would not commit murder or steal, but would bribe because that is the only way they can run business. The phenomenal growth of black money in the country is a result of our taxation laws. On the other hand, the recent experience of ITC shows that even the so-called multinationals or professionals will also indulge in practices like Hawala as that was the way to get things done, thanks to the FEMA. The solution to the FEMA problem may be ultimately a fully convertible rupee on the capital account also. Perhaps this is not still possible in this country. But if we are looking at the whole issue of corruption from a structural point of view and want to eliminate corruption, perhaps to make a judgement between checking corruption, Hawala and the issue of foreign exchange control before taking a decision. What I want to highlight is that a lot of corruption exists in our system because of our red tape.

The critical issue is whether the vested interests that are benefiting from red tape would be willing to eliminate it. Force may have to come from outside. Industry, trade associations and voluntary agencies like common causes should come up with proposals about simplifying system. There can be a widespread debate that demystifies the governmental process and builds up public opinion for speedy decision-making. It is said that human beings are rational but they will do the rational thing only after trying everything else. When we are dealing with corruption and changing systems, we are dealing with vested interests that stand to benefit immensely from the present system.

The fourth root of corruption is the archaic law. Shakespeare pointed out in Measure for Measure that laws are like scarecrows; they are set up to scare the birds. However, once the birds realize that the scarecrow is only a dummy, they start building their nests on it. We should adopt the principle of sunset laws as in the United States right across our legal system. Automatically there will be pressure for reviewing laws and finding out whether they need to be on the statue book. There is always a tendency to keep some archaic laws on the statue book because they may come in handy when somebody is to be harassed. Making laws up-to-date by building in a sunset principle will be one method of ensuring that this part of our system is not prone to corruption.

We can take each and every law made in our country and we will find that virtually every law breeds corruption. I come from Gujarat. The greatest defenders of prohibition there are bootleggers. For every law vested interests thrive and therefore amendment of the law is the problem. We all remember how when Shri Chidambaram liberalized the import control regime, people from CCI & E's office went and attacked his room.

Another aspect of our legal system, thanks to the various judgments of courts and administration tribunals, is that the corrupt in our system get much protection. There are so many cushions of protection for a corrupt person that bringing him to book is very difficult. What is needed is a systematic review of these cushions and sees how they can be removed. The path to hell is paved with good intentions. Many of these cushions have been the result of such good intentions being exploited by the corrupt. I do not know whether in any department/ organization such a review has been made.

In fact we can adopt from Singapore, the physical punishment of lashes to set an example. However mighty the corrupt person may be, the fear of public lashing may be an effective deterrent. This is one punishment, which the rich corrupt person cannot delegate to someone else on his behalf.

Prof. P.V. Indiresan says in article that when he was director of the IIT, Madras he adopted the strategy of minor punishments but promptly given, like stopping the increment as a method of bringing discipline. Perhaps this strategy is useful.

Credit must be given to T.N Seshan for focusing the nation's attention on political corruption especially relating to elections. We see today the launching of cases under the Prevention of Corruption Act against members of Parliament.

I find that when the law brings people under its purview, those who are powerful want to escape the clutches of the law by amending the law itself. The present description of the FERA as a draconian law and attempts to amend it are an example. One of the trade associations has called for an amnesty for foreign exchange stored aboard. Another example is the debate going on about providing an escape route to members of Parliament and members of Legislative Assembly by saying that they are not public servants and will not come under the definition of the Act. While no decision has been taken on of either these are excellent examples of how those with influence can amend the law to exempt themselves from activities considered illegal.

We must look at the whole systems and procedures and do what is fashionably called business process re-engineering to eliminate corruption. To make the system moves fast, we should also move towards a more open and transparent system by amending the Official Secrets Act. We should also employ the modern technology of computer and communication, information technology, to speed up the whole process, so that delay, which is the breeding ground for corruption, is eliminated.

Excessive obsession in the context of economic liberalization with corruption may be counter-productive, especially in the public sector enterprises. We will have to look at the entire issue of vigilance afresh. So far as the PSEs are concerned, they have to function now more on commercial lines and follow business ethics. Efficiency, productivity, quality, customer services etc. should be their watchwords and they should able to ensure that the investments made in the PSEs bring excellent results. It is now more important to do the right thing than do the thing rightly.

We can have a new beginning to the entire issue of vigilance by evolving a code of conduct, which can be the basic frame of reference for deciding what is proper and ethical behavior in public sector. Interestingly, the government notification of 3 March 1987 constituting PESB is to advise the government on formulation and enforcement of a code of conduct and ethics for managerial personnel in the PSEs.

My opinion about the PSEs gives an impression that merely having a code of conduct and ethics for the PSE employees is inadequate. At least to the extent it is relevant, the administrative ministries concerned also must be covered because the general complaints of the executives of the PSEs have been about lack of autonomy, interface and back seat driving by the administrative ministry and difficulties in taking purely commercial decisions, and so on. The role of the government directors also has been very much commented upon. In this context therefore if we are able to evolve a code of conduct, it may help bringing a change in the overall level of ethics in the PSEs and also bring a more responsive, responsible and businesslike work culture. The former Chief Election Commissioner Seshan has shown that with a code of conduct, which does not have even legal backing, could be conducted with less ostentation. It should be possible therefore to evolve a more effective, transparent, easily understood code of conduct for the PSEs and the administrative ministries.

"*Oscar Wilde said that the thief is the artist and the policeman only the critic*". It has been well said that it is difficult to make anything foolproof because fools are so ingenious. Therefore, while we redesign the system we can never afford to relax and rest on our oars.

Perhaps voluntary agencies or consumer activist group can come up with model laws and mould public opinion. In these days of judicial activism so that the system can get reformed. Merely complaining that scams are a result of systemic failure is no excuse.

CORRUPTION IN THE FINANCIAL SECTOR

In the ultimate analysis, business is based on trust. Honesty is the best policy. After all, business is a win-win exercise. Business flourishes when they is greater transparency, honest and trust in business transactions. When trust fails and fraud occurs, business suffers. Being aware of the potential for business frauds and also detecting them in time and preventing them therefore becomes an essential condition for success in any business.

Business frauds are basically white-collar crimes. The fraudster is always the creative person and flag the initiative. *So when we talk about business frauds, we are talking about a group of intelligent knowledge workers who are crooked and who can always think of innovative methods of beating the system and committing frauds.* So the main challenge before those who would like to ensure a clean transparent accountable business is how to first increase the awareness about the potential for business frauds, detect them and prevent them.

The nature of frauds is constantly, changing. One of the important developments in recent times is the increasing application of information technology and computers, which has provided opportunities for a new generation of crimes, which can be called cyber crimes. We lack a basic legal framework for the electronic business.

The insistence on computerization in banks is with a view to ensure that the corruption cases are reduced. There are people who challenge this idea saying that at best computerization can help in detection of corruption and not prevent them. In this context it is worth noting what bankers says:

As regards the question whether computerization would help banks in prevention and early detection of frauds can be classified as (a) frauds in con-credit areas and (b) frauds in credit areas. In non-credit areas mainly frauds relate to fraudulent encashment of cheques, withdrawal slips, refund orders, demand drafts, bankers' cheques, misappropriation as also fraudulent transaction in the books of branches put through cheques, misappropriation as also fraudulent transactions in the books of branches put through by the bank's own staff. Existing computerized system and upgradation thereof will help in prevention as also early detection of frauds, which will save bank's precious funds as also will protect the long-term interest of bank employees who unwittingly become prey to the design of unscrupulous elements. Following are the areas where full-fledged computerization will have salutary effect in prevention and early detection of frauds.

Fraudulent encashment of cheques bearing forged signatures occur because the passing officials do not find it convenient to verify the signature stored in signature card cabinets requiring manual location of the signature. If specimen signatures are captured in the computer, it will facilitate easy verification and provide security against tampering.

Stop payment instructions received from account holders with regard to lost cheques can be put in computer so that a caution signal would be available a lost cheque is presented for payment.

Manipulation of books unscrupulous staff interalias casting of wrong balance and making wrong credit entries can be either prevented or detected promptly because the computerization would enable tallying/balancing of books on daily basis.

The reconciliation of transaction relating to drafts issued and paid through computerized system would help early detection of fraudulent payment.

Frauds relating to local clearing operations may be minimized through prompt reconciliation of number and amount of cheques through computerized system.

Attempts of unscrupulous staff to perpetrate frauds by raising fake credits through inter-branch accounts may be thwarted through computerized system for reconciliation of entries between originating branches and responding branches.

By introduction of passbook writing machines frauds relating to misappropriation of cash receipt by cash department staff can be prevented or early detected.

There is increasing trend in payment of lost /fake DDs presented by fraudulent means. Computerization and continuous updating of data related to stolen/lost drafts on the system can help in reducing this. Officer's signatures captured in the computer can be used to verify whether the DDs are signed by the concerned officer.

As per the guidelines of RBI, MICR cleaning and electronic clearance system has been introduced at Metro Centres to take care of corporate clients. The Service Branches does the work of intermediately between the local branches of the bank and cleaning house. Lack of proper reconciliation of number and amount of cheques sent by branches to the service branch/main branch and vice versa on a daily basis has facilitated perpetration of massive fraud. A software system for daily reconciliation, if introduced, can be used to avert/ detect such frauds.

As regards advances, in credit related frauds, it would help banks if computerized database of parties enjoying credit facilities from different banks in the same centre is available to avoid double financing, to know the state of affairs of the existing account, and to ensure that the same persons do not enjoy facilities under different names or firm.

Database of information of fraudsters, willful defaulters with photographs of the proprietors/partners/directors etc. will help the banking system.

Quick exchange of information relating to transactions in corporate accounts, remittances, clearance of instruments, payment of divided warrants, interest warrants, refund orders and reconciliation thereof, etc. will enhance customer service and help prevent frauds.

A fraud essentially involves either the initiative of an individual or collusion among many people. When it comes to the individual initiative,

I am reminded of what one of the bankers said. He is afraid, he said, of the loyal workers than the sincere worker works sincerely, may be puts in long hours, he never takes leave. So he is able to run parallel accounts and play with the system. Because he knows the system through and through, he can wreak havoc on the system. When it comes to collusive type of frauds, it involves more than one person. In order to prevent this happening, we must be able to make our entire system processing is transparent as possible and also building in check and balances to prevent frauds.

One of the issues that is expected to rise especially in the context of greater use of information technology is the danger from hackers. Hackers are those who are able to cut through the security cordon through encryption in the installed software and are able to break codes. There is therefore need for focusing on building up healthy and vigorous encryption systems. Especially in the context of the prohibition of the United States permitting export of really effective encryption systems, it is necessary that we develop our own indigenous systems so far as encryption is concerned.

One method of ensuring that frauds do not take place is to also have effective punishment systems. Our legal systems are so dilatory that many a time the guilty escape and even if the punishment is meted out, it takes a long time. Many a time when financial frauds are committed, the fraudster has so much resources at his command, he can engage the best legal brains and quibble his way through the entire process to freedom. We should therefore have a look at the punishment is quickly meted out to the corrupt and the guilty.

Technology also can help many a time in cheering frauds. Apart from the general issue of computerization we have seen above, with the increasing use of credit cards, which are used on the magnetic strip, I am told, it is possible within 10 minutes, to duplicate the strip and exploit the credit cards. I understand that companies like *VISA are losing nearly $5 million per annum on such frauds and they have taken this loss as a part of their occupation hazard*. Of course better technological methods are being evolved to ensure that such frauds do not take place.

How do we evolve systems which can detect and prevent frauds/ probably the best example is the old adage "set a thief to catch a thief." While we cannot engage fraudsters to detect frauds, just are in the murder cases where one of the accused turns approver, it may be worthwhile to tap the brains of the fraudsters and also build up wide database about the modus operandi. Thus not only preventive measures can be installed but also the awareness all through the organization can be enhanced to prevent frauds.

Ultimately it may boil down to a question of specialization. In England, there is the Serious Fraud Office and some other countries may also have similar systems which can look into economic offences and particularly frauds. This sort of building up of expertise and domain of knowledge in different areas of business frauds is a vital institutional framework needed today. Especially when our economy is getting closely linked with the global economy there is every possibility that in future the frauds need not be only national but could have international ramification also. Building up knowledge of fraud awareness, detection and prevention, therefore, becomes vital.

OPTIONAL

Role of IT in Controlling Corruption on the Financial Sector. The financial sector consists of the banks, the financial institutions and the capital market. Forty per cent of the cases that come of the Vigilance Commissioner relate to bank frauds. We may therefore start by examining the corruption dimension in the banking sector. Corruption has its root in greed. Ultimately the level of corruption in the banking sector or for that matter in the financial sector will depend upon the quality and the nature of the people operating in these sectors.

One glaring deficiency is the fact that in this age of information technology (IT) and the shift towards digital economy, our banking system is hopelessly in a manual made. Out of 65,000 branches only 5,000 are computerized. I am told may be about 25,000 to 30,000 branches deal with nearly 80 per cent of the business. It may not be possible to computerize the rural branches. But in a city like Mumbai, one of the greatest scams in recent times, the Harshad Mehta scam took place because in the Public Dept. Office of the RBI, there was a manual system. A fifteen-day float was available and that was exploited. Like locking the stable doors after the horse fled, I understand the computerization of the Public Debt Office was done after the scam broke out. The government's explanation, if I remember right, is that the scam took place because there was a systemic failure. So, it is obvious that we have at the system and improve it.

Some would say that funds would be a problem for computerization. But I understand the World Bank has been able to help some banks. Even otherwise, I would suggest that the customer in this country deserves a better treatment and there is no reason why outstation cheques should take two weeks to get enchased. Computerization incidentally will also have the benefit of increasing the velocity of business and reducing to some extent the working-capital needs of industry. As CVC my responsibility is only restricted to the vigilance angle. From the purely vigilance angle there is an urgent need for computerization. The issue had so far got bogged down between the trade unions and the management and the pace of computerization was low. But today, after the CVC's order the choice before the public at large is: Do we want computerization or do we want corruption in banks? Stated so simply the quibbling about the difficulties of computerization will disappear. No one even the greatest beneficiary of our corrupt system will dare to openly say that he is in favour of corruption.

A number of problems are posed by those opposed to computerization. The first is the availability of hardware and software. So far as the hardware issue is concerned, the National Task Force on Information Technology (NTFIT) has already given valuable recommendations, including rapid depreciation to the extent of 60 per cent in the first year itself for investments made in computers. Especially when we have a national goal like India becoming an IT superpower, we cannot afford to have the banking sector crippled by a manual system.

Another important aspect in the banking sector is the need for secrecy and safety. This will care for excellent encryption systems. In this connection Dr. Vidyasagar of the Centre for Artificial Intelligence unit of the DRDO in Bangalore has brought the following to my notice.

It is not enough merely to computerize the operation of each bank branch—it is imperative also to computerize the transaction between branches and between banks. In other words, both intra-branch and inter-branch (as also inter-bank) transactions must be through a computer network so that the opportunities for fraud and delay are greatly reduced if not eliminated. Once the computerization of banking is adopted as an objective to do attained at top speed, we must all squarely confront the issue to be addressed namely (1) the security of the network itself, and (2) the security of the traffic carried on the network. The first item involves protecting the network against "hackers" who will try to disable the network, while the second item involves preventing anyone from using tools such as encryption and decryption, digital signatures, message authentication etc. Unfortunately, most of the "firewall" products sold by commercial vendors for network security incorporate only very rudimentary packet level filtering, and can be compromised very easily. Indeed it is not an exaggeration to say that by providing a false security these weak firewalls are worse than having no firewall at all. As for the security of the traffic, you may be aware that, by U.S. export law, no encryption software products can be expored from the U.S. if they are too strong to be broken by the U.S. National Security Agency. To put it bluntly, only insecure software can be exported. When various multinational companies go around peddling "secure communication software" product to gullible Indian customers, they conveniently neglect to mention this aspect of U.S. export law. Another related point is that when we buy an imported software product that is a "black box" to us, we cannot be sure that the software package does not contain a time bomb of sorts, to cause havoc to the network when an external command is issued by a hostile nation.

The only way to guard against insecure or booby-trapped software products is to write our own software and to develop our own hardware. It so happens that both network security and traffic security are core competencies of DRDO and to this centre in particular. We have now (1) evolved a set of software tools give protection at several layers and thus provide much greater security than simple packet level filtering. As for providing secured communication between computers, fortunately the mathematics for encryption algorithms is well known and the ideas themselves are either not patented or else in the public to write our own code for encrypted communication. With the assistance of another DRDO laboratory (SAG located in Delhi) we in this centre have begun to develop secure communication tools, and hope to have a prototype in place in three months time. The encryption part of the software is already complete and only the communication protocols remain to be written. Since the software has been written by ourselves there is no upper limit on the security level provided by the encryption in contrast with software exported from the U.S.A. Moreover, we can guarantee that the software is not booby trapped which one can never do with imported software.

Now I come at last to my purpose in writing to you. I believe that, as the CVC, you must make it mandatory for vital institutions such as banks to adopt indigenously developed and tested software. Without such strong and coercive administrative action, our Indian institutions will have a tendency to succumb to fancy marketing brochures and put in place a network and communication tools that are easily compromised.

Another problem is connectivity. Fortunately the RBI has already taken the initiative and set up the hub in Hyderabad and has ordered 438 VSATs. I was fortunate in that I could persude Dr. Kasturirangan, Secretary, Department of Space to make available half a transponder, which was needed by the RBI. The RBI has also brought out another important era where frauds take place, namely the listed companies' cash transaction, especially relating to dividend, etc. the order at Annexure also lies down that with immediate effect all listed companies' should make their payment transactions using the electronic system. This is another method of using technology to check the possibility of fraud.

At the same time, I am acutely conscious that while use of IT may be helpful in checking the frauds in the manual system, use of IT itself will bring in a new set of computer frauds. We have also to move urgently to get the cyber laws enacted so that use of computerization is not delayed for want of appropriate legal cover.

Yet another aspect of computerization is the availability of computer-literate manpower. In the order at Annexure we have indicated that the percentage of direct recruitment at the entry as well as senior levels, which has been agreed to between the banks and the unions, can be utilized to induct computer-literate staff. Thus apart from training the existing staff, there will be adequate technically skilled manpower available with the banks to operate the computer systems smoothly.

One of the most important questions in handling the issue of corruption in banks is whether we are bale to punish the corrupt in banks effectively and simultaneously encourage honest people. An off-repeated complaint in the banking system is that because of the CBI there is a fear complex at the cutting-edge level. Honest bank officers find that their career can be ruined by one or two procedural mistakes, which may lead to CBI raid, and all the attendant negative consequences.

To tackle this problem, a new chapter on banks has been introduced in the Vigilance Manual from 1 January 1999. The chapter takes into account the need for giving suitable assurance to the honest bankers. One feature of the chapter is that while in the case of direct frauds in deposit accounts, the CBI will directly go ahead with investigation, in prosecution in cases of decisions relating to loans and advances, the CBI will consult the central advisory board in the case of officers of the level of GM and above and bank specific advisory boards for junior officers. The present advisory board constituted by the RBI will become part of the infrastructure of the CBI. So far as bank-specific boards are concerned, they will be constituted as early as possible and will consist of retired district judge, retired DIG and a retired banker of the level of GM. The advisory boards are expected to give their comments within a month and if they do not give their decision, the CBI will be free to take further action. To expedite departmental proceedings, the CBI at the time of seizing documents will make authenticated photocopies available with four days. Authentication means the charged officer will also sign them. Many a time it is the charged officer who indirectly contributes to the delay by continuously asking for adjournments or examination of more and more documents.

Complaints are made many a time that political pressure or outside pressure is brought in loan cases. In such cases, I have already told the bankers that they can directly complain to me and I would write a formal letter to them saying that the decision must be taken on merits. I will also send a similar communication to the Secretary, Department of Baking. This will at least remove the excuse today given that because of political pressure or outside pressure, wrong decisions are taken.

The juniors sometimes complained that the seniors are corrupt and they are protecting the corrupt and they are forced to do corrupt things. In such cases, I have already issued an order on 18 November 1998 that if the juniors initiate a case, which will result in a vigilance case, they can send a copy directly to me.

In other aspects of the financial sector like insurance companies, SEBI and capital markets and financial institutions, these organizations may first peruse the chapter on the banking sector. If this would meet their requirements, we can simply extend its applicability to them also. Alternatively we can think of dedicated chapter in the vigilance manual to these organizations.

From a macro point of view, another cause of corruption in the financial sector is the system that governs advance to industry. We find that industry, which draws funds from the banking system, may become sick but the industrialist does not become sick. He becomes sick only when the CBI raids him. Among the factors, which probably help unscrupulous industrialists to cheat the banking system is the Sick Industries Companies Act (SICA). I have therefore requested the Banking Secretary to examine whether SICA should be scrapped and BIFR abolished so that one part of our financial sector which institutionalizes opportunities for unscrupulous people to exploit the system and indulge in corrupt practices can be eliminated.

EMPHASIS ON GOOD CORPORATE GOVERNANCE

With the growing emphasis on good corporate governance to attract FDI in the context of globalization and the shock of the currency crisis in the Southeast Asian economic tigers, thanks in part due to corruption, cronyism, the failure of sound financial system, there is an increasing realization that honesty is, after all, the best policy.

Perception about corruption in the country has a direct bearing in global business today. The experience of the Southeast Asian countries like Indonesia, Thailand and South Korea shows that if there is no proper corporate governance, and the financial sector is not regulated properly and is subjected to crony capitalism, investments may result in disaster.

When the chips are down in global trade today, integrity and corporate ethics count. According to one World Bank estimate, if a country is perceived to be more corrupt, the FDI goes down by about 35 per cent and it is to be perceived generally corrupt, it goes down by 25 per cent. From a purely bottom-line and financial point of view companies who have a reputation for integrity and best corporate behaviour stand to gain in this context.

In a highly competitive business environment, the trust of the investor and the consumer becomes a very valuable commodity. This is why one hears so much talk about brand equity today. But if we analyse what lies behind brand organization which find that ultimately it is the reputation of the organization which gives to the current and the potential customer a sense of reassurance in terms of quality, transparent behaviour and value for money. Reputation and brand equity are becoming increasingly important as competition increases. We can, therefore, see that the issue of corporate ethics is directly linked with adding a competitive edge to an enterprise apart from other aspects like good corporate management, productivity, quality, customer orientation and so on.

Competitive organization, today, market by the increasingly closed technology-finance-people loop. In discussing ethics and corporate integrity, we are focusing on the people aspect of this loop. If an enterprise is perceived to be an honest, straightforward, transparent enterprise which practices the highest values. It helps greatly to improve the company's morale. This in turn is translated in building a sense of loyalty and trust for the employees towards the organization. In this aspect, the responsibility of the top management and, particularly, the CEO becomes very important. It is necessary that the CEO and the top management are able to walk their talk. There are various parameters by which companies are being constantly ethics, if the top management do not practice them. There are various parameters by which companies are being constantly judged in different form. Industry associations and business ethics magazines are coming up with various criteria for judging, listing and ranking companies. Perhaps, as business ethics will increasingly emerge as an important factor, determining the performance of an enterprise, especially, in the listing of the most admired countries, this factor will become very significant. The more a company is admired because of its business ethics, the more it is likely to attract the right type of people and retain them.

CONCLUSION

As a whole solution of corruption is lying in Vedanta and only the Vedantic Philosophy and can give the permanent solution of the corruption. So to say that we have to go for the permanent settlement for the solution and uprooting of the corruption from the different level and for these we need proper environment right from the childhood level for making a man complete moral and ethical. The seed of corruption is being sown at the early stage of the life and parents are much more responsible for creating the great environment by which the children are been influenced and affected and grow up as a corrupted being. Now what we need is to resist and to get corrupt-free nation we should start at the early stage of every individual life by giving proper education through the Indian Tradition of moral and ethical systemic approach by which one can grow up with the corruption and ailment-free habits and behaviors. For this we need to change the complete education system into the avenue of Indian Traditional system with proper modern and Technological Education. We have to leave the habit of imitating the West and tendency to be the slave of the West.

11

COMBATING CORRUPTION

Shahnawaz ul Rahman
Dept. of Public Administration,
University of Lucknow, Lucknow

Corruption is a phenomenon, which has affected the welfare and development in India, in such a drastic manner that it has hampered the overall socio-economic progress of the country and is ruining our dreams of a prosperous and self-sufficient developed nation. Corruption is not a new phenomenon; neither is it something, which can't be understood. It is as old as our civilization is. We find written traces of this acute problem in the Kautilya's *Arthashastra*, which is considered as the first systematic work on Public Administration, at least in India. We all know what corruption really is, and this has been well brought under the ambit of various statues and laws, and has been well defined therein.

From the ancient India, to the present day administration, corruption has never been an absent entity. It has always affected our lives, mostly in a very adverse manner. But present day situation is far worse, because as any other poor developing country, we also have the task of speedy socio-economic development with scarce resources at our disposal, and an imperfect, if not, incompatible administrative machinery. But all prevalent corruption disallows us to accomplish these objectives. It is a hard fact that efficiency and economy cannot be brought in, unless this problem is cured or at least controlled in manageable limits.

The dreams of developed, prosperous and self-sufficient India will have to wait until then.

The problems in curing and curbing corruption lie in the fact that our approach towards its elimination has more often been legal. It needs to be remembered that rules and laws can only work when they become, or they are accepted as social norms. If the society at large thinks that corruption is inevitable and a part of the system, then the laws for curbing it become useless entities. So, the need is to focus more on social, cultural, psychological and environmental factors.

Some of the reasons, which are very often put forward for the prevalence of corruption in India, are inequitable distribution of national wealth and the gap between the socio-economic needs and the actual earnings. But if we analyse the problem with a holistic approach, we find that the poor is lesser prone to get corrupted than his rich counterpart. Although the circumstances are such that he is the one, who has to become a part of this process, being the most vulnerable and easy victim of this draconian problem. When an analysis is made of various big scams which have shaken India regularly since independence, starting right from the Rs. 216 crore Jeep Scandal in 1949, involving Krishnan Menon, the then India's ambassador in UK, to the recent Stamp Paper Scam (Telgi Scam), which involve a large part of the Maharashtra's politico–administrative class. It is easily inferred that those involved, belong to the highest strata of the society and there are no reasons, such as scarcity, behind their corrupt behaviour and practices. For these highest strata of the society the reason can be the limitless economic aspirations, not the economic needs.

When we talk about the very common citizenry in India, the society at large has accepted corruption as a norm, and laws and rules regarding its cure, as forgotten and meaningless statements of the law books.This is the most unfortunate, drastic and urgent problem to be addressed. The mentality, thinking and approach of masses are not shaped in a day, or a fortnight. It evolves over a long period of time. Since many centuries, the political and the adminstrative class in one way or other has duped common man. Thus, today they are compelled to shape mentality that corruption is necessarily a functional aspect of administration. From executive to the judiciary, everything is on sale. One can manage a fake arrest of his enemy by the police, or can get a non-bailable warrant issued, even against the first person of the country. In such a situation, how can a persn believe to get justice if he stands and talks against this menace?

Although, not only one, but the most important organ which has promoted corruption is politics. It has abetted corruption by virtue of its linkage with criminals, big contractors, industrial and business class, undue interference in administration, irresponsible behaviour towards society, huge election expenses, horse trading at the time of government formation and then pumping money to keep this government alive. It is well said statement that power corrupts and absolute power corrupts absolutely. The impact of this corrupt politics also fall on administrative machinery that sees its masters playing money games and which necessarily requires their interference too. This alters their behaviour to a large extent, although they also have their own individual sets of narrow interests to jump into this practice. But in democracy, the people who must be accountable and feel the responsibility are our elected representative. Otherwise democracy becomes a useless phenomenon. The practice and process of corruption has diversified and complicated in such a huge proportion that a common man finds himself a helpless creature and gets entrapped into this net.

Fallout of corruption are numerous and very dangerous and are the reasons, for why today we find ourselves in the distressed position of illiteracy, unmanageable population, bad health conditions, poverty, inefficiency in administrative machinery, low degree of technology and specialization, low level of resource utilization, poor delivery mechanism and huge economic losses. To fight and cure corruption thus needs an urgent, well-focussed, and honest approach. It has to be dealt with an integrated approach, which can visualize all factors ranging from the very basic factors to the complex ones. Although legal provisions in this regard have their own very important place, but they are not the ultimate solution to the problem. The ulimate solution lies in awakening the people, empowering the citizenry through value-based education, imparting political education, providing right to information and setting up sound grievance redressal machinery. Public opinion against corruption needs to be changed and this requires democracy to be strengthened.

Making the people aware about the value of their vote and politicians the fear of electoral decision; will do this. This can be done when people are educated and have an enthusiastic approach towards real democracy. There are various measures, which need to be taken to bring this menace of corruption in control. Some of the important ones can be listed as:

1. EDUCATION

Education is the first requirement to curb corruption. Only the educated and enlightened masses can realize and then stand against corruption. The education involves, the basic school education, the value education that contains in its ambit the lessons of morality and character, the political education to make people aware of their basic rights, and the various politico-administrative processes. People should be well informed of the various government policies, the mode of their implementation, various administrative mechanisms and the officials responsible.

2. RELIGION AND CULTURE

India is the land of religious and cultural people. Here the people are deeply associated with religion and traditions. It is the universal truth that every religion talks against corruption and all those practices, which promote corruption. Also our Indian cultural values have to place for this. But today, a tendency is in practice to point out the shortcomings of other religions than to introspect and to get to the truth of the religion. World's greatest religious philosophies have originated or propagated in India at one point of time or other. But today Indians are deviating from those chapters of morality and character building, which their religion and culture teaches them. In pursuit of western style of living we are forgetting and losing our values and traditions in a blind manner. The need is to instill the messages of integrity in the masses, who still have great association with their religion and culture, and which can make the fight against corruption, a success.

3. BETTER DEMOCRATIC CHOICES AND STANDARDS

Democracy is meant for the welfare of the people. But if governed by the corrupt leaders, this makes no good to the society. If our representatives are corrupt then it is a direct indication of the shortcomings and weaknesses in our democratic system. The need is to provide political education to the people, and instill in them a sense of political responsibility. Democracy needs to be based on values and vision and not on money and muscles. This requires a strong initiative from the public, which can put pressure on the corrupt politicians to correct their behaviour. There are various problem areas, which need to be addressed. Some of them may be mentioned as, the politics-criminal and politics-industrialist linkages, high election funding, horse trading for government formation and the money games in coalition politics. General public needs to stand against such corrupt politicians and oust them from the positions of power. This again needs a strong public opinion.

4. ADMINISTRATIVE DEVELOPMENT

Administrative development is essential in developing societies, like ours. The administration needs to be made more capable and compatible. Undue interference of politicians need to be curbed. The main support for corruption in administration comes from the complexities involved in various administrative processes. This gives a chance to the corrupt officials to dupe the common public. Red-tapism is another aspect, which puts pressure on the citizens to become part of this game to get their work done in time. If the processes are made simpler and transparent, a big hurdle in curbing the corruption in administration will be crossed. Popular monitoring groups need to be formulated to keep an eye on various administrative processes and point out the gray areas. These problem areas should then be brought in notice of the elected representatives in a commanding and not the feeble voices. It needs to be remembered that in democracy, it is the people who are the ultimate power and not the leaders.

5. SOUND GRIEVANCE REDRESSAL MACHINERY

Sound grievance redressal machinery needs to be in place, where the grievances of the citizens may be easily and timely redressed. Where the people affected by the corruption can get speedy justice. We in India, are trying to bring ombudsman system in the form of Lokpal, since last forty years. But the goal is still not reached. This shows the callous approach of the politicians and a weak public opinion towards the problem. The other systems formulated for the purpose, such as

Lokayukta at the state level, are suffering from their own shortcomings. Moreover people at large are unaware of such provisions, which make these systems ineffective, if not useless.

The measures stated above, cannot be claimed to be the ultimate formula for curbing corruption but they can prove to be very effective. Above all it is the public opinion, which needs to be transformed and then strengthened against corruption. For this very purpose, society is required to be instilled with confidence and a positive outlook towards the system. Their psychological approach needs to be changed. People are required to stand against such a disastrous problem because in democracy they are themselves responsible for their bad or good. Situation requires action, an action with an honest and focused approach. If we do not address this problem today, tomorrow will be very late.

REFERENCES

- *Eradication of Corruption and Restoration of Values* by Kashyap, Subhash C.
- *Corruption in India: Agenda for Action* by Guhan S., Paul Samuel.
- *Corruption In India: The Roadblock to National Prosperiy* by Vittal, N.
- *India from Midnight to Millenium*, by Shahshi Tharoor.
- *Public Administration in India* by Fadia, B.L.

12

SUGGESTIONS TO CHECK CORRUPTION

C.S. MISRA
Department of Computer Science
Bankey Bihari College of Technology, Agra, (U.P.)

Corruption is a global phenomenon. It is a factor part and parcel with the human being having its root with the origin of the man. It is omnipresent and is a bad hidden power within the man. It is a slip from the good deeds and the fact of life. It is a low-risk and high-profit business for those who can afford to be corrupt. The dictionary defines it as MORAL DETERIORATION (BRIBERY). The law defines it as "A Departure from what is pure-corrupt or from the original". The religion defines it as wrong behavior. Corrupt means Tainted with vice. What is corrupt in one religion may be pious in other religion. This is somewhat relative term difficult to define. The general meaning may be "the act which is against religion, morality, law, society, nation, race or human being etc. is corruption."

Now coming back to the theme of this seminar the meaning may be restricted to the act against the law, society, religion, morality or ethics. With the origin, growth and development of human being the corruption also grew simultaneously. It is in India as well as in the entire world. Globally, no country is free from corruption. It is the greatest enemy of national growth, development and freedom of any country. In India it exists in the govt. sector as well as in private sector.

REASONS OF CORRUPTION

Following may be the reasons –

(1) Deterioration of the religious values.
(2) Lack of morality due to the first reason above.
(3) Removal of fear from the GOD due to the reason first and second above.
(4) Love for the material world.
(5) Poverty
(6) Lack of knowledge or ignorance.
(7) Change of goals of life.
(8) Scarcity of goods and services.
(9) Red tape and delay.
(10) Lack of transparency.
(11) Delay in courts' judgements.
(12) Lack of accountability.

SUGGESTIONS TO CHECK CORRUPTION

I would like to mention some suggestions to check corruption from the society and the Government.

(A) *Role of Information Technology in removing corruption from the society—*

The information technology has very wide applications in every walk of life. Computers are used to process the data with a very tremendous speed and sending the information globally. Many types of corruption grow because of ignorance, lack of knowledge and non-availability of data. If we have the facts or data in hand or we have the full information nobody will dare to befool us and we will not be paying illegally to get our work done.

Sometimes money is taken illegally with the assurance of doing a job which has already completed. With the help of internet we can download the global information in a fraction of seconds and update our knowledge (The lack of knowledge or lack of transparency give rise to corruption).

Following *tools* are important to access many types of information:

(1) Global e-mail.
(2) Remote login (TELNET).
(3) Views and News (USENET).
(4) File Transfer Protocol (FTP).

(5) Information Servers – Navigators.

(6) Gopher (Menu-driven Browser).

(7) Archie (Global Librarian).

(8) Hytelnet (Hypertext Browser for the telnet accessible sites)

(9) Window Area Information System (WAISE – program search dozens of data bases in one go).

(10) World Wide Web (WWW – most advanced browsing and searching system on the internet based on the hypertext paradigm.

(11) NIC-NET (National Information Center Network).

(B) SUGGESTIONS TO CHECK CORRUPTION FROM EDUCATION SYSTEM

Privatization of higher education has brought the commercialization of education. Since the government has failed to impart higher education with its own resources, it has helped in privatising the higher education. Many big businessmen have started opening schools and colleges and earning money without maintaining the quality of education. Degrees and Diplomas are being sold without teaching. This has brought the concept of educational corruption.

There are many deemed universities giving affiliation to many institutes having sub-standard educational infrastructure including classrooms, laboratories and workshop, insufficient and non-qualified teachers.

FOLLOWING ARE THE SUGGESTIONS

(1) Govt. should have control over such institutes and deemed universities and affiliation process should be made difficult and after due inspection and verification.

(2) The process of the de-affiliation should be strictly applied to such institutes and universities who have insufficient infrastructures.

(3) Frequent checking and inspection should be made to ensure the quality of education.

(C) SUGGESTION TO REMOVE CORRUPTION FROM THE GOVERNMENT

Tehleka.com has exposed how in sensitive areas like defence purchases there are people who are willing to compromise and sell their soul and the security of India.

E-GOVERNANCE IS ONE OF THE ANSWER

The present govt. system has many types of corruption relating to the budget and welfare policies. The govt. funds are highly misused and the intended beneficiaries are not benefited by the various welfare schemes which are being implemented for them.

The funds allocated by the ministries for the welfare of the public, ultimately go back to ministers who are making such schemes through various channels. The answer to this corruption is the e-Governance. Some terms are important to understand the topic.

Electronic Govt. (E-GOVERNMENT) is simply the ability of a govt. to provide access to services and information 24 hours a day, seven days a week (24 × 7)

E-DEMOCRACY

Electronic (E-lek-tro-ik) adjective, by computer using or controlled by a computer or computer network or relating to the use of computer in an activity.

(*Source*: Microsoft Encarta online encyclopedia, 2003)

Electronic democracy (E-lek-tron-ik dE-mok-ra-see) noun, the use of computer and computer network by the people of a country to rule their country through any form of govt. their majority chooses to establish. (Source: Majority voice. Com Online freedom 2003)

DEMOCKERY (dE-mok-er-e) noun, a deceptive system of govt. which resembles democracy and is frequently called democracy even though it has no laws which make it a democracy but which actually enslaves the people while enriching an elite few.

(*Source*: Majority voice.com Online freedom, 2003)

E-democracy represents the use of information and communication technologies and strategies by democratic actors (Govt., elected officials, the media, political organizations, citizens/voters) within political and governance processes of local communities, nations and on the international stage. To many, e-democracy suggests greater and more active citizens participation enabled by the internet, mobile communications and other technologies in today's representatives as well as through more participatory or direct forms of citizens involvement is addressing public challenges. (Steven Clift).

E-GOVERNANCE

(1) E-government is the transformation of public sector internal and external relationship through net-enabled operations, information technology and communications to optimise govt. service delivery, constituency participation and governance.

True E-Government requires transformation of all the system involved in processing a transaction not just those facing citizens and business… "if you just process print outs from the web, all you have done is to build a great big remote E-Controlled typewriter. (Christopher Baum).

(2) E-Governance seeks to realize processes and structures for harnessing the potentialities of information and communication technologies (ICTS) at various levels of Govt. and public and sector and beyond for the purpose of enhancing good govt. E-Governance is the commitment to utilize appropriate technologies to enhance governmental relationship both internal and external, in order to advance democratic expression, human dignity and autonomy, support economic development encourage the fair and efficient delivery of services. (Rogers W'o Okat-uma).

In its simplest sense, e-governance can be said: 'the use of emerging information and communication technologies to facilitate the processes of govt. and public administration.' In reality though, e-governance is really about choice. It is about providing citizens with the ability to choose the manner in which they wish to interact with their govt. as it is about the choice govt. make about how info and communication technologies will be deployed to support citizens choices. E-governance is not just a website on the internet. It can be elaborated what it is exactly.

EXAMPLES OF E-GOVERNMENT

http://www.parliament.to.ug

http://www.gov.za/

http://www.govt.nz.

http://www.ukonline.gov.uk.

http://www.govonline.gov.au

http://www.fiji.gov.fj

http://www.gta.gov.zw

http://www.gov.sg

There are certain problems in implementing the E-Governance in India due to political and social reasons like lack of cyber laws, budget, corruption, piracy, bureaucracy, misuse of power, lack of majority in parliament, language, IT-literacy etc.

Mr. Arun Shouri the then Central Minster for Communication an Infotech has said that the govt. has chosen ten areas where e-governance could be implemented in months.

NASSCOM, the apex industry association of software and service companies in India made the statement that the e-governance market in India in gaining grip but still there are challenges. The E-Governance growth is Rs 1400 crores in size in 2001-2002. Its market grew by 18 per cent in 2002-2003.

NASSCOM feels that the govt. should first focus on giving efficiency in governance by better use of technology. The govt. should also analyze project champions who can push e-governance in govt. dept. and states. NASSCOM has also given phased recommendations from year 2003-2005.

The question is—Should the corruption be Legalized?

The Times of India poll on 7-5-2002 showed that corruption is perceived number one problem in India. It is anti-national, anti-economic development and anti-poor activities. Legalising it means legalizing all these, activities which none of us would like.

REFERENCES

* Newzealand, Singapore and Fiji Govt.

* Official websites of NASSCOM, http://www.nasscom.org
* E-governance in developing countries: Michiel Backus
* http:// *www.licd.org*
* http:// *www.publicus.net*
* http:// *www.worldbank.org/publicsector* /egov
* majority Voice.com
* Article by Shri Gaurav Kumar, Dept of Magmt, Kurukshetra University, Haryana.
* "*Corruption in India*" Book written by Mr. N.VITTAL.

Part - 2

CORRUPTION IN CONTEMPORARY INDIA

13

CORRUPTION, DEMOCRACY AND GOVERNANCE IN INDIA

J. Laxminarasimha Rao
Osmania University,
Hyderabad

If there is any activity that has been continuing since the dawn of civilization it is the misuse of public office and corruption. Kautilya recorded in his seminal work that misuses of official position and deviant conduct among officials were common in ancient India. In the modern times, Machiavelli observed that any human being put in a position of public office and commanding public obedience is tempted to use official power for personal advantage or for the good of his kith, kin and friends. Today, the scholars argue that corruption is prevailing everywhere and is common to all societies. The only difference is degree rather than its kind. It is rooted in human nature and part of human vices such as greed and lust for power and wealth.

There is no clear definition of corruption. There is no objective and uniform means of identifying it as it thrives on darkness and invisibility and it is also anonymous and immeasurable. However, it is generally identified with the use of public office for private gains. It can range from illegal cash transactions to seats in legislature, and from dishonest judicial decisions to bureaucratic promotions. It may include money-laundering, capital flight as a result of official kleptocracy[1]. It means any act of commission or omission by a public servant for securing any material gain can be treated as corruption.

In day-to-day life the problem is more complex. It is viewed differently in various societies as its form and incidence takes many shapes. For instance, Europeans view nepotism as part of corruption whereas in India it is not and favoritism in the form of region, caste, creed is common at the time of recruitment and promotions. In the US, taking bribe from the citizens is considered as corruption but if a company pays bribe to foreigners to get a contract that company gets tax concessions. Corruption manifests in a variety of shapes and various forms in the private sector. In India, on a petty scale it is rampant in the form of milk vendor adulterating milk, the grocer using false weights and the contractor doing a shoddy job of road construction etc. In developing societies it is a product of the way of life where 'money talks,' where what 'works' is justified and where people are judged by what they have rather than what they are. Thus, corruption has become habitualized, indeed institutionalized both in public and private life. Throughout the globe people are socialized into its way and become so accustomed to it that they no longer even recognize it. They cannot conceive any other way of conducting public affairs much differently. Attempts to change the situation and things are defeated mostly. This is more so in the developing world. That's why the issue gets more attention and receives publicity in media.

Corruption comes in many forms. There is high-level corruption and low-level corruption, and there is predominantly political and predominantly bureaucratic corruption. There are mutually reinforcing networks of complex, indirect and subtle transactions; and simple, direct and bilateral transactions. Gerald Gaiden enumerated commonly recognized forms of corruption. There are[2]:

1. Treason; subversion; illegal foreign transactions; smuggling.
2. Kleptocracy; privatization of public funds; stealing.
3. Misappropriation; forgery and embezzlement; misuse of funds; unaudited revenues.
4. Abuse and misuse of power; undeserved pardon and remission.
5. Deceit and fraud; cheating and swindling.
6. Perversion of justice; false evidence; unlawful detention.
7. Non-performance of duties; desertion; cronyism.
8. Bribery and graft; extortion; illegal levies; kickbacks
9. Tampering with elections; vote rigging.
10. Misuse of inside knowledge and confidential information.
11. Manipulation of regulations, purchases and supplies; bias and favoritism in decision-making.

12. Tax evasion; excessive profiteering.
13. Acceptance of improper gifts and entertainment.
14. Illegal surveillance; misuse of mails and telecommunications; improper use of electronics and computers.

Above list provides the understanding that any illegal transaction carried out by an individual either in public life or in private life can be considered as corruption. From this certain generalization too can be drawn regarding corruption.

1. Corruption can be found in all political systems, at all levels of government, and in the delivery of scarce public goods and services.
2. Corruption varies in origin, incidence and important in political, economic and administrative context.
3. In assumes different patterns and guises.
4. It is directed at real power, decision and discretionary authority. It commands a price for access to decision-makers and influences in decision-making.
5. It persists as long as its perpetrators can coerce participation, public attitudes toward it vary and it greatly benefits a few at the expense of many.
6. Unstable polities, uncertain economies and unequal access to wealth facilitate it.

CAUSES OF CORRUPTION

As there are varieties of corrupt behaviour, so there are multitudinous factors contributing to curruptoin. Many of the officials fail to live up to expectations, because moral standards are set too high and the personal gains are too tempting. Further the chances of being caught are less and punishments are lenient thus making the people indulge in corrupt practices. Thus, there are many causes of corruption.

Human Nature: By nature human beings are not perfect but selfish, egotist, greedy. They are not cared about others. They exploit and victimize others to get ahead and to come out as winners. In course of time they get sucked themselves into corrupt practices. Thus, psychologists point out that the roots of corruption can be found in the defect human nature.

Economic Scarcity: Economic scarcity is the important source of corruption. Any shortage forces people to compete with each other and in the process men become worse. A failure to gain access to goods and services means deprivation. Developing countries lack sufficient resources to fulfill their subjects' aspirations and desires and governments are also poor to provide sufficient public goods and services. Same cake has to be distributed for all ensuring scarcity and unequal access. Thus, the mad rush for limited resources and under payments to ensure to get one's share.

Lack of Transparency in Administration: Bureaucracy is all-powerful and it determines the personal fortunes of large segment of society by its decisions. The more important the official's decisions, the more necessary it is to influence them. Thus, corruption reaches out key officials in charge of most important decisions when public office is confined to a narrow elite; extraordinary means are employed to reach and influence them to obtain desired concessions. In other words more the discretion on the part of the public official, greater the possibility of favoritism and red tape. The delays in the decisions make the concerned parties to bribe the officials to get their works done as the delay increases the costs. Either way it benefits the both.

Complicated Legal Procedures: Legal procedures are long and complex. Any delay in delivering justice makes the people go for shorter routes. Similarly, complex laws involve lot of time in taking justice to the needy. This provides for a safety cushion to search for faster justice through various means available to public. Thus, corruption enters into the judicial department.

Technological: In a globalised and informatised world, technology is deciding everyone's life. Faulty technologies are also responsible for corruption as they permit those inclined to remain unseen and unknown. Mechanization lends to backstage manipulation by technocrats. Insiders can exploit loopholes known only to them. Modern day technologies are conferring undue discretion on technocrats by giving them a monopoly of specialized skills and knowledge which in turn providing them absolute power on their own and placing them beyond public accountability. Thus, greater the society's dependence on technological complexity, the greater the propensity toward corruption based on monopoly and discretion.

Whatever may be the reason, whatever may be the form, corruption is a profitable thing for those who indulge in it. Through it officials can accumulate power and exercise it with fewer restrictions. They can lead privileged life and amass huge private fortunes. They can do whatever they want to do and prevent others from achieving anything.

Corrupt officials display contempt for others. This may lead to monstrous crimes where people are considered expendable. It deviates from the search for a good society. It also exhausts governmental legitimacy and supports wrong kind of public leadership.

In the contemporary times the awareness of corruption and its impact on the functioning of governmental institutions, development and governance have increased. A number of international agencies such as Transparency International and the UN Development Program operate special websites giving information related to corrupt practices and efforts are made to combat them around the globe. Even the World Bank admits the prevalence of corruption in different countries related to misuse of the loans given by it.

II

Corruption, it has been recognized, is a universal phenomenon and has global appeal. In today's globalised and informatised world it reached monumental proportions. Hardly, there is any aspect of human life not touched by it. To reduce its impact, efforts are made to reduce it to a more tolerable level. In the West, institutional changes are brought in to reduce the opportunities for corrupt practices and to reinforce the changes that condemn corruption and support moral behaviour. The Law with effective law enforcement and with easy access backs the changes to remedial organizations.[3]

The scholars have argued that there is a direct correlation between corruption and the extent people are empowered. Where people participate in governance, the ruling elite has greater difficulty hiding their immoral practices. In open societies corrupt practices of leaders and officials get exposed in the media and the judiciary may scrutinize the charges. In this way, efforts are made to cleanse the society even though corruption is not totally erased.

In the developing world corruption has become a part of social fabric. People are socialized into its ways from the early years. Everything goes on in conduct of public affairs. Indeed it has become institutionalized. Any effort to reform the public life is seen as an attempt in vain. Arrival of new technologies further complicated the situation. New technologies are lending backstage manipulations by technocrats.

The case of India is no exception. Here, corruption has become a part of day-to-day life. Hardly, there is an institution, which did not come under the influence of corruption. Mahatma Gandhi used to cite that corruption is one of the main causes of India's backwardness. His relentless battle against it could not improve the situation. In the post-independence period many scandals have seen the light of the day. Emergence of new source of wealth and power in the form of expansion of the public sector, regulation of industrial activity and private business enabled the politicians and bureaucrats to patronage a few resulting in multifold increase of corruption in public life.

The phenomena of corruption triumphed over every resolve, every ideology and every political movement. Institution after institution has succumbed to the temptation of easy money. Bending of rules for private gain has become common. Political elite across the parties and ideologies and civil servants has come to collide in perpetuating corruption beyond manageable level.

Successive governments both at the center and at state level used corruption as an instrument of state policy to win over dissidents, to co-opt turbulent and disaffected groups and left-wing and ethnic insurgents by offering ministerial berths, gubernatorial positions and bribes. The legitimized use of all such practices by governments helped making society at large immune to their detrimental long-term effects.

In the post-independence period, corruption spread to all walks of life in all the government departments. As the state taken up various developmental and welfare programs and schemes, the government penetrated into diverse sphere of social and economic activities which brought more and more people not only into the programs but also within the ambit of corruption. It almost became that more the developmental activities and greater the role of state mean greater the incidence of corruption in India. Slowly the illegal activity transformed itself in the creation of a parallel economy, which undermined the state structures and apparatus. It is roughly estimated that the parallel economy is more or less to India's GDP.[4] The rise of parallel economy also resulted in the criminalization of politics and the rise of new social crimes such as destruction of environment, adulteration of food, manufacture of spurious drugs and medicines and other crimes against human life. Thus the international agency, Transparency International, which studies corruption and emanates information related to corrupt practices at global level rated India as one of the most corrupt countries in the world. Its corruption perception Index ranked India at 69 out of 90 countries in the year 2000.[5]

Political corruption, it is observed, is at the root of other types of corruption in India. It is said that even democracy in India is based on corruption. Almost all the political parties collect party funds through backdoors. Most of the money is unaudited. As a result every party makes compromises and offers favours to different groups and industrial houses while in power. This means black money intersects will all sectors of life in India.

The highest political institutions have come to be dominated by the vested interests of the corrupt and criminal elements. These elements are detrimental to the functioning of the democracy and they breed contempt for law of the land. They not only subvert the functioning of the institutions but also ruin the very ethos and character of the nation. At present the corruption culture vitiate all the public institutions from judiciary to administration to police. In some cases they are converted to private boroughs of the vested interests. As a result the state has drifted away from the 'soft state' to 'failed state', being unable to address the problems of the citizens.

The manner the political institutions work in the public domain in India made the former Prime Minister, A.B. Vajpayee, to remark that every MP elected to the Lok Sabha begins his parliamentary career by making a false statement about his election expenses. Given this reality, it would be impractical to expect scrupulous honesty from parliamentarians, as dishonesty was build into the system.[6] A poll survey conducted a few years ago also revealed the same. A study of 100 MPs of the 10th Lok Sabha of the years 1991-96 revealed that 94 per cent of the parliamentarians conceded that the high cost of elections, combined with a 'farcical' ceiling on election expenses has a corrupting influence on India's law-makers.[7] A former minister also explained the nexus between the politician and vested interests and how the parliamentarians converted their public office into a business. A former minister in the NDA government and the BJP MP from Bombay, Mr. Ram Naik, pointed out that those who successfully contest elections by taking money from businessmen or spending huge sums from their own pockets, "try to recover their expenses in the first two years. What they get in the next three years is a bonus. MP-ship is reduced to a business".[8] The Tehaika.com exposure focused attention on the issue of political fund raising in India. It raised the issue that to what extent an Indian politician can go to and how easily they can be managed for private gains. The exposure may be a tip of an iceberg in the Indian political system.

At the state level the spread of disease of corruption far more. Hardly, there is a state, which has not come under the influence of corruption since independence. Starting from Pratap Singh Kairon to fodder scam in Bihar, many chief ministers and other ministers used official position to serve personal ambition and personal interests or their family's interests. That's why a member of his own family always succeeds a minister. The politician and administrator nexus helped the both in plundering the budget provided funds leaving not much to the development of the people. The case of Bihar fodder scam is the finest example of the politician-bureaucrat nexus in embezzling the public funds. In no other fraud officials were so dismissive of rules as in this scam. Confident that they would never be caught, the bureaucracy submitted accounts that are breath taking. For instance the account books submitted to the CBI has shown that a sum of Rs. 253 crores were spent on the purchase of fodder for 959 sheep, 5,664 pigs, 40,504 hens and 1,577 goats in one year against the allocated sum of Rs. 105 crores.[9] Yet, another monumental falsehood in the case was that the administration has shown that two buffaloes were transported from Haryana to Bihar, a distance of about 1000 kilometers by a two-wheeler scooter. The reason for the falsehood, given at a later stage, was that panicky officials while filing the accounts in the animal husbandry department were at loss to explain the vast amounts pilfered from the public exchequer. Apparently, while making fictitious entries they spotted a scooter through the window and entered its registration number in the file, as they had to furnish the registration number of a vehicle that transported the buffaloes. While committing such a mistake the concerned officials could not anticipate that the CBI would cross check it.

The fodder scam may be one among many such thousands of cases in India. It could have seen the light of the day because of peculiar circumstances and judicial intervention at the highest level and its constant monitoring. Thus, the BBC correspondent in India,

Mark Tully in his seminal work 'India in slow motion' observed that "the [political] system, which is rotten…, is being used by not only politicians but also bureaucrats in order to behave in a rotten way themselves". He further commented on the necessity of "radical reforms in administrative structure, a radical limitation on the powers of politicians to interfere, a radical limitation on the powers of bureaucracy and a radical reform in the police service"[10] for good governance in India.

III

The President of India, A.P.J. Abdul Kalam while inaugurating the UNDP seminar on April 25, 2003 called for a corruption-free India for achieving India, a developed nation by 2020. He also desired that "It is essential that the three pillar of democracy—legislature, executive and judiciary—are strong in structure, pure in form and uncorrupted and unblemished in conduct".[11] Unfortunately the three pillars of the Indian democracy have come under the influence of vested interests. All the institutions have become subversive from within and sabotaging from outside that rendered our democracy a farce. Misuse of power reduced democracy to serve the personal aspirations and ambitions of some people. Electoral verdict is used for pursuing personal ends, plundering people's money and perverting the institutions in the name of democracy.

In a democratic set up governance depends upon legislature, executive and judiciary. Since governance is a process by which policies of a state are implemented, effective functioning of state organs and administrative institutions are a prerequisite necessity. In the developing countries state plays a major role in bringing effective change in society through the implementations of various development programs. Hence, good governance is necessary for achieving the full benefits of various development schemes and programs.

Corruption comes in the way of good governance. It hinders human development, deepens poverty levels, undermines economic development and growth, lowers investment, decreases government's resources and increases injustice in the society and undermines the legitimacy of state. In fact, when corruption becomes entrenched, it can devastate the entire political, economic and social fabric of a country.

In India human development is not taking place as per planning because corruption is coming in the way of limiting access to basic services provided by the state. Core services are restricted with the intention to make the corrupt elements gain. Low level of human development has been contributing to an environment breeding more corruption worsening governance further. Thus, we hear the instances of a government doctor deliberately refusing to admit a patient until he is paid bribe and storing away free medicines, a police official denying to file a FIR unless paid a kickback and a teacher engaging tuitions at home for a price rather teaching at school. Since access to these services involve illegal payment corruption is also increasing the price of these services. The former Prime Minister, Rajiv Gandhi, once remarked that every rupee spent by the government for poverty alleviation, only fifteen paise is reaching to the beneficiary. Another forty paise may be spent on administrative overheads and the remaining forty-five paise lost in corruption.[12]

Corruption reduces economic growth. It reduces efficiency on which economic performance depends. Under its influence the choices that are chosen may not be optimal. Non-creditworthy firms secure loans by bribing the financial institutions' managers and workers may perform routine tasks. Innovativeness, creativeness may be lacking which are important in increasing production and productivity. On the other hand the government officials who have control over scarce resources may not use them for public welfare but divert them by abusing their power. There is a possibility of further wastage in using the resources.

However, sometimes, in the developing countries like India, corruption is not seen as an evil for faster economic development. It is argued that since India is an underdeveloped country the process of modernization and development have to pay same price for faster progress. If a project is completed on a fast track by spending lavishly, the economic benefits accruing from it are greater than the small leakages here and there. Such an argument is untenable as the human behaviour is complex and unpredictable. Even if such an argument is acceptable there is no guarantee that the work, completed speedily, would not be shoddy. A vested interest may develop in making the projects expensive, so that one gets a larger slice. Thus one finds increasing costs of projects from time to time between planning and completion in India.

Similarly corruption also hinders investments into the economy. An empirical study has shown that corruption lowered investment both domestically and internationally. It revealed that corrupt practices prevailed in the economy is likely to reduce aggregate investment levels by five per cent points less and per capita growth rates half a per cent point less.[13] As per the UNDP Report of 1999, the GDP of India could grow by 1.5 per cent and the foreign direct investment could increase by 12 per cent if the corruption level in India comes down to that of Scandinavian countries.[14] It is also observed that corruption acts as an additional tax on investment by lowering the potential return. The World Bank identified the sources of economic corruption in the form of bribery in purchasing government contracts, licenses, evading customs duties, taxes, misappropriation of public funds, party financing.

Corruption also reduces the government resources and hence its capacity for investment. It can also shift government expenditure from priority sector spending to areas where the opportunities for illegal money are greater and the possibilities of detection lower. Similarly the possibilities of corrupt gaining from spending on new program are greater than expenditure on the maintenance of existing programs. Perhaps this explains the despair many school and health centers in rural India falling short of funds whereas many new mega projects being undertaken in urban areas. This is so, because allocating funds to mega projects is more attractive to corrupt officials and political leaders than spending the same money for rural reconstruction. Similarly there may be a greater temptation to choose complex hi-tech technologies than the simpler and appropriate technologies of development.

The Mazdoor Kisan Sangharsh Samiti in Rajasthan highlighted corruption in IRDP Programs. The public distribution system is designed to provide food security for those living below poverty line. However, the program saw many loopholes and goods reached the black market at the implementation stage. It has been admitted in parliament that 31 per cent of the food grains and 36 per cent sugar disappeared from the public distribution system.[15] This amounted to rupees 5000 croers and taken away by the corrupt shopkeepers, official and politicians.

In recent times the scale of corruption seem to have increased. The reasons for this boom is the deregulation and privatization of markets, mushrooming of opportunities for economic transactions between innumerable actors across the globe and the acceleration of information technologies that can move money instantly anywhere in the world. Thus one comes across men like Harshad Mehta, Ketan Parekh, and Hawala exposure and links between political leaders and terrorist groups.

Thus corruption is a major challenge being faced by the humanity. It is undermining the efforts of good governments, challenging good governance, distorting public policies, changing the allocation of resources and priorities from top to bottom. Thus half a century planned development in India did not dent the poverty of the poor. The development processes have been aborted by the endemic corruption. The administrative corruption coupled with political corruption without a check has deprived the downtrodden of the possible development through education and health. In the process the judiciary either has become a spectator or sometimes colluded with the other two. The Human Development Report on India has observed that "corruption is the most endemic and entrenched manifestation of poor governance in India" today, so much so that it has almost become "an accepted reality and a way of life". Corruption hijacked development, which survives largely in form.

REMEDIAL MEASURES

Political corruption is the root cause of other forms of corruption in India. Politics is neither an art nor a science of government but a national obsession. Every aspect of national activity—agriculture, industry, commerce, and administration—has a political projection. The result is the emergence of professional politicians who depend upon politicking for income and livelihood. Over the period attraction for politics has grown among the ambitious either take to politics or seek alliance with politicians. This resulted in a growing rapport between politicians, businessmen and criminals. And also politics has become the preserve of those who cannot make headway in any other walks of life. Such people's motive is to make only personal advancement by illegal means. Unless such a nexus in broken it is almost impossible to bring other form of corruption under control.

Similarly the nexus between political corruption and administrative corruption is too strong in India. To bring bureaucratic malpractices under control, it is necessary to break the matually convenient relationship between politician and administrator. The first Chief Vigilance Commissioner, N. Sreenivasa Rao, opined that without tackling political corruption it was not possible to root out dishonesty from the administration. He told a press conference on July 29, 1966, "Without a proper machinery to deal with at the political level vigilance commission would not be able to function with full effectiveness".[16]

To reduce the scope of corruption at administrative level rules and procedures have to be simplified. Greater transparency can check the official corruption. As more discretionary powers with bureaucracy leads to greater corruption at the official level, such powers are to be minimized with greater accountability. The feeling among officials that they would be never caught and even if caught would escape punishment because of judicial delays or bribing the higher ups can be eliminated with speedy trails and greater transparency and public empowerment.

The legal and the judicial system have also to undergo transformation to reduce the level of corruption in India. The judicial system is having many antiquated laws, failing to implement formal statutes. Often the judiciary is corrupt itself does not enforce laws fairly.

There are also several laws in India whose purpose seems to be creation of opportunities for corruption by the officials. For example, in Mumbai it requires 47 different approvals to construct a building and a small-scale entrepreneur has to handle 36 different inspectors each month and 46 different documents.[17] Such provisions give scope for corruption among corporation people as they have the discretionary power to give permission or not. There are also agencies that perpetuate corruption rather than eliminate it. There are instances where officials did not become part of corrupt practices are promoted less frequently, or transferred to relatively unimportant departments.

Thus to reduce corruption a bold and concrete agenda need to be worked out not only at political and administrative level but also at civil society level. Such an agenda must involve all sections of the population; evolve a gradual strategy, sensible approach in tacking the problem. In this effort the press and media can play positive role as channels of protest, naming the individuals and agencies participating in corruption. People's right to protest against corruption can be a preventive force.

The quality of governance can be satisfactorily improved once the corruption can be brought under control. Then development in its true sense can become a reality.

REFERENCES

1. *Human Development in South Asia*, 1999, Karachi: Oxford University press, 1999, p. 96 and Gerald E. Caiden, O.P. Dwivedi, and Joseph, eds., *Where Corruption Lives*, Connecticut: Kumarian Press, Inc., 2001, p. 1.
2. Gerald E. Caiden, '*Corruption and Governance*' in Gerald E. Caiden et al., op cit., p. 17.
3. Ibid, p. 3.
4. Chandan Mitra, *The Corrupt Society: The Criminalisation of India from Independence to the 1990s*, New Delhi: Viking, 1998, p. 24.
5. Quoted in N. Vittal, '*Corruption*', A paper submitted at the 5th Annual National Conference of NEPASI on "Governance for Development: Issues and Strategies" organized by IGNOU between 24-25 August 2001, New Delhi, p. 1.
6. Chandan Mitra, *op. cit.*, p. 111.
7. A. Surya Prakash, *What Ails Indian Parliament: An Exhaustive Diagnosis*, New Delhi: Indus, 1995, p. 278.
8. Quoted in Chandan Mitra, *op. cit.*, p. 112.
9. Ibid, p. 150.
10. *The Hindu*, December 15, 2002.
11. Quoted in Capt, K.V. Reddy, *Corruption Subverts Democracy*, Hyderabad, 2002.
12. Quoted in N. Vittal, *op. cit.*, p. 1.
13. Paolo Mauro, 'Corruption: Causes, Consequences and Agenda for Further Research', *Finance and Development*, March 1998. Quoted in *Human Development in South Asia* 1999, Karachi: Oxford University Press, 1999, p. 98.
14. Quoted in *Human Development in South Asia* 1999, p. 98 and R. Gandhi,

'Combating Corruption: A National Agenda', A Report prepared by the Indian Merchants Chamber and Mckinsey's, December 21, 1997, Bombay.

15. Quoted in N. Vittal, *op. cit.*, p. 2.
16. See G.S. Bhargava, *India's Watergate: A Study of Political Corruption in India*, New Delhi: Arnold Heinemann Publishers Pvt. Ltd., 1974, p. 34.
17. Quoted in *Human Development in South Asia*, op, cit., p. 102.

14

CORRUPTION: GENESIS, CAUSE AND CURE IN INDIAN PERSPECTIVE

Ashootosh Sharan
Dept. of History, Govt. P.G. College
Uttarkashi – 249193. U.A.

Corruption means deviation from the standard practice whether it is language usage, social custom or administrative behaviour. In the administrative field corruption may be defined as "Deliberate and intentional exploitation of ones position, status or resources, directly or indirectly for personal aggrandisement, whether it be in terms of material gain or enhancement of power, prestige or influence beyond what is legitimate or sanctioned by commonly accepted norms to the detriment of the interest of other persons or the community as a whole".[1] Extravagant expenditure of public money practicing patronage in public employment and misuse of government machinery in elections etc. too are corruption.

HISTORICAL BACKGROUND

Corruption has been known since the inception of administration. The Rigveda refers to social corruption. The implied meaning of the 'Ramarajya' may be that corruption had been prevalent elsewhere. The Arthashatra States "just as it is impossible not to taste the honey that finds itself at the top of the tongue, so it is impossible for government official not to eat up at least a bit of kings revenue". Kautilya refers to judicial corruption too and prescribes that integrity of judges should be periodically tested by agent provocateurs. Vishnu

Smriti prescribes banishment and forfeiture of all property for a judge found guilty of corrupt practices.[2] Miscarriage of justice due to official corruption has been well illustrated in the 'Little clay cart'. Majority of medieval texts state that the one-third revenue actually amounted to one-half in practice for cultivators[3] because of corrupt revenue officials. Cornwallis' reforms were primarily directed towards checking corruption among the official ranks.[4] Afterwards the upper stratum of British administration was largely free from corruption till independence.

The twenty-eight months of the Congress rule (1937-39) too was riddled with the charges of corruption. It went for bogus membership, careerists entered its ranks and many Congressman give way to casteism in search for power. The Left even accused the Congress regime of Madras of using the CID against the political adversaries.[5] Gandhi welcomed the resignation in the wake of the Second World War as it would help cleanse the Congress of the 'rampant corruption'.[6]

But since independence, the administrative efficiency has touched a new low. The entire administration seems reeling under corruption. Reasons are not for to seek:

1. THE SECOND WORLD WAR

The war efforts saw the massive transaction of money. Various supplies and contracts presented unprecedented opportunities for amassing wealth. Wartime scarcities and controls provided opportunities for bribery, corruption and favoritism. The tendency got established by the post-war flush of money and consequent inflation. The partition of the country witnessed not only the exodus of population but departure of officials too. British and Moslem civil servants left the country enmasse leading to the promotion and recruitment of the officials of unproven integrity. They were inexperienced too. It bred the corruption further.

2. THE CONFLICT OF VALUES

Presently values are at a conflict in India. In the expanding economy, the old moral code of plain living and high thinking has been weakened under the growing influence of urbanisation and industrialisation. Consequently there is no agreement as to what amounts to corruption. At times it is even taken as just as means to overcome the belly problems and hence should not be acted against. Corruption is becoming a normative. People are judged by what they have and not by what they are. This resulted in the emergence of white collar jobs and economic crimes and rendered the enforcement of law, not sufficiently deterrent in themselves, even more difficult. The gap of income among the officials is very large[7] and the trend continue even after the implementation of the recommendations of the fifth pay commission. It is disproportionate to qualification and ability.

3. GOVERNMENT STRUCTURE

Rules are still very complicated and complication breeds corruption of interpretation especially in depts. like customs, central excise, import & export. The failure of the Enron project resulted from such complications. Corruption requires persons willing to corrupt and the corruptible. This interpretation requires speed money to be over-powered. The industrial and mercantile class is willing to pay. Complication has prevented many major FDIs in India. India's share of 1 per cent global FDI compared with Hongkong's 28 per cent is startling.[8] The rank of corruption has been further swelled by the speculators.

4. PROTECTION TO PUBLIC SERVANTS

The Constitution has laid down that an official can not be dismissed by an authority lesser than one that appointed him or her [Art 311 (1)]. The process of action for wrong administrative decision too is a very complicated one. Corruption thrives under this protective shield.

5. THE PROBLEMS OF A DEVELOPING NATION

In general, in developing states, rules are not observed with uniformity. Patronage has a long sequence. The ruling troika favours the 'haves' and ignores the 'have-nots'. Administrative decisions are based on incrementalism and not principles. Prohibitive laws are respected more in violation than observation, e.g. rules of town planning. In policy decisions, religious, social and familial considerations overshadow the actual problems and principles.[9]

6. THE DEMOCRATIC PATTERN IN PRACTICE IN INDIA

Corruption is a disease in which the infection essentially travels down the order. The politicians at the top brass first require corruption. The nature of our political parties has undergone a sea change with the stepping up of the role of money and muscle power in our democracy especially elections. Earlier political parties were content with the black money donations from the industrial houses in addition to some foreign funds. With the growing elections expenses came the technique of using kickbacks in large commercial deals to finance the ruling party. Now even the kickbacks are not sufficient. The monetary supply is now largely contributed by smugglers, drug traffickers and criminal gangs. This makes corruption more pervasive. Bureaucracy comes under constant pressure to ignore law. There are bureaucrats ready to cooperate in this sinister act. Honest officers become submissive for the fear of a punitive transfer or getting their promotional avenues affected. That is why, we see that T.N. Chaturvedi's record, as Union home secretary had been different from his record as the C.A.G. of India. The extraordinary boldness that T.N. Sheshan displayed as the CEC was never visible when he was a secretary.

Corruption in India is taken as normative. Dismissal of corrupt officials will affect their children and dependents and hence rendering cooperation in the act of dismissal is regarded as sin. As such, salary is always regarded as inadequate. It is like a full moon, which loses its size every subsequent day and vanishes in the middle of the month.[10] So other avenues must be explored for income. So the battle against corruption becomes the lone fight of the victim. The machinery to tackle corruption is not accessible and cost of legal battle makes the victim prefer corruption over court.[11] "The commission share is fixed on the top, collected from down the order and sent to upper rungs, revealed some. P.W.D. officers on the request of anonymity".[12]

Corruption has been found proportionate to the opportunities available in the concerned department. However corruption is becoming rampant even in the service sector. Here money is changed for 'not derelicting the duty'. It was found that for police department, possible recruits would queue even if the posts were declared on honorarium basis because, the department is capable of eliciting money directly from the market itself.[13]

On the whole, the CVC identified some 27 modes of corruption prevalent in India.[14]

THE EXISTING MACHINERY TO TACKLE CORRUPTION

As early as 1941, Especial Police Establishment was set up to tackle corruption. The govt. enacted in 1947 the Prevention of Corruption Act which defines the scope of corruption in regard to public servants. Later the Rules of conduct were laid down for all India Services in 1954, for Central Services in 1955 and for Railway Services in 1956. Besides many enquiry commissions were set up of which two merit especial mention Railway (Kriplani) Enquiry Committee 1953-55 and Committee (Santhanam) on Prevention of Corruption 1962-64.

On the recommendation of the Kriplani Committee, the Central Vigilance Commission was set up in 1955 and many states established State Vigilance Commission. A Supreme Court judgment had made the CVC an autonomous body and given it more teeth but there has been no considerable scaledown in the level of corruption. Another institute of repute, CBI has a dubious fame in cases of corruption where political bigwigs are involved. From Mundra deal to Jeep scandal, from Maharashtra Cement scandal and Churhut Lottery scandal to Animal Husbandry-scam, and share-scam, the CBI seemed helpless. Perhaps, the orginisation has wilted under the political pressure.

The Santhanam Committee recommended the setting up of an institution patterned on the office of the Parliament Commission of New Zealand, i.e. the Lokpala. It is yet to become a reality. The ARC Rajasthan (1963) recommended for a state ombudsman, i.e. Lokayukta. Many states have got Lokayukta, but its power stands too circumscribed to address citizens grievances. In Bihar, Maharashtra, Rajasthan etc. they redress the grievances of the public officials themselves.

WHAT SHOULD BE THE RADICAL MEASURES

Economically India has been fast changing in the last one and a half decade. Liberalisation has brought opulence, though sporadic. The graph of economic crime is rising and the problem of corruption is becoming even more complicated. The change requires some radical measures.

In the 1st five year plan itself, the insidious impact of corruption was realized, "It not only inflicts wrong which are difficult to redress, but undermines the whole structure of the administration and confidence of public in administration. So there must be a continuous war against corruption".

I conceive a three-pronged strategy of the aforesaid war: (1) Reducing the red tape and making the bureaucrats accountable for results, (2) the coordinators and mentors of corrupt bureaucrats, i.e. politicians too should be denied many of the immunities enjoyed by them presently and (3) the role of the government itself should be reduced.

Art. 311 (1) of the Constitution provides strong security of tenure to bureaucracy against dismissal or demotion. The judiciary has interpreted the article in a way, which has made action against the corrupt even more difficult.[15] Even the confidential rolls are not touched by the superiors unless they are in a position to adduce overwhelming evidences. Under the rules of procedure, permission from the govt. is necessary for prosecuting an officer for corruption. This must go away and the permission clause should be limited for the 'act of negligence' only. 'Good error of judgment' too should be made fit for prosecution if it appears deliberate prima facie. In the judicial services of the state, officials have been dismissed by the High Court for judgments which violated the sound principles e.g. removal of Mr. Anant Pd. Shrivastav for granting bail to M.P. Shahabuddin and removal of 16 Judicial officers on the charges of corruption on Chattisgarh in Sept. 2004. Similar rules can be set for regulatory civil servants. In the recruitment process, there should be a fair scope for character assessment. The present system is heavily weighed in favour of academic excellence. Even the recently mooted idea of recruiting future bureaucrats after the 12th class has not given any considerable thought on the soundness of character. Recruitment should have an enhanced role for the psychologists.

Though appreciated by the western philos, the Indian democracy is actually far from maturity in more than one sense. Here the criminals, politicians and bureaucrats combine to make a fatal triangle. This triangle needs to be broken to check corruption. Bureaucrats are scared of unfavourable posting or delay in promotions. Therefore, they become subservient to the nefarious designs of the politicians and even patronise the criminals associated with the politicians. Politicians in turn, wink at the inefficiency of the bureaucrat and combine with them in eating of the govt. purse. Of late, it has been reported in the newspapers that in many states, bureaucracy not only used its officials position, but contributed monetarily also in organising state rallies by the ruling parties. The caste affiliations of the bureaucrats and politicians have further worsened the situation. Election manoeuvring has become easier. It would require many radical measure to change.

The election machinery presently working under the control of the D.M. should be brought under the DJ. The latter works under the control of the H.C. and can therefore be free from fear of political repercussion.

Secondly, the transfer and posting of the govt. servants especially gazetted ones should be assigned to independent commissions designed on UPSC or SPSCs. It may be given to the State Administrative Tribunals, which should formulate a policy of transfer and posting. Our bureaucracy is an impersonal order and the personal choice of the politicians must be done away with.

The noose around the politicians should be tightened directly too. The recent limiting of the size of the council of minister is a welcome move in this direction. For prosecution of the MPs and MLAs in criminal cases should be rid from the 'permission of the speaker' clause and no gubernatorial permission should be required for prosecuting a minister on criminal charges. Presently, the judiciary can not question the acts of commission and omission of the legislators inside the House. It should be conditioned with "not amounting to corrupt practices". In the JMM bribery case, the Supreme Court observed that public representatives where drawing from the public money and were hence, public servants. A natural corollary of this observation is that they can not assume the office unless the criminal cases pending against them has been disposed of. It would require a parliamentary legislation. It is difficult as it has been observed that the selfishness of the public representatives knows no bounds. "On the last day of the sitting of the 9th Lok Sabha, the MPs unanimously voted for ensuring their pension, and at an enhanced rate... without caring to see that a bill or motion having a financial liability could not be introduced without the president's recommendation", (Art 117).[16] The check on such irresponsible act we perceive an extended role of the judiciary, the PILs and NGOs.

One radical solution suggested to check the political corruption has been the substitution of the Parliamentary form of govt. by the Presidential form because instability too breeds corruption. But such a change may not be tolerated by the Supreme Court so long as the thirteen judge dogma that "Parliamentary democracy is a basic feature of our Constitution" is not superseded by a larger bench.[17]

In the end, I shall come to limiting the role of the government itself. Greater the number of tools of corruption, bigger the scope of corruption. The power of discretion makes the scope for corruption and discretion creeps despite precisely laid down rules. Officials use this discretion emanating from the loopholes of legislation, e.g. in automobile what makes a complete knocked out kits and what is an assembled one. The economic reforms since 1991 has tried to reduce the red tape and the power of discretion associated with it. But the first few years of reforms have brought a deluge of corruption. Industry was particularly affected; controls were eased but were not fully replaced by a system that reduces the human interface or cuts the middleman fast enough. Transparency is still conspicuous by its absence. Enron debacle was just one instance. The political and civil bureaucracy tends to utilize to maximum the opportunities, which are never going to come up again, once a regulatory regime substitutes their role. This psyche can explain the reason behind recent scams.[18]

India is presently passing through a transition phase. The transfer is not smooth. The present sales of govt. equities are done mainly to acquit the govt. of the BoP deficit without inciting public ire. Presently the power obtained from privatization is not shifted to the market but to politicians and bureaucrats.[19]

Though heightened corruption in an adverse fall out of the transition from govt. to market-oriented economy, it won't be a misplaced optimism to think that the bureaucrats and politicians in post-liberation India would be less corrupt.

REFERENCES

1. Awasthi and Awasthi – *Indian Administration*, p. 358.
2. A. L. Basham – *Wonder that was India*, p. 117.
3. Harishchandra Verma – *Madhyakalin Bharat I.*
4. Grover & Grover – *A New Look at Modern Indian History*, p. 123.
5. Bipanchand – *Freedom struggle – 28 months of the Cong. Rule.*
6. Ibid.
7. Railway Enquiry (Kriplani) Committee – 1954-55.
8. Report of UNCTAD, *H.T.* New Delhi – 23.09.04.

9. F. W. Riggs.
10. Premchand Dhanpat Rai, '*Namak ka Daroga*'.
11. (K) Santhanam Committee – 1962-64.
12. Ibid.
13. N.P.C. 1977.
14. Awasthi & Awasthi – Indian Ad. p. 369.
15. Ibid.
16. D.D. Basu, *Introduction to the Constitution of India* -394.
17. Kesvanand vs State of Kerala, A, 1973, SC, 1461.
18. Vito Tanzi: *IMF Corruption, Govt. Activities & Market.*
19. Ibid.

15

CORRUPTION IN INDIA – CAUSES AND SOLUTION

Abhay Saxena

Dept. of Computer Science,

Dev Sanskrit Vishwavidyalya, Haridwar, U.A.

PRESENT SCENARIO

Various steps had been taken by almost every country of the world to counter the corruption but unfortunately the roots are so deep, it looks as if the corruption is immortal. In Indian society it looks like.

- Corruption while applying for Gas/ Electricity connection…
- Corruption in getting the berth while travelling on Indian Railway.
- Corruption while getting the driver's license/vehicle's paperwork.
- Corruption when you are stopped by traffic policeman.
- Corruption in the local govt. while registering birth/death, or work related to any real estate papers.
- Corruption /harassment when you are going out/coming back in India by immigration or customs officer.

CORRUPTION

Corruption is defined as a platform where we use public office for private gains. Scales of corruption can be grand, middling or petty and payment of bribes can be due to collusion between the bribe taker and the bribe giver, due to coercion or even anticipatory. In other words, it is an offering, giving, soliciting or acceptance of an inducement or reward, which may influence the action of any person.[1] It looks that the desire to get things done at any cost, in forces the person to adopt this tactic.

REASONS

Existence of corruption implies that there are corrupt people, there are also corrupt practices, and there is a corrupt system. Therefore, all the three have to be fought simultaneously to eliminate the vice of corruption.[1] The fact that money is being demanded directly and openly by the corrupt is a clear indication that the corrupt persons are confident that no worthwhile action can be taken against them.

Cause for corruption is certainly containing not 'low salary' of those indulging in corruption. It is the lack of effective deterrence in the form of punishment to the corrupt and the lack of adequate supervision. Among the several causes of corruption the important ones are greed, circumstances, opportunities, misconception, petty excuses, special temptations.

In many cases the citizen is not even aware that the practices can be classified as corrupt for example when patients are directed to specific pathological laboratories for conduct of tests.

PEOPLE OPINION

Indians think that corruption can't be eliminated in India—at least not in their lifetime. This pessimistic and cynical perception of the people is largely an outcome of confusing corruption with all kinds of illegal actions like dishonesty, cheating and duping etc.

As per perception of the people, police is the most corrupt sector. However, the impact of corruption is on a much larger scale in the health and education sectors involving far greater number of population.

WHY CORRUPTION IN INDIA?

It is infact not confined with the politicians or the government machinery but it is now spread over in almost every section and every level of society. Education, Police System, Telephone, Power, Land and Building, Administration, Railways, Judiciary, Ration and Politics are the key most areas where corruption has taken an utmost height.

A shortage of basic decent human life in India has forced a common person to be corrupt. It is impossible for a common man to own a roof, provide good education to his children and hope for a peaceful retirement in India using normal and honest means.[2] One has to bribe someone to get good education, to get a deserving job and to avail services, which one is entitled as being a citizen of India.

- The Transparency International (TI) Corruption Perception Index (CPI), 2002 ranks 102 countries in terms of the degree to which corruption is perceived to exist among public officials and politicians. It is a composite index derived from 15 different polls and surveys from 9 independent institutions carried out among business people and country analysts. Finland the least corrupt country and Bangladesh came into the worst affected corrupt country.

(Corruption perception index and rank of India, 1995-2002)

Year	*No. of countries*	*Rank*
1995	41	35
1996	54	46
1997	52	45
1998	85	66
1999	99	72
2000	90	69
2001	91	71
2002	102	71

- World Competitiveness Year Book, 2000 also ranks India amongst those countries where bribing and corruption is very high.

CORRUPTION IN INDIAN HISTORY

Corruption is as old as Indian history. Right from Satyug, Treta, Dwapar and now in Kalyug, corruption is flourishing very rapidly. Causes were different in various time-periods but the bottom line was to make the job done at any cost–consequence by *Sam* (love-affection), *Dam* (cost), *Dund* (punishment) or *Bhedh* (divison). Some of the popular scam during last decade are as follows:

- Petrol power Scam
- Jain Hawala Scam
- HDW Submarine
- Churhat Lottery
- Fodder Scam
- Bitumen Scam
- Anantnag, Transport Subsidy Scam
- Tansi Land Deal
- JMM
- Nagarwala
- Sukhram Telecom Scam
- Urea Scam
- Bofors Scam
- Sugar Scam

The Unit Trust of India (UTI), the largest government-run mutual fund in India, duped millions of investors out of their hard-earned money. But what was the stand of Government? It bailed out UTI for the second time by injecting fresh funds into the company. And these fresh funds came from the taxes paid by the people to bail out UTI. Isn't this one of the most hideous forms of corruption?[5]

RELIGIOUS MENTALITY OF INDIANS

The irony is that India is still considered to be a very religious country and it is still widely believed that the religion is the basis of Indian life, thoughts and actions. This is obviously true, considering the fact that there are hundreds of temples, churches and mosques spread all over the country and they are all densely visited day in and day out by the feverishly praying Indians.[4]

Is not religious ethos contrary to corruption and dishonest practices? The unfortunate situation in India is that those who call themselves most religious are often found to have indulged themselves in dishonest practices on many occasions. Several of the religious centers, of all religions, are suspected to be steeped in nepotism; as such incidents have been repeatedly published in the press.

THE FUTURE OF THE INDIAN SOCIETY IN SUCH CONDITIONS

It can only be frustration, chaos, unrest and even bloodshed in the not too distant future.[4] This kind of corruption in the national polity and public and private life cannot go on forever, without disturbing the overall peace in the society.

COUNTERING CORRUPTION

Government Act and Policies

The common perception is that Government can eradicate corruption and responsibility of eradicating corruption is that of Government only but this is absolutely wrong.

To deal with corruption amongst public servants India enacted Prevention of Corruption Act, 1988, replacing Prevention of Corruption Act, 1947. PCA 1988 incorporates provisions of chapter IX of the Indian Penal Code to deal with Public servants and those who abet them by way of criminal misconduct and provides to enable attachment of their ill-gotten wealth obtained through corrupt means.

In PCA 1988 Public Servant and Public duty have very wide definitions covering every person who is in the actual possession of the situation of a public servant and discharging public duty which the state, public or the community at large has a interest.

PUBLIC EFFORTS

Though there exist a high level of expressed concern on the scale, pervasiveness and consequences of corruption, there has been no effort to translate it into effective action. The daunting nature of the problem tends to generate a feeling of helplessness and apathy. This, in turn, is often rationalized in terms of cynicism or in arguments that tend to acquiesce in corruption.

Fundamental changes in Constitution, through going deregulation and privatization of the economy and emphasis on moral values and character are some of the counter checks for this everlasting problem. Unfortunately all these have their own limitations in terms of scope and feasibility is concerned. Some preventive, punitive and promotional steps will only curb the corruption.

Preventive aspects will include electoral reforms, especially in the matter of campaign finance; an optimal balance between the roles of the state and the market involving appropriate deregulation and privatization, curtailing the role for discretion in government decisions; decentralized governance strengthening transparency and accountability.

The **punitive** aspect will consist of strengthening laws, rules and mechanisms for the effective detection, pursuit, punishment and deterrence of corruption.

The **promotional** aspect will involve the encouragement of value-based politics and administration, respect for laws and a culture of compliance with them.

Our sincere and collective efforts will only be a solution for combating corruption. Each one of us has to fight on his own level to eradicate this evil from our Globe.

REFERENCES

1. www.ti-bangladesh.org/ti-india/documents/corrlnd-pt3,doc (a South Asia survey)
2. www.india-reform.org/articles/corruption.html
3. *Corruption Perception Index*, Transparency International, Berlin
4. www.pucl.org/Topics/Human-rights/2002/corruption.html
5. www.strike–the-root.com/4/das/das2.html.

16

CORRUPTION IN INDIA: NATURE, CAUSES AND REMEDY

Ashok Kumar Singh

Dept. of Political Science, Y.N.College, Chapra, Dighwara (Saran) (Bihar)

INTRODUCTION

Corruption is surely the oldest malady afflicting public administration. It existed before the State came into being perhaps would outlast State-based public administration.

History is replete with instances of corruption in its multiple forms. For example, practice of bribery as a form of corruption had found reference in Old Testament (1200 BC), in Babylon (120 BC), Roman Empire (67 BC), Manu Smriti, etc. Although pace of corruption was low among Greek officials, yet by fifth century bribery become common among its officials. In Rome too, corruption was not very significant initially, but it went up with raise in State's earnings. In India Kautilya (in his Arthasastra) gave a detailed account of corruption being very widespread. Even modern States, like USA, is seriously afflicted as corruption has established itself as a way of life.

DEFINING CORRUPTION

Because of myriad forms in which it manifests itself, it is very difficult to define corruption. Let us, nevertheless take a look at some of the important definitions of corruption. Huntington (1968) has defined corruption as follows: "corruption is a behaviour which deviates from the formal duties of a public role because of private (personal, close family, private clique) pecuniary or status gains".

Susan rose-Ackerman has defined corruption as "an illegal payment to a public agent to obtain a benefit that may or may not be deserved in the absence of pay-off" (The Costs of Corruption for Private Business).

OECD Working Group defined corruption as, "The promise or giving of any undue payment or other advantage, whether directly or through intermediaries, to or for the benefit of a public official to influence the official to act or refrain from acting in the performance of his or her official duties in order to obtain or retain business".

Robert Klitgaard through his equation, defines corruption as follows:
$C = M + D - A$

Where

C = corruption:
M = monopoly
D = discretion; and
A = accountability.

According to Alatas, corruption is "abuse of trust for the sake of private benefits".

According to Dr. Mahathir Mohamad (Prime Minister of Malaysia, who authored a book entitled *The Challenge*) "corruption is understood as giving something to someone with powers so that he will abuse his power and act favouring the giver".

To Francis Beaumont, "corruption is a tree whose branches are of immeasurable length, they spread everywhere and the dew that drops from thence hath infected some chairs and stools of authority".

To Bouvier, corruption "is an act done with an intent to give some advantages inconsistent with the official duty and the rights of others".

As per World Bank definition, "corruption occurs when a function, whether official or private require the allocation of benefits or the provision of a good or service. In all cases, a position of trust is being exploited to realise private gains beyond what the position holder is entitled to".

Admittedly, it is difficult to resist the temptation of quoting from Kautilya's *Arthashastra* as his definition has ironically greater relevance to our own 'times'. He wrote about corruption as follows; "...what is entered earlier is entered later on; what is realised later is entered earlier; what ought to be realised is not realised, what is entrusted is of another, what is realised from one source is shown as realised from another, what is payable is not paid; what is not paid is often when paid is paid untimely; small gift made large gifts; the real job done is one while the person entered as done is another; what has been taken into (the treasury) is removed while what has not been credited to is shown as credited; commodities of greater value are treated for those of small value; what is of smaller value is bartered for one of greater value; prices of commodities enhanced in consistency with transaction carried on with personal supervision; income through making of false weights and measures".

Although Kautilya has defined, in addition, several other kinds of corruption, yet forms of corruption today far exceed any description because people indulging in such practices have adopted means which are far beyond the pale of imagination.

As is evident from the definitions given above, corruption dilutes established processes and procedures of control in administration to the extent of rendering them totally ineffective thereby jeopardising the ability to govern. In the developmental context too, it adversely affects both policy-making as well as implementation levels allowing thousands of crores to go down the drain.

Before moving further, it would be necessary to differentiate between "corruption" and "maladministration" for conceptual clarity. Comparatively speaking, corruption is a narrow term but maladministration is a much wider term ranging from laziness to broader infringement of administrative integrity. Corruption is a phenomenon which has existed for such a long time and it would not be wrong to surmise that almost everyone has a rough idea about its nature and Universality.

TYPES OF CORRUPTION

Alatas has classified corruption as follows:

1. **Autogenic** —It is self-generating and involves only the perpetrator as in the case of leakage of information by a person dealing in inside trading.
2. **Defensive** —It is compulsive in nature. A person in dire need of a service is compelled to pay bribe otherwise his interests would suffer. The person pays bribe in self-defence.

3. Extortive — It is a compensation in exchange of service.

4. Investive — It is undertaken with a future reward in view. There is no direct favour at the present.

5. Nepotistism—It is giving preferential treatment or unjustified appointments to relatives/friends in violation of accepted guidelines.

6. Supportive — It involves money or immediate gains to protect the existing corruption. Examples of it will be preventing appointment of an honest and capable person for fear that his acts might be probed by such a successor.

7. Transactive —It exist where two willingly participate in the corrupt practices to the advantages of both of them just as payment of a bribe by a businessman to an official for getting a contract.

To this classification of Alatas, the following have been added by Bhure Lal (Corruption: Functional Anarchy in Governance).

1. **Collusive Corruption:** In this form, the corruptees are active participants and use corruption as an instrument of inducement to allure the authorities to do a wrong /illegal activity. The benefits accruing from it are far greater than the cost of corruption.
2. **Coercive Corruption:** It is victimization and is forced upon corruptee by those in authority and power. The authorities take undue advantage of their position and the miseries of the victims.
3. **Non-Conjunctive Corruption:** In it, the victim does not come to know of this victimisation. The benefits are obtained by the corrupt at the cost of some one.

As was the case with its definition, the scheme of classification given above, despite covering a lot of ground, is not exhaustive.

After familiarising ourselves with the nature of corruption, it is clear that corruption is multi-disciplinary and nearly all pervasive. It touches all aspects of life of man living in a modern society–democratic or otherwise. It surely is a negative phenomenon. The democratic form of government was supposed to have an effective check on corruption to a great extent, but unfortunately this has never happened. To our dismay, as reality prevailing in democratic institutions unfold, we discover that with degeneration of democratic values among those manning these institutions, the accountability aspect has evaporated allowing these very institutions to become breeding grounds for corruption of newer varieties.

CAUSES OF CORRUPTION

Major causes of corruption are:

1. **Underdeveloped civil society:** Power is exercised in the government system in the absence of any checks in the form of watchdog groups, advocacy society organisations, healthy mutually balancing political party system, independent labour unions, strong business organizations, educated and informed public opinion, and independent media with positive approach.
2. **Enjoying of wide powers:** Both the political executive and bureaucracy have been enjoying wide powers in the existing governmental framework. Despite elaborate structure of rules and regulation, further reinforced with discretionary powers, there is hardly any worthwhile check to deter them from improper discharge of authority or using their discretionary power as an effective corrective measure.
3. **Evaporation of Accountability:** In the absence of transparency, and prevalence of the principle of anonymity in governmental functioning, accountability has taken a severe bearing. Hardly any institution exists to effectively hold the executive responsible for its misdemeanour.
4. **Weakening of Institutions like Ombudsman:** Abuse of transparency decision-making coupled with weak or non-existing system of checks and balances, non-vibrant court mired in their own dilatory procedures, and weak ombudsmen offices have together helped corruption to proliferate in an unrestricted manner.
5. **Cynicism Towards System:** Because of prevalence of public cynicism towards government authority, common man has over the years acquired an anti-system attitude. This has adversely affected common man's adherence to Rule of Law. As a result, Rule of Law has now been replaced by promotion of personal loyalties for unduly gaining mutual advantage.

Corruption today is all-persuasive or omnipresent. Its tentacles have spread to economic, political, administrative, social religious, technological, cultural, educational, institutional and environmental spheres. Narayanasamy, Borain and Jeyaraju (eds) in their book (*Corruption at the Grassroots: The Shades and Shadows*) have enlisted a more recognised common features of corruption which manifest in following acts;

- Taking bribe
- Giving bribe
- Misusing facilities
- Giving improper access
- Stealing things
- Letting others steal
- Allowing undue favours
- Diluting quality of work
- Taking undue favour
- Accepting poor quality.

17

CORRUPTION IN INDIA: MAGNITUDE OF THE PROBLEM AND POSSIBLE SOLUTION

Jogendra Kr. Das
D.K College, Mirza, Kamrup, Assam

Corruption is a world-wide phenomenon and no country is free from the trap of corruption and bribery. But corrupt practices are especially much more pervasive in the contemporary developing societies including India which absolutely disrupts economy, polity and administration to a far greater degree than in the case of developed western societies. Corruption now becomes almost institutionalized in the Indian society, politics and administration which eats into the vital of our national life and society. We often finds corruption reports in the newspapers but the corrupted persons do not care and got off scot-free. The Indian people now take it as a natural phenomenon and therefore, it becomes almost legitimate. Corrupt disorders becomes the order of the day and it seems, corruption is also inherent in our culture and morality.

In the present paper we propose to deal with this problem, its magnitude, causes and possible solutions. We have also tried to trace out the various forms of corrupt practices, and some factors which promote corruption. It is however, not possible to make an intensive investigation of the corrupt practices at the individual level which may necessitate nationwide major research projects. Corrupt practices are so extensive and complex that even it may be difficult for an economic detective too to exactly trace out the corruption evidences at the micro-level. In the absence of dependable data and non-availability of accurate statistics, the present paper may suffer from limitations. We only restrict our discussion to corrupt practices which involve government and administration, the most pervasive aspect of corruption in India today.

(II)

The Committee on Prevention of Corruption (1964) defines corruption as 'Selfish exercise of power and influence attach to a public office or to a special position one occupies in public life.' The *Concise Oxford Dictionary* defines corruption as the illicit gain of money and employment and the use of public resources to further private interest.' *Collins Co build English Language Dictionary* defines corruption as dishonestly and illegal behaviour by people in position of power and authority. Andriski considers it as the use of public power for private advantage in ways which transgress some formal rule or law.[1]

J. Nye states that corruption denotes the abuse or misuse of public offices for personal gains.[2] Thus, comprehensively, we can define corruption as the misuse of pubic power for private or personal profits by violating the laws and deviating from the accepted norms of the society. Corruption is spread as an epidemic disease in the form of the bribe, nepotism, misappropriation, patronage, commission, and favoritisms.[3] There is the high level corruption occurs at the law making level that involves politicians, ministers, bureaucrats, economic elites and at this level political elites extort money to consolidate power. Moreover, corruption also occurs at the level of law-implementation that involves the lower echelons of the civil and public services where petty officers, employees and contractors would busy in corrupt practices.

(III)

Corruption has a historical root in India. In ancient times also corrupt practices were endemic. Kautilya has referred in his *Arthasastra* to embezzlement by government servants out of the state fund.[4] During Ashoka's regime and in medieval society the scope of corruption was minimum.[5] During the British rule both the Indian and the British officers were involved in corruptions. During the first ten years of independence, corruption was not sky-high, but after 1960's new political elite started to involve in wanton corrupt practices. Since 1970's onwards several central and state ministers including the Prime

Ministers were alleged to have been involved in corruptions of several forms including nepotism. There were major signals in the Nehru era that political and administrative corruption, including large scale tax-evasion was beginning to burgeon.[6] During the fifties the tentacles of corruptions were not yet far-reaching and major barriers to it existed in the form of a political leadership and cadre with their roots in the freedom struggle and Gandhian ethos, a largely honest bureaucracy, and a judiciary with high integrity. Nehru took up individual corruption cases but no strategy was evolved. As a result, the scale of corruption went on increasing as the government began to assume a larger role in the life of the people. Over the years since independence, the Indian political system began to fall pray to corruption. With added fillip provided by political patronage, rampant and all pervading corruption began to engulf and corrode the whole administration. Not only the politicians and bureaucrats are corrupts, but no section of society is free from it, the media, press, academia, professionals, judiciary all tainted and polluted buy it.

(IV)

A major source of corruption during post-colonial period, among others in the Indian political system since late 1960's, is the funding of elections. Elections have been becoming costlier by the day giving unfair advantages to these, backed by moneybags and black money. Today expenses for running a Lok Sabha or State Assembly seat run into several hundred thousand rupees. Despite the existence of prescribed statutory limits, the expenses incurred by political parties and their candidates are grossly underestimated when returns are filed. Most of their money was financed by black money-holders and those who required political patronage to obtain economic concessions at the cost of the public exchequer.

After the elections are over, those who willed political power are actively involved in corrupt practices. Ministers, parliamentarians, legislators, officers and bureaucrats are prone to purchase government land for personal use at one-fourth its real worth, purchase costly flats in cities and led uncommon, isolated and luxurious life. Many politicians, bureaucrats, engineers and officers are arrested on corruption charges, cases are filed against them in the courts but nobody was found in central prisons. As a result corruptions by the elites are going on unabated.

(V)

We assume that the root cause of corruption in India lies in the capitalistic path of development that India has adopted to shape the post-colonial society and politics. Corruption, nepotism, bribery and misappropriation are the features of capitalistic system and the Indian ruling elites and their petty followers have openly practiced these clandestine means to engulf public resources for personal gains. The Indian political elite, after 1970s worked only on the basis of the some vested interests. Their policies are interest-based. These selfish bureaucrats also encouraged the bureaucrats to practice corruptions. The economic policy of the government is also highly defective for which scandals are very frequently reported in the media. In the absence of clear and transparent rules, the ministers and bureaucrats take into corrupt practices by arbitrary decisions. Corruption is also caused by scarcity and due to the decline of morality, honesty and values in the minds of the administrators. Lack of vigilance enormous powers to the ministerial staff, unaccountability, defective information system give ample scope to officials not only to be corrupt, but also remain unaffected even after following corrupt practices. Thus, social backwardness, unaccountability of officers, administrative delay, clumsy handling of corrupt cases, and lack of public forum to oppose corruption, may be cited as some factors of corruption. Besides, the old institutional arrangements where our politicians and bureaucrats, and inefficient role of the media, popular indifference, rapid expansion of governments activities involving huge outlays, stringent regulations of the private sector, poverty and ignorance of the people and extreme individualism are also responsible for the increase in corruption in our country.

(VI)

Here it would be important to cite areas where corruptions are most prominent. The greatest farce of our legal system is the defamation cases. Defamation cases always safeguard the corrupt echelons and indulge them to continue the very malpractices. When allegations have been raised in the newspapers, against the leader politicians, they are prone to file defamation cases in the court. Due to lack of proofs, the allegations vanished. This type of legal provisions is known as Strategic Lawsuits Against Public Participation (SLAPP) in the USA. By frequent application of SLAPP in the USA, corruption of all forms have been almost legitimatised. In India too, Public Interest Litigation are often liquidated by applying similar techniques. Recently, the Center for Science and Environment had raised an allegation against PEPSI, a foreign Cold Drinks company, that PEPSI cold drinks are found poisonous in the laboratory and inadequate for drink. But PEPSI was proved innocent by the Court possibly because PEPSI had a nexus with the big Indian leaders.

We have already mentioned that general elections of India is the most vulnerable field where corrupt practices are rampant and unchecked. T. N. Sheshan, the former Election Commissioner said on the 10th Lok Sabha elections that... ceiling limits on election expenses have been violated extensively.[7] He further said, cash, crime and rampant corruption are the three pillars on which Indian democracy stands today.[8]

There are at least four ministries in the Union Government where corruption is rampant such as Defence, Petroleum, Power and Communication. The Defence Ministry spends Rs. 40,000 crores on defence purchage every year where 15-40 per cent are spent on commission.[9] Lot of money is also involved in giving drilling rights, fixing pipelines, opening of petrol pumps in the Petroleum Ministry.[10] The Power Ministry spends 4 crores per year which provides opportunities to its officials to accept kickbacks."[11]

Corruption is also rampant in PWD, Police, Excise, Revenue and Railway departments. In many establishment, while awarding contracts fixed percentage is taken as a form.[12]

Corruption is also noticeable not only at the top it percolates all way down. Assistant and junior engineers, middle and low rank officials in all the government departments both at the central and state level clerks in secretariats and education departments, junior staff of the railways accept bribes in return for favours. Gifts giving is a major form of corruption in cities and this affair occurs between officers, doctors and the secretaries or the ministers. In Assam fake jobs are sold in the unemployed market for crores of rupees during the last 20 years, but no actual appointment was noticed. Speed money is a common type of corrupt practice particularly in matters relating to grants and sanctions.

Share of kickbacks keeps on shooting up every few year. The Preparatory Committee for Alternative Economic Policies has conducted research in kickbacks.[13] It estimates that the kickbacks shot up from Rs. 3036 crores in 1980-81 to an astonishing Rs. 19,414 crores in 1990-91.

Registered number of cases of corruption in India under the prevention of the Corruption Act, 1947 varied from 300 to 500 between 1981 and 1987 but after the enforcement of 1988 Act the number varies between 1700 and 2100 per year.[14]

Needless to state that leaders and politicians are most corrupt persons in India. On the basis of top-brass corruption evidences, India is ranked as the 7th most corrupt country in the world by a non-government German organization called "Transparency International."[15] There are very few honest and socially responsible politicians in the country. Once they grasp political power they spontaneously involve in corruption. Even in India, the most corrupt persons can easily come to the seat of power by virtue of money and muscle power and with the help of established dishonest leaders. They can go scot-free, unharmed and unpunished. During the post-independent period some of the persons who were appointed as Ministers at the center and the states, should have been in jail but instead, they managed to strut on the political stage as honest leaders. During the last 55 years, several scandals and corruption allegations have been reported in the country. Mostly the Chief Ministers, Ministers, leaders, holding important political position, bureaucrats and big business were reported to have been involved in multi-crores scams. But no effective steps were taken against these culprits on the plea of inadequate evidence. Some of the much publicized notorious scandals were the Bofors Gun Deal (1986), the Hawala Scandal (1990), the Animal Husbandry Scam (1990), the Telecommunication Scam (1996), the Bitumin Scam in Bihar (1996), the Jharkhand Mukti Morcha Scandal (1993), the Indian Bank Scam (1991-95), the Cement Scandal (1982), the Sugar Scandal (1994), the Treasury Fraud Scandal in Assam (1995), the OIL Pipeline theft scam in Assam (2003-04), and finally more than three dozens scams against a former Tamil Nadu Chief Minister, who latter successfully blackmailed the BJP-led government during 1998-99. These and many other scandals have involved corruption of thousands of crores of rupees. Corruption is also very common in central and state civil services. When complaints are received against highly place officials, inquiries are held, vigilance agencies are set in motion to pacify the people and the media, but rarely the accused officers are punished. A whopping amount of money are spent in central and state general elections, parties and candidates spent crores of rupees in the election, expropriated from big capitals as black money and crores of rupees are spent in Horse Trading in the country.

(VII)

Thus, we find from the above discussion that corruption and nepotism is inherent in India. It has cancerous consequences on the nation. It makes our democracy a mockery and the democratic governance disfunctioning and it deceived the people at large, from getting their bigotted economic and political share in the democracy. It has created violence, artificial resource crunch, financial crisis and lawlessness. The big bosses who are most corrupt can easily influence the law-givers, law-makers and the judges. Corruption has given birth to ugly casteism, linguism, communalism and it gives upper hand to the blackmarketeers and big capitals for concentration of surplus resources and black money as such. It has destroyed political morality and societal values. It heightened inefficiency, nepotism, smuggling, bribery, mutual discontent, and created indiscipline in all fields of administration. It has destablised governments, both at the center and at the states. It create shortage of public resources which led the governments to become uncapable of paying monthly salaries to the employees and to liquidate jobs. Corruption compels government to abolish existing government posts and compels the policy-makers not to create new jobs, which results in unemployment. Hence, corruption badly infects the healthy functioning of our large democracy specifically, the large scale corruption of the big political leaders has to a large extent, lowered the image of our democracy.

The delay in catching the culprits, the manner of functioning of rules in state, does delay the prompt rectification of this gigantic menace. The legal procedures are often so time-consuming that it taxes on the public patience. The law of proof is so ineffective against those accused of the guilt, that the common people is frightened about the outcome. Thus, political parties as such, have to be supplemented by a vast network of non-official activities organizations to undertake the task. A mass social and political movement should be launched under leadership of the progressive middle classes and the students to combat it. The delay in dealing with corruption may often lead to the flagging of the public interest to generate a cynical view that those involved in serious allegations of corruptions in public are seldom punished.[16]

Experience has shown that the anti-corruption police and the CBI have largely failed to investigate and initiate actions against the corrupt leaders, politicians and the bureaucrats. Many times the CBI officials have confessed to political pressures on them. The Central Govt. has set up the following 4 (four) department as anti-corruption measures:

(i) Administrative Vigilance Division
(ii) Central Bureau of Investigation
(iii) Domestic Vigilance Units in the Ministers/Departments/ Public Undertakings/National Banks
(iv) Central Vigilance Commission.

But it remains in the dark whether these anti-corruption departments are active, vigilant in combating and controlling corruption. Besides, the Govt. of India has set up more than 25 commissions to inquire into the charges of corruption against politicians and public companies. The United Front government introduced Lok Pal Bill in the Parliament in Sept, 1996, which was not passed even by the former BJP led Govt. The real hurdle in passage of the bill was the lack of political will. There is no substitute for Lok Pal the jurisdiction of which has to be confined to investigate into the corruption charges against those holding high offices including the Prime Ministers. But uptill now fresh initiative from the present Govt. has not been noticed to pass the Lok Pal Bill. It should be stated that the Lok Pal can be moved by anyone to start a case by filing an affidavit.

From the above discussions we can infer that the Indian democratic governance is severely affected, injured and plagued by the growing menace of corruption. Unlike the western democracies, where corruptions are prevalent only among the top level echelons In India, corruptions are endemic everywhere from top to bottom. Corruption has been institutionalized and becomes a natural phenomenon. Our policy, economy, society and the democratic governance, are eroded by wanton corruptions. Especially, democratic governance in the country has become impossible to carry on to the benefit of the common people. Today, the government has lost credibility, viability, confidence and legitimacy in governing the state for the top-brass leaders and politicians, who are freely involving in corruption. It destroys the mutual trust between representatives and the people and underestimates confidence in the democratic process to the point where people may not think democracy worth defending.[17]

(VIII)

Now, we confront with this very pertinent question as to whether it is possible to root out this dreaded evil for the consolidation of a corrupt free Indian society. We are living at a time and in such a society where corruption has become a way of life for the leader-politicians and bureaucrats under whose authority, Indian state machinery runs. Today most of the corruption cases remain unreported. Though we have a galaxy of responsible and enlightened citizens, they fear to report corruption cases to the media with an apprehension that the corrupt forces may to harm to them. Those who declare crusade against corruption may face physical assault, attack and punishment from the corrupt elements. In the western countries legal protection are given to those who intend to bring the corruption cases into light and make people conscious against corrupt practices. But in India, it is still a distant dream. No body can secure the life of the citizen who wish to raise allegations against corruption, even here the lives of the journalists are also not secure. On the other hand, most of the people are either indifferent or pessimists regarding corruption. Today much of the corruption exists because of people's tolerance or complete lack of public voice against it, as well as the absence of strong public forum to oppose it. While many intellectual, educated social scientists, well-informed and articulate citizens remain worried about this monstrous problem in the country.

What is basically more important is the increase of accountability and transparency of our government to at least minimize the magnitude of corruption to a tolerable limit. Many Indian leaders declare their firm determination to eradicate corruption, but soon after assuming power, they become the worst corrupts and the slogan of a corruption free-society, becomes a good political game for the leaders. But it is the earnest necessity for the nation to treat corruption very seriously and efforts should be made to minimize it, even if it can never be completely eradicated.

(VIII)

In order to facilitate a near corruption-free democratic society and governance, we have suggested the following measures to be adopted:

(i) To minimize corruption at all levels, we have to focus on appropriate law, procedure and responsible administration. Bad, harsh, complicated and ambiguous laws may lead to corruption.

(ii) Artificial shortages, which facilitate illegal gratification have to be controlled.

(iii) Vigilance should be increased so that sudden checks could be carried out at vulnerable point of corruption.

(iv) Election expense should be strictly controlled and the Horse Trading business should be totally banned, the Anti-Defection Law, 1985 should be amended and properly implemented.

(v) Liberalization Policy should be very carefully introduced. Here we like to note that capitalist countries like the USA, Japan, South Korea, Thailand, Malaysia, Italy etc. are considered as most corrupt societies where China has become able to minimize corruption in spite of injecting liberal policy into the communist culture in recent times. The Chinese deal corruption very seriously.

(vi) Co-operation of the people has to be obtained for successfully controlling corruption.

(vii) Mass media should be free from political bias and should come forward to highlight corruption before the public.

(viii) Strong public opinion should be created against corruption.

(ix) Corruption charges should be dealt with properly and vigorous punishment should be given to those who are proved to be indulged in corruption.

(x) Public organizations should act as watch-dog bodies for democracy to save it from corruption ailment.

(xi) Political parties have to be supplemented by a vast network of non-official non-govt. activists, organizations to undertake vigilance against corruption.

(xii) Student bodies, Youth organizations and NGO's etc. also should aware to stop corruption.

(xiii) Governmental measures to deal with corruption should be vibrant and strong.

(xiv) The state funding of elections like Germany, Norway, Sweden and some other advanced countries of Europe yield good results; this practice may be tested in our country which may reduce corruption to a large extent.

(xv) Lok Pal laws are necessary to look into the charges of corruption at the highest levels.

(xvi) Women organizations, including all educated women should come forward to raise strong and rigorous protests against corruptions.

(xvii) The government of India should initiate actions against corruptions by creating special departmental anti-corruption vigilant cells, for each departments separately, so that the department cells could scrutinize the behaviour, activities, assets and liabilities and corrupt role of the officers and employees of the department and accordingly initiate tough actions.

(xviii) Necessary legal protection and security should be given by the state to the persons who reveal corruption evidences, report to the media and bring corruption cases to the notice of the concerned authority.

(xix) Close and cordial relationship should be established between the people and the administration.

(xx) Police and CBI should be made active and vibrant.

(xxi) Income Tax reports should be published.

(xxii) Nexus between political parties and big business houses should be banned so that political parties can't accept huge donation/ contribution/ gift from them.

(xxiii) Departmental anti-corruption vigilant cells may be introduced both at the center and in the states and in the government corporations and boards to manitor corrupt activities of the high echelons, middle and lower-ranked officers and the employees.

(xxiv) All the autonomous enquiry and investigative organizations, commissions and institutions already set up, including the Courts, should be made free and independent of political interference so that they could catch the culprits.

(xxv) Special Anti-Corruption Vigilant Department should be created to look into the properties, assets, liabilities, all known sources of income of Ministers, Parliamentarians, Legislators, leaders, Politicians and Bureaucrats.

(xxvi) People should socially boycott those who have been proved to be involving in corruption, nepotism, favoritism, bribery and misappropriation.

(xxvii) A strong anti-corruption democratic movement under leadership of University and College students is necessary.

(xxviii) Value-based education containing anti-corrupt morality should be imparted to our children in the educational institutions.

Finally, we can say that if the above mentioned methods and any others not mentioned, have so far been applied, corruption may be minimized. Already India is tortured by communal and caste riots and have been initiating hooligans into politics. As a result of communalism, casteism, laxity in enforcement of law and order, corruption and the use of money and muscle power in elections, criminalisation of politics have been completed with a nexus developing between politicians, businessmen, bureaucrats, police, criminals and gangsters. Now, to conclude, it is not at all possible to completely root out corruption which is deep rooted, but it is certainly possible to roll it down within tolerable limits. Corruption is a dreaded and cancerous evil and the people of India must fight against it. It is now high time containing corruption is taken up by dedicated political rulers and the political parties. If we fail to eradicate corruption even to a considerable extent, India's democracy may be hijacked from within. We must also say, it is not desirable to invite an alternative totalitarian system to combat corrupt, but it is suggested that corruption, crime, violence, nepotism and misappropriation of public money and resources could be contained within democracy by democratic methods.

REFERENCES

1. Machael, Clarke (ed). *Corruption: Causes and Consequences*, Francesis Publishers, London, 1983, p. 214.
2. Nye, J. 'Corruption and Political Development: A Cost-Benefit Analysis,' *American Political Science Review*, 1967, p. 410.
3. See for a discussion Ahuja, Ram. '*Society in India: Concepts, Theories and Recent Trends*', Rawat Publications, New Delhi, 1999, p. 403.

4. Ibid., p. 404.
5. Ibid., p. 404.
6. Chandra, Bipan. *India After Independence* Vikash, Penguin Book India, New Delhi, 1999, p. 484.
7. "Cash, Crime Ail Political system." *The Tribune*, Chandigarh, Feb 1, 1994, quoted in Shukla, S.K., 'Democracy in India: Issues and Problems," The *Indian Journal of Political Science*, Vol. IV, No. 4, Oct-Dec, 1994.
8. Ibid., p. 404.
9. Ahuja, Ram, op.cit., p. 402.
10. Ibid., p. 402.
11. Ibid., p. 403.
12. Ibid., p. 403.
13. Choudhury, P.C. "Corruption", in *Seminer*, No. 421, Sept, 1994.
14. Santhanam Committee Report on Prevention of Corruption, Govt. of India, 1964 (Sunday, Calcutta, Dec 3, 1994), quoted in Ahuja, Ram, *op. cit.*, pp. 408-409.
15. *The Hindustan Times*, May 5, 1996.
16. Chakraborty, Nikhil. "Introductory note" in Jean Beachler '*Democracy: An Analytical Survey*', UNESCO Publishing Hose, New Delhi, 1995.
17. See Beetham, Devid and Boyle, Kavin, "*Democracy, 80 questions and Answers.*"

    National Book Trust India UNESCO Publishing, New Delhi 1995, pp. 67-69 for a discussion of multi-dimensional affects of corruption.

18

CORRUPTION IN INDIA: AN EXERCISE IN PERPETUITY

Bhawani Singh and Vibhuti Singh Shekhawat

Deptt. of Political Science, University of Rajasthan, Jaipur.
Deptt. of Humanities & Social Science, Malviya National Institute of Technology, Jaipur.

An irate and angry crowd, a pent up mob consisting of women in distress, fully worked up, determined and decisive enter a Nagpur court and create a bizarre event. A history sheeter convict Akku Yadav, wanted in many cases ranging from rape, molestation and murder, kidnapping and extortion, was attacked with sharp weapens by women protestors, in full view of police and public, lawyers and judges. The dreaded tormentor was lynched and done to death in court premises, unmindful of consequences, fear of arrest or apprehension of punishment. It was not a preplanned, pre-meditated attack. It was a spontaneous outburst of pent up public rage against an outrageous offender who for years was committing open assaults on women, the police and the administration being hand in glove with the tormentor left the suffering women with no choice except to take the law into their hands and to do collectively in a fit of rage what the police, administration and law enforcing agencies could not accomplish in years. That he was allowed to dodge the police and judiciary and continued with his individual acts of lawlessness and highhandedness, ultimately induced or even forced the weaker sex to rise in revolt as one person and beat the offender to death and thereby exposing the utter hollowness and complicity of our law enforcing agencies to protect the law abiding against law-breakers. A similar incident happened on September 2, 2004 in Bareilly where an irate crowd killed a history-sheeter Islam.[1]

With the public lynching of Akku Yadav, and Islam curtain fell on a tortuous judicial process of police remand, examining the witnesses many of whom turn hostile for fear of reprisals, and finally greasing the palms of police personnel involved, settling the fees of lawyers and making ancillary "arrangements" to secure conviction which in most cases would not be available and offenders will be released scot-free for lack of evidence and other factors. Can there be worse example of corruption completed and compounded in such a brazen manner that offender in publicly flogged to death by members of weaker sex in Nagpur. It was spot justice and the culprits so-called refused to run away from justice, abscond or attempted to destroy evidence. In fact bail was granted to them for lack of evidence against them.

Will Nagpur and Bareilly repeat itself in other parts of the country where identical situations prevail or will these remain an isolated occurrences, a once in a century incident is a moot point but there is no denying this incident exposes the police-criminal nexus which is the cause for despair and despondence among victims who apprehending miscarriage or total denial of justice ultimately resort to self-protection and self-defence and are compelled to take up the cudgels themselves to mete out spot punishment. Let all those who talk of corruption and its eradication take a clue from these gruesome and bizarre incidents that justice delayed is truly justice denied and the aggrieved and the assaulted will not indefinitely wait for justice to drop from heaven like manna dews on expectant mouths and may be forced to take law into their hands—the law which denied them protection, deprived them of justice and became a handmaid of the high and the mighty in society be it mafia, the law-makes or law-breakers. The need of the hour is to ensure that these incidents are not erased from public memory as nothing hampers the pursuit of justice more than public amnesia.

Corruption today is a hydra-headed monster whose one head you chip and the other springs up thereby creating a continuum, an eternity of corruption. The legendary demon king of Lanka, Ravana was blessed with ten heads and had thereby a degree of finality about his death that the chopping down of tenth head would herald the ultimate solution and proclaim his death. But the modern Ravana of corruption is a multifocal universal eternity of Indian system which knows no bounds and is endless as eternity, universal as the cosmic system, constant as the polar star, permanent as the star galaxy and perennially saltish as sea water full of brine. Needless to say that its area of operationalization is too wide and comprehensive and includes all branches of administration. So wide is gamut and extended the canvass that it covers practically every organ of government and the germs have penetrated deep into our veins and arteries which appears beyond detection of even laser surgery. Since the polity is headed by people of dubious integrity and unflattering renown, barriers of rectitude do not hamper their pursuits. Governed by unalterable rules of moral turpitude and backed by a decadent and remorselessly shameless law-enforcement agency, the sentinels of public interest are enveloped in the thick fog of putrid depravity and feel emboldened to continue with their depredations without fear of penal action. This is because nothing succeeds like success and as the old saying goes "Seek ye first the political Kingdom and all things shall be added into you."[2] Once this is achieved, all things happen automatically. A person in power, his naivete and dubiety apart, his tawdry twaddle about future notwithstanding, can ladder his way to the top through only route and that is the one of rampant and unabated corruption. Its perpetrators are cloven-hoofed people with an outward saintly visage. Since the system is an ongoing one, its outcome though uncertain is still predictable and despite being dubious is definite and has acquired a rare degree of durability and permanence. The important thing is that it is not a single individual's cloistered virtue but a multilateral effort of several participants who together receive their share of spoils that makes corruption institutionalized and market worthy.

The difficulty in organizing a debate on corruption stems not from limited options but from unlimited avenues and opportunities concerning it. This is because every aspect of national life is tainted by corruption and the problem is one of selectivity to decide where to begin with and which aspect to choose for a dialectical diagnosis. There is a plethora of factors encouraging corruption and one is at his wits ends to decide which factor is seminal and which is a booster and finally one has to settle for a conjunctional perspective only. Not every factor can be discussed or else the narrative would run into volumes. Only a few factors can be identified to highlight the impact of corruption.

Corruption destroys liberty and subverts democratic institution. In the words of John Stuart Mill. "A people may prefer a free government; but if from indolence, or carelessness, or cowardice, or want of public spirit, they are unequal to the exertions necessary for preserving it; if they will not fight for it when directly attacked; if they can be deluded by the artifices used to cheat them out of it; if by monetary discouragement, or temporary panic or a fit of enthusiasm for an individual, they can be induced to lay their liberties at the feet of even great man, or trust him with powers which enable him to subvert their institutions—in all these cases they are unfit for liberty."[3]

As stated earlier, corruption is multivariate and has affected every aspect of national life—public, private or corporate. A corrupt coterie, a degenerate cabal of time servers and place hunters promotes corruption through genuflexion. Unforgettable in this matter was the presumption of Congress Party President Dev Kant Barua who coined the spacious slogan Indira is India. Little bid he realised then that in the election that followed in 1977, has party would met its nemesis and collapse like a house of cards. The election result was a fitting finale to the political myopia being exhibited by this corrupt-political class which during the infamous emergency employed the medieval methodology of running a paper-logged administration which was full of political naivete and administrative dubiety; and was manned by self-doubting Thomases who were gripped in their self-created political allergies. The new political class was bereft of ideological moorings and suffered from dialectical illiteracy at the apex level. Its dependent cronies given to gullible evasiveness and spoilt by induced megalomania become intolerantly indifferent to the life-saving pharmaceuticals of a democratic polity—the time honoured systems of checks and balances and thereby deprived the polity of its functional limbs.

The result was that during emergency the system failed to receive political oxygen through a democratic feedback mechanism resting on free speech and a non-captive press. Defending its parvenu performance, the new political class began using ballet-proof attire forgetting that such an outfit only ensured security against physical elimination but provided no protection against political blunders. The sycophants reluctance to undergo performance audit only strengthened the cult of personality and created of hallowed ring master in a political circus unmindful of the impending disaster of 1977 election, which proved that genuflexion is no substitute for good governance or inspired public service. It only augments the foundation of the edifice of corruption and promotes political illiteracy resting on self-created amnesia of its own wrong doings.

FUNCTIONAL REQUISITES OF TAINTED ADMINISTRATION

One may now begin an inquest into the causal factors that facilitate the growth of corruption below.

1. EROSION OF RULE OF LAW

Maintenance of law and order through compliance with rules, orders and edicts serves as a bulwark against corruption. The Indian administrators are too prone to exhibit legal pedantry and constitutional logomachy to hoodwink the unillumined but take no steps to prevent an erosion of rule of law by cunning politicians and their crafty mentors. A distinct proclivity to subvert legal norms to polevault over the deserving and the meritorious is discernible in this country which insulates one against parliamentary and judicial scrutiny and frees him from the control of invigilatory, interogatory and auditory mechanism. This induces circumvention of accountability and powers remain securely tied to pro-tem incumbents of authority who ensure the integrality of system through an invented mechanism of spoils sharing which takes care of every single political player. Corruption thus is a unifying factor, a bridge between the carpet-beggars of politics.

The most egregious form of political corruption is our rulers penchant for circumventing the law-breakers "de facto amnesty in exchange for political support."[4] In such a situation, nation-building becomes a "handsome neo-classical building in which political prisoners scream in the basement"[5] and legal system becomes the first casualty.

2. EXTENSION IN THE RANGE OF RESERVATIONS

It is a new mantra to create societal schism by pole-vaulting some communities over others similarly placed to create a vote bank whose shaky foundations are mired in political corruption. Birth, no administrative acumen or still being the criterion of recruitment, the list of OBC faithfuls keeps changing with every changing in government and competitive populism resting on the requirements of vote bank politics determines the range of hopefuls. What was intended to be reverse discrimination to provide justice to the hitherto neglected sections of society has become an instrument of appeasement and creating greater discrimination in society. The incumbent in OBC list today include, some of the most affluent sections of society such as Jats and Yadavs whose claims to OBC membership rest more on convenience and political chicanery than on social status and economic needs. Policy of enhanced reservations has become a fulcrum of power politics today.

3. UNHOLY ALLIANCE BETWEEN THE POLITICIAN AND THE BUREAUCRAT

Corruption is rampant in a system run by the uninitiated and the unillumined political leaders because their proven incompetence and immaturity creates infantile disorder. But the moment the greed of the politicians receives overt and covert support of the bureaucrats, corruption becomes institutionalised and rule-based and this inaugurates a regime of sleeze by power-hungry opportunists and upstart adventurists whose lack of rectitude in public life has always been pet subject of gossip columns, public debate and wall writings. Any epistolary confrontation between the two mega-functionaries would hit them both hard and hence both invent institutional props to provide legitimacy to their deeds and treat each other with worshipful finality to extract their pound of public flesh. They know the value of old maxim—united we stand and divided we fall. When sinners unite, the people get divided and fall. The rights of the people are consigned to the star chambers of mounting corruption.

4. TYRANNY OF POWER-BROKERS

This class is necessary component in a system of spoils sharing. These people swear by trite traditionalism of the Westminster system but in practice, they are free from the slavery of this genetic code. They are an invisible empire within the empire and liasionise with apex rulers by offering them the mess of ballot pottage. It is difficult to brush aside these power-brokers through dilettantist devices or self-serving resolutions. Their credentials are not sacrificial but instrumental. They did not make any sacrifice during the freedom movement but they know the utility of political institutions such as state and governments where can be used as instruments for self-aggrandizement and private welfare. They are not the unsullied charioteers of public weal but skilled players who draw political and economic mileage through their involvement in dubious deals, treacherous transactions and sordid bargains. In the name of altruistic acts of public charity, they petrify the purpose for which public institutions are created and by social pacification through acts of moral turpitude, economic sleeze and political bargain they taint the system. No one epitomises institutionalized corruption more than class of power brokers.

5. STAR WAR

Corruption receives institutional boost when two rival infallibilities such as the President and Prime Minister clash. When two apex functionaries indulge in an unseemly tussel to settle constitutional niceties such as Presidential thirst for sharing sensitive classified information matched by an equal resistance by the office of Prime Minister to conceal information because of the cult of suspicious secrecy. Sometimes it may lead to litigative battle between the two with the judiciary playing the honest broker as being the guardian of the Constitution. This is the time-honoured caveat against interpretutional unwisdom by either apex ruler to establish the inerrancy of constitutional status of both or either. After all, one has to pay the price for retaining power. Jawaharlal Nehru, in his work Price of Power said:

"In the world of politics and economics there is a search for power and yet when power is attained much else of value has gone. Political trickery and intrigue take the place of idealism, and cowardice and selfishness the place of disinterested courage. Form prevails over substance, and power, so eagerly sought after somehow fails to achieve what it aimed at".[6]

With despair deepening and constitutional edifice shaking owing to this gubernatorial confrontation, the croonies of either rulers flock around their chosen leader and make necessary noises to exhibit their loyalty and strengthen the personality cult by demeaning and debasing the rival centre of power. In such as unseemly wrangle between apex rulers, the corrupt flourish under the protective shield of their apex patron promoters.

6. POLITICS OF VOTE BANK

With the disintegration of one-party dominant system enshrined in the Congress party, India has entered an era of coalitional politics and this calls for competitive populism to acquire votes. Different political formations have their own vote bank composed of castes or religious followings and a scramble is on to appease and accommodate them through doling out largesses or offering political posts that carry power and pelf. How important these groups have become for political parties can be seen through in an inept remark of Dev Kant Barua, who speaking about the importance of Bangladeshi Muslims and tribal plantation labourers for success at the hustings for the Congress party in Assam once said "...so long as the Alis and coolies are with the Congress party, it did not care for anybody".[7] Statements such as this opens the floodgates of corruption through minority appeasement.

CAVEAT FOR FUTURE

Identification of a variable that facilitate corruption is not the end of the tunnel. It is only an ominous beginning and the list remains only illustrative, not exhaustive as new causes spring up that promote corruption. It is like damming water on one hand, only to see it burst forth at another end and inundating vast untapped areas. It is like a raging fire which if one tries to extinguish at one place, erupts at another place and consumers everything that comes its way: Corruption is thus characterized by both continuity and change, the change only supporting and sustaining the sinews of corruption instead of eradicating it. There may be optimists who hinge their conviction on some time worn archaic traditions to come to our rescue in this fight against the demon of corruption. This is because tradition may strengthen and solidity superstitions, it cannot reform anyone. Engels was right when he said "Tradition is a great retarding force, the vis inertiae of history."[8] Over the years, the Indian Constitution, our Deed of Destiny has undergone nearly a hundred revisions but the basic framework supporting traditional wisdom and conventional morality remains unchanged and the phenomenon to torrent of corruption unleased in the earlier years of its promulgation still remains.

Thus the search for a solvent of corruption still remains incomplete and illusive. The cynical view is that alternative to corruption is greater corruption and one accepts it as a part of system. The optimist's view is that make corruption unrewarding and unremunerative. Let not the corrupt swim incognito, unnoticed, undetected and unpunished. Make penalties larger than the ephemeral gains of corruption. While the cesspool may take indefinite time to completely dry up, in the meanwhile some efforts can definitely be made to control the breeding of its germs. Hence, despite deepening despair all around, one may still hinge one's hopes on those who stand to suffer most on account of this surging wave of corruption—the common people of India, the vast pool of suffering humanity, the neglected teeming millions who form the electorate. To quote V.R. Krishna Iyer, "That our political cosmos is not all that dark, that our democracy not all that brittle, that our constitutional parchment not that easy to pulverize, that personality cult has poor purchase at general elections, that the imperatives of Independence and the Preamble to the Great Charter still conscientise Indians in their millions, is heartening contemporary history."[9]

REFERENCES

1. *Rajasthan Patrika*, Jaipur, dated Sep. 9, 2004, p. 5.
2. Quoted in V.R. Krishna Iyer: *The Indian Presidency*, Deep & Deep Publications, 1998, p. 11.
3. Ibid., p. 1.
4. Sanjib Baruah, *India Against Itself*, Oxford University Press, New Delhi, 2001, p. XXI.
5. Ibid., p. 1.
6. V.R. Krishna Iyer, *op. cit.*, p. 14.
7. B.P. Shukla, *What Ails India's North East*, Suruchi Sahitya, New Delhi, 1980, p. 24.
8. V.R. Krishna Iyer, *op. cit.*, p. 11.
9. Ibid., p. 15.

19

CORRUPTION IN INDIA: CAUSES AND REMEDIES

S.S. Tiwana

Corruption in all societies is as old as power itself. It is, therefore, common in all countries, irrespective of their stage of development. However, its nature, volume and dimensions differ largely from country to country and from one environment to another. India is not free from the evils of political and bureaucratic corruption.[1] Many scams and scandals that took place in India are enough proof of this rampant and wide-spread corruption due to near total lack of effective vigilance. Corruption is rampant in administration of welfare schemes, public distribution system, police, revenue, excise and taxation and irrigation departments, and several other sectors where people come into contact daily with administration. Corruption at lower levels takes the form of speed money for expediting approvals or providing legitimate services, or bribes for twisting rules. A matter of great concern is the vertical integration of corruption at various levels of government between officials and politicians and the inability of top functionaries to check the prevalence and growth of corruption. In fact, corruption has now been institutionalised and has become a commonly accepted way of life.

The purpose of this article is to trace the historical legacy of corruption in India and to analyse major factors contributing to corruption. Endeavour has also been made in this paper to analyse the action plan adopted by the Government to combat the galloping corruption in India.

DEFINITIONS OF CORRUPTION

It is not an easy task to define corruption, as it is not a unified phenomenon. Corruption has many forms with different types of participants, settings, stakes, techniques and cultures. L W J C Huberts has distinguished corruption from fraud.[2] His observation is based on the results of a survey in which 257 experts from 49 countries participated in 1994.

Clear legal definitions were put forward earlier in the United Kingdom by the Royal Commission on Standards of Conduct in Public Life (1974-76)[3] following the case of John Poulson who corruptly penetrated high levels of the British Civil Service, the National Health Service, a number of local authorities and other bodies. The offence of corruption, as defined in the United Kingdom Public Bodies Corrupt Practices Act, 1889 and the Prevention of Corruption Act, 1906 consists of three main ingredients.[4] It has to be shown:

1. that a gift of consideration was given or offered by party to another;
2. that the gift or consideration was given, or received as an inducement or reward for services to be rendered or already rendered in relation to official duties; and
3. that the transaction took place corruptly.

The first ingredient is the objective and is the basic fact – the *actus reus* – which the prosecution have to prove, the second ingredient in respect of relevant gifts and considerations in the United Kingdom Acts involves bribes. For an offence to be committed, bribes need not actually pass hands; soliciting or agreeing to accept them are offences as much as their acceptance and offering to give bribes is as much an offence as actually giving them. The second and third ingredients involve a mental element or *mens rea*.

Other definitions of corruption, such as those adopted by L.W.J.C. Huberts, draw on the knowledge of eminent political scientist, like Carl Friedrich, Samuel Huntingdon and J.S. Nye. Before putting forward his own interpretation of public corruption, Huberts distinguishes not only between public corruption and fraud but proceeds to differentiate between political corruption and administrative corruption as follows:

"When public corruption or fraud is committed by politicians, it is called political corruption or fraud; when civil servants are involved, it is administrative corruption or fraud... both mean the misuse of public power for private gain – [that is, are] related to private instead of public interests".[5]

Public integrity by contrast, stands for acting and deciding according to prevailing norms for public behaviour. One norm for public behaviour, Huberts maintains, is that private interests should not interefere with political and administrative responsibilities.

The term corruption, then, may be used in its strict legal sense, as defined in any particular country or group of countries, or it may apply loosely and broadly to unethical activities which may be on a spectrum from the criminal offence of corruption involving inducements to unethical activities, such as fraud or the misuse of political influence.

HISTORICAL LEGACY OF CORRUPTION

India inherited a legacy of corruption from its ancient rulers who always expected some gifts (in the form of nazarana) from their subject. One of the important aspects of the employers function in those days were to milch the common folk to enrich the treasury of rulers. Appointments to key positions were made on family considerations. Most often, a Prime Minster's son succeeded his father, a Government's son the Governor, a judge's son a judge, a village Headman's son the Headman. Replacing relatives in good positions, irrespective of merit gained merit in the eyes of the People.[6] Thus nepotism as an evil was an alien concept in those days and the vocabulary had no proper word for it.

Chanakya's famous statement in *Arthasastra,* many centuries ago, testifies to the durability of the phenomenon of corruption. He said, "Just as it is impossible not to taste the honey or the poison that finds itself at the tip of the tongue, so it is impossible for a Government servant not to eat up at least a bit of the Kings's revenue. Just as a fish moving under water cannot possibly be found out either as drinking or not drinking water, so Government servants employed in the Government work can not be found out [while] taking money [for themselves]. It is possible to mark the movements of birds flying high up in the sky; but not so is it possible to ascertain the movement of Government servants of hidden purpose."[7]

Kalidas in *Abhigyan Shankuntalam* and the twentieth century poet, Kshemendra, have mentioned about the prevalence of corruption. It germinated in pre-colonial and colonial India when the rulers representatives (gumashtas) made exorbitant demands from helpless peasants.

CORRUPTION DURING SECOND WORLD WAR TIMES

Corruption was rampant in 1937 when Congress party got an opportunity for the fist time to form Minister at the state level. Mahatma Gandhi took a serious note of the growing corruption in Congress ranks and lashed out at it in the columns of *Harijan*. In May 1939, he told Gandhi Seva Sangh workers, "I would go to the length of giving the whole Congress organisation a decent burial, rather than put up with the corruption that is rampant."[8] Jawahar Lal Nehru felt more or less the same way. In a letter to Gandhi on April 28, 1938, he lamented: "What is for worse is that we are losing the high position that we have built up with so much labour in the hearts of the people. We are sinking to the levels of ordinary politicians who have no principles to standby and where work is governed by a day- to-day opportunism."[9]

Gandhi was much relieved when Congress Ministers resigned in October, 1939 on political issues arising out of Britain's entry in Second World War. The problem of corruption in administration and public services became more glaring during Second World War years (1939-45).

CORRUPTION IN POST-INDEPENDENT PERIOD

The position, however, changed radically after independence and assumption of power by the elected leaders. The launching of economic development Five Year Plans from 1951 onwards phenomenally increased government spending. Banking, insurance sectors came under government control. Numerous large and medium size PSUs were set up. Licence, Quota and Permit Raj came into being in areas of economy left open for the private sector. The increased authority for 'licensing', 'control' and 'regulating' has earned the government the nick name of "licence, permit and quota raj."[10] This has provided umpteen opportunities for corruption, bribery and affluence through ill gotten wealth.

Numerous 'middle men' and peddlers of influence too emerged to facilitate corruption and to share the booty at the cost of the public exchequer. Many kinds of 'White Collar' or economic offences in violation of the numerous new fiscal laws, like the Foreign Exchange Regulation Act (FERA), The Import Export (Control) Act, the Customs and Excise Act, The Income Tax Act, The Industrial Licencing Act, etc., provided additional avenues of corruption. The higher level economic offenders of these years established nexus with higher categories of politicians and bureaucrats due to the bigger sizes of their illegal transactions. Their corrupt activities could not be adequately dealt with by the existing law enforcement agencies, like the CBI, the Directorate of Enforcement, or the various Income-Tax, Customs and Excise Authorities. These authorities were all under the control of the executive wing of government and seldom dared to set the appropriate laws in motion against persons holding high political offices even when any of them were duly suspected to have made illegal gains. As a result, huge, unaccounted wealth was amassed by dishonest ministers and high officials without much fear of detection and punishment. Many were suspected to have kept such money in secret Swiss Bank accounts.[11]

MAGNITUDE AND INTENSITY OF CORRUPTION IN INDIA

It is argued that corruption in the Third World tends to differ from that in industrialised countries in its scope and intensity. For example, in India where goods and services provided by public authorities are in short supply, it is not uncommon to see people paying a small sum to a minor official for reserving a seat in public transportation, for being admitted to a hospital, for having a telephone connection or licence. Scarcity of public resources and almost unlimited demand by the community give rise to such corrupt and unethical practices. As the craving for material goods continues to increase, public officials in charge of the provision or regulation of such services face temptation and may try to take advantage of whatever opportunity their position provides. In turn, their actions confirm to the prevailing public view that officials, generally, are corrupt. And, as R.B Jain states, "nothing is so corrupting as a suspicion of corruption."[12]

It is very difficult to identify and measure the magnitude and intensity of corruption due to its *modus operandi*. The *modus operandi* of corruption can take three forms. First, there is a collusive corruption, a form of corruption that involves the willing and planned cooperation of the giver and the taker. Political corruption, scams involving large contracts and other favours belong to this category. Secondly, there is extortionary corruption that implies forced extraction of bribes or other favours from vulnerable victims by those in authority. This tends to work when people who seek certain services or decisions are in a tight corner, with very few options. Thirdly, there is anticipatory

Table Comparative Statement of Cases of Corruption taken up by CBI during the years 1990, 1991, 1992, 1994, 1995, 1996.

	1990 (31.8.90)	1991 (31.8.91)	1992 (31.8.92)	1994 31.8.94)	1995 31.8.95)	1996 31.8.96)
No. of cases registered (total):	629	786	833	975	1011	1129
(a) against public servants.	518	639	676	796	764	996
(b) against private persons/firms.	111	147	157	179	247	133
No. of Gazetted Officers involved.	664	600	557	717	752	933
No. of cases handled by CBI including cases pending at the beginning of the year.	2019	2028	2203	2078	2145	2490
No. of cases sent for trial.	251	233	258	314	332	334
No. of cases decided by the courts.	167	178	172	199	204	222
No. of cases which ended in conviction.	92	105	103	117	121	122
No. of GOs involved.	26	26	20	23	34	33
No. of cases which ended in acquittal/ discharge or otherwise disposed of.	75	73	69	82	83	100

No. of cases reported to the administrative authorities concerned for departmental action or for suitable action.	276	319	344	258	222	225
No. of cases in which departmental proceedings concluded.	317	370	424	308	312	388
No. of cases which resulted in punishment	230	254	300	254	262	334
Amount of fine imposed (Rs.)	7,55,900	19,61,400	7,99,05	38,18,750	28,24630	1495,500
Amount of recoveries made in departmental action (Rs.)	6,52,336	71,688	20,600	10,000	22,500	1,15,558

Source: Government of India, Ministry of Personnel, Public Grievances and Pensions, Annual Report, 1996-97, New Delhi, 1997

corruption, the best example of which is the tendency among some people to pay a bribe or present a gift in anticipation of favourable actions or decisions from those in authority. Those who engage in such practices seldom question them having been brought up in a tradition (mamool) that considers it the right thing to do.[13]

Those who engage in collusive or anticipatory corruption are unlikely to complain about it, at least not openly. Collusive corruption will not come to light unless uncovered trails are held or some clever persons sniff it out. It is only in cases of extortionary corruption that protests or leakage of information are likely to occur.

Official report of the Central Bureau of Investigation are the only formal source that provides information about the magnitude and intensity of corruption in India. A comparative statement of the cases of corruption taken by the Central Bureau of Investigation during the years (1990-96) makes it clear that the volume of cases of corruption taken by the CBI during this period has increased.

The number of cases registered by the CBI was 629 in 1990, while in 1996, the number increased to 1129. The number of cases prosecuted in court was 251 in 1990 and 334 in 1996. Number of cases which ended in conviction was 392 in 1992 and 122 in 1996. The number of cases that resulted in punishment was 230 in 1992 and 334 in 1996.

MAJOR FACTORS CONTRIBUTING TO CORRUPTION

Following are some of the causes responsible for the emergence of the menace of corruption in India.

(a) **Government Monopoly:** Government performs many monopolistic functions which cannot be subjected to competition. Absence of competition tends to create opportunities for corruption by restricting supply deliberately or through withholding information. This tendency can occur in both public and private sectors. When people have no other option, they are more vulnerable to the pressures of monopolistic regulators and service providers. Monopoly is natural in some sectors for reasons such as economies of scale (e.g., water supply). Regulatory activities have to be managed by authorities designated for the purpose and cannot be left to competitive forces (e.g., licences for buildings, oversight of infrastructure, etc). The point to note is that the inherent monopolistic nature of these functions create a fertile environment for arbitrary decisions and corrupt practices that an individual citizen easily monitor or fight.

(b) **Discretionary Power:** The second contributory factor is the discretion that government and its monopolistic public agencies enjoy in their decision-making and allocative roles. If, for example, the rules and criteria are simple and unambiguous, the validity of their decisions and actions can easily be checked by citizens. When multiple criteria are involved and all cases are not alike, use of judgement becomes necessary. But this situation also creates opportunities and incentives for those involved to engage in corrupt practices. Often the decision-makers, their supervisors and clients collude, taking advantage of the freedom to use discretion. Here again, the remedy may not lie in the elimination of discretion, but rather in clarifying and demystifying the decision-making process, disseminating information on rules, specification of criteria, and providing for greater transparency and the right of appeal.

(c) **Lack of Accountability:** The third factor is the relative lack of effective accountability in government except in the nominal sense of presenting annual audited accounts and reports to Parliament or answering questions in Parliament, holding periodic elections, etc. When those who are expected to supervise their subordinates are themselves party to collusion with the latter, the enforcement of accountability becomes extremely difficult. The problem is exacerbated by the difficulties in measuring the performance of the staff and the outcome of their decisions. The lack of proper reporting systems and supervisory controls add to the severity of the problem. Furthermore, accountability is viewed as hierarchical, with little attention paid to the need for accountability towards the customers (citizens) being served.

(d) **Role of Information Barriers:** Fourth, the role of information barriers is another contributory factor to the rise of corruption in India. Corruption involves both givers and takers. In the public sector context, the givers are mostly citizens or other users of services who have limited information about the rules of the game and the standards of service they can expect from public agencies. Service providers may behave opportunistically because they have access to information that citizens do not have. Existing legislation in India contributes to this phenomenon as public agencies are not required to divulge information concerning specific decisions or actions to the public. Citizens, having been brought up in this traditions, are not used to demanding information and often are unaware of their vis-à-vis public agencies and of the remedies available if justice is denied to them. Under these conditions, information barriers tend to create a setting in which the incentives and opportunities for corruption gain strength.

(e) **Episodic exposure of the average citizen to corruption**. Fifth, the exposure of the average citizen to corruption in the public sector tends to be episodic. Everyone does not experience corruption on a daily basis. If a person does not encounter the problem frequently, it is unlikely that he will invest his time and resources in systemic reform. This, indeed, is a major reason why it is difficult to organise effective collective action against corruption.

(f) Other factors causing corruption among public servants are job scarcity, insufficient salary and ever-increasing powers being given to them by the state to regulate its economy and affairs. This increased regulatory authority creates various opportunities for money making as for instance in connection with development planning permits, contracts for construction, granting import-export licenses, collecting customs and other duties and strict accounting for foreign exchange.

All these factors, when taken together, to explain a substantial part of the phenomenon of corruption in India. They no doubt interact with the tolerance to corruption in our society.

REMEDIAL MEASURES—SANTHANAM COMMITTEE REPORT

(a) **Santhanam Committee Report**: The Committee on Prevention of Corruption, popularly known as Santhanam Committee, in its report gave special attention to create a machinery in the government which should provide quick and satisfactory redress of public grievances. For combating corruption among officials, the Committee stated that absolute integrity on the part of Ministers at the Centre and the States is an indispensable condition for establishment of a tradition of purity in public services. It thus gave priority of prevention of political corruption. To tackle the problem of rising corruption among Ministers, the Committee recommended that specific allegations against any of them should be promptly investigated by an agency whose findings would command respect.

(b) **Central Vigilance Commission:** The Central Vigilance Commission was created by an executive resolution of the Union Council of Ministers in 1964 on the basis of the recommendations of Santhanam Committee for dealing with grievances involving corruption and lack of integrity on the part of government servants. It advices the Government on all vigilance matters. It has jurisdiction and powers in respect of all matters in which the executive powers of the Union Government extends. Its role is advisory in nature like that of Union Public Service Commission. A statement outlining the activities of the Central Vigilance Commission during the period of 1996-97 is given in Table II.

Table II. Work done by the CVC during the period of 1996-97

1.	Complaint received*	725
	Action decided	569
2.	Investigation reports	
	(a) Received from CBI*	753
	(b) Advice tendered	439
	(c) Received from CVOs*	2955
	(d) Advice tendered	2055
3.	Reports of inquiries submitted by CBIs	
	Reports submitted*	616
	Advice tendered	509
4.	Major/ minor penalty cases received from	
	CVOs for second-stage advice Received*	1116
	Advice tendered	632
5.	Other advice cases** Received*	858
	Advice tendered	611

* Including cases carried forward from the previous year.

** Includes reconsideration, appeal stage, difference of opinion and other miscellaneous cases.

Source: Government of India, Ministry of Personnel, Public Grievances and Pensions, Annual Report, 1996-97, New Delhi, 1997.

Central Vigilance Commission proved to be an inadequate institutional advice to eradicate corruption. Its performance has remained for from satisfactory and has failed to inculcate a sense of confidence among the citizens that their grievances would be justly and duly remedied.[14]

(c) **Lokpal and Lokayukta:** The Administrative Reforms Commissons (ARC) in 1966 recommended the creation of Lokpal to investigate the alleged cases of political corruption against ministers at the centre. Six attempts were made in the past (i.e. in 1968, 1971, 1977, 1985 and 1989) by successive Governments to enact some kind of Lokpal Bills, but could not become an Act for a variety of reasons. The seventh and latest Lokpal Bill of 1996 is still pending in the Parliament. The new Bill provides for a very weak and inactive Lokpal which may turn out to be a protector of the corruption charged politicians instead of punishing them. In the proposed law, this Lokpal has been made a crippled institution, a toothless tiger and at a later stage a white elephant.[15] The States seem to have done fairly well in this field; legislation pertaining to Lokayuka and Upalokayukta has been adopted in several States. Maharashtra and Orissa were the first two states which adopted Lokayukta Bill in 1971. They were followed by Rajasthan (1973), Bihar (1974), Uttar Pradesh (1975), Madhya Pradesh (1981), Andhra Pradesh and Himachal Pradesh (1983), Assam and Gujarat (1986), Punjab (1995) and Haryana (1997).

ACTION PLAN TO ERADICATE CORRUPTION IN INDIA

A conference of Chief Ministers was held at Delhi on May 24, 1997 to determine action plan for effective and responsive Government. The conference felt the urgent need to tackle corruption and the increasing erosion of moral values in public life. The recommendations which have emerged in this regard has been explained as under:

(a) Elimination of corruption in pubic services should address preventive, surveillance and deterrent punishment, and deal ruthlessly with the nexus of officials with criminal elements and venal political functionaries.

(b) There should be no scope in the rules for any interference in the prompt prosecution and punishment of corrupt public servants, and permissions for such prosecution should be given within a prescribed period to investigating agencies like the CBI where prior approval has been stipulated. At the same time, clear norms should be laid down to prevent the demoralization of public servants on account of frivolous complaint or enquiries.

(c) The investigating agencies and vigilance machinery should be strengthened. It should have adequate staff, powers, resources and independence, accompanied by proper accountability for results. The preventive aspect of corruption in government or the public sector depends on an independent and well staffed vigilance set-up.

(d) Amendments should be enacted to relevant rules on the lines of those proposed in the rules relating to All India and Central Services to provide for the premature retirement of officials at a reasonably early stage of employee careers to weed out elements which are either inefficient or of doubtful integrity. It is further necessary to amend the relevant Service Rules to enable the review of integrity and efficiency of officials at any stage during their career and to provide for the premature retirement of officers to doubtful integrity in the public interest.

(e) Attachment and forfeiture of properties (movable or immovable) acquired by public servants by corrupt or illegal means not only in their own names but also in the names of their relatives and other under their control can be considered, through provisions modelled on the Smugglers and Foreign Exchange Manipulators (Forfeiture of Property Act, 1976); and prompt penal action in respect of proven holding of assets disproportionate to known sources of income.

(f) Areas of discretion available to various levels of administration should be curtailed to the minimum, along with steps to prevent their arbitrary use. Equally urgent are steps for deregulation, procedural simplification, elimination of unnecessary controls, decentralisation and delegation, monitoring of service delivery through citizen groups, greater transparency in all areas of public interface and corruption prone agencies, and the review of the rules and procedures governing procurements, contracts and quotations, as these would bring down the incidence of speed money on the one hand extortions at the decision-making level.

(g) Objective and transparent criteria for the transfer and promotion of officials in order to insulate them from political influence in actions taken according to law and in public interest.

(h) Strengthening the role and powers of Audit in the identification of financial and procedural irregularities to be followed by investigation for possible corruption.

(i) Close networking of different agencies like Lokpal /Lokayukta, CBI/ CVC, Income Tax authorities, Enforcement Directorate and CAG, in terms of sharing information and intelligence, and coordinated investigations.

(j) Encouraging the adoption of Code of Ethics not only by civil servants but public functionaries, media, professionals, and the corporate sector based constitutional principles and moral values.

(k) Assuring adequate remuneration, congenial working conditions and access to housing and health care for the employees.

(l) Mobilising public opinion against corruption, increasing awareness of avenue of complaints and investigation, and supporting efforts of citizen groups and NGOs in this respect.

(m) Encouraging officials at all levels to bring irregularities or suspected corruption to the notice of the Chief Secretary, and to reward such officials in cases where the fraud reported by them are established.[16]

To conclude, corruption has spread its tentacles in almost all spheres of the administration. The rot started with the need and demand of money by politicians at the time of elections. The permit-licence-quota system made industrialists and businessmen vulnerable to the demand of money and the politicians took full advantage of that vulnerability. It is alleged that political corruption has invariably acted as the foster-mother of administrative corruption. When Ministers started amassing money for themselves, it would be unrealistic to think that those in the administration under them would not get afflicted with the same malaise. The result has been that many of those in higher echelons of administration which at one time projected an image of high integrity, have acquired unsavoury reputation. Fighting corruption is not just a question of moral imperative. It is highly practical necessity for a political system to function in a democracy. Though the eradication of this canker is not easy task, it can certainly be minimised by removing public apathy, creating a strong public opinion against it and by bringing about all-round transparency and accountability in administration.

REFERENCES

1. R.B. Jain, "Political and Bureaucratic Corruption in India: Methodology of Promoting Ethical Behaviour among Administrators," *Indian Journal of Public Administration*, Vol XLI. No. 3, Delhi, The Indian Institute of Public Administration, July-Sept 1995, p. 402.
2. LWJC Huberts, "What can be done against public Corruption and Fraud; Expert Views on Strategies to Protect Public Integrity" Paper delivered at the Ethics in Pubic Service Conference, Brisbane, Queensland, Australia, August 5-9, 1996.
3. Royal Commission on Standards of Conduct in Public Life (1974-76) Chairman Lord Salmon, Report, London, HMSO, Cmnd. 6524 July 1976.
4. Ibid., pp. 17-18.
5. LWJC Huberts, n. 2, p. 4.
6. Khushwant Singh, "Are We a Corrupt People?" in Suresh Kohli (ed) *Corruption in India,* Delhi, Chetana Publication, 1975, p. 10.
7. R.B. Jain, "Public Service Ethics: An Indian Perspective" Paper delivered at Ethics in Public Service Conference, Brisbane, Queensland, Australia, August 5-9, 1996, p. 2.
8. Jai Narain, "Political Corruption: Reversal of Gandhian Legacy," *The Tribune.* Chandigarh, June 30, 1996, p.10.
9. Ibid.
10. F. W. Riggs, *Administration in Developing Countries: The Theory of Prismatic Society*, Boston, Houghton, Mifflen, 1964,
11. U.C. Agarwal, "Galloping Corruption: Need for Effective Vigilance", *Indian Journal of Public Administration*, Vol XLIII, No. 3, Delhi, The Institute of Public Administration, July-September, 1997, p. 436.
12. R. B. Jain, n-6, pp. 6-7.

13. Samuel Paul, "Corruption Who will Bell the Cat?" *Economic and Political Weekly*, Vol XXXII, No. 23, Bombay, June 7, 1997, p. 1350.
14. S. S. Tiwana, "Machinery for Redress of Public Grievances in India". *Administration Change*. Vol XXII No. 2, Jaipur, January –June 1995, pp. 155-167.
15. *The Hindu*, February 26, 1997.
16. *Action Plan for Effective and Responsive Government*, Delhi, Ministry of Personnel, Public Grievances and Pensions, 1997, pp. 51-53.

20

CORRUPTION IN CONTEMPORARY INDIA—A SOCIOLOGICAL APPRAISAL

Raj Singh

Dept. of Sociology C.C.S.,
Haryana Agricultural University, Hisar- 125004.

PRELUDE

It is a well established fact now that the most serious problem plaguing the developing societies is corruption. It refers to the abuse of trust in the interest of private gain. Books definition of corruption is the intentional misperformance or neglect of a recognised duty, or the unwarranted exercise of power, with the motive of gaining some advantage more or less directly personal including nepotism. To make the concept more clear corruption is characterized by the following situations; a betrayal of trust; deception of public body, private institution or society at large; deliberate subordinations of common interests to specific interests; secrecy of execution except in situations which allow powerful individuals or those under their protection to dispense with it; involvement of more than one person or party; the presence of mutual obligations and benefits, in pecuniary or other forms; the focusing of action on those who want definite decisions and those who can influence them; the attempt to camouflage the corrupt act by some form of lawful justification; and the expression of a contradictory dual function by those committing the act. It is also a fact that the problem of corruption is trans-systemic; that is, it inheres in all social systems—feudalism, capitalism, communism and socialism. It affects all classes of society; all state organizations, monarchies and republics; all situations, in war and peace; all age groups; both sexes; and all times, ancient, medieval and modern. The study of corruption is like the study of a disease. First we should know the nature of the disease, then its host, next its distribution, causes and conditions, then its effects, and finally its cure. The war and the independence of Asian countries from western rule figure prominently in the growth of corruption. Under colonial rule there was also corruption, but its dynamics and phenomenology took a drastic turn following independence.

K. Santhanam committee noted that the immence war effort 1939-45, which involved an annual expenditure of hundreds of crores of rupees for war supplies and contracts, created unprecedented opportunities for the acquisition of wealth by dubious means. Before the war, according to the Committee's report, corruption was prevalent among low-grade officials but higher ranks were comparatively free from it. Rapid urbanization brought about the weakening of rural values. Social controls which maintained frugality and simplicity of life were replaced by those encouraging materialism, impersonalism, status-seeking, greed for money and power, and an unwillingness to adhere to moral values. In this climate the business and commercial classes, whose ranks were swelled by the speculators and adventures of the war period, exerted their corrupt influence. The salaried classes meanwhile, experienced a decline in real income. The large part of them belonged to the government service and this formed a fertile soil for the growth of corruption. These gave to 'speed money' corruption in the working of government offices.

Dr. S. Radhakrishnam, then President of India said, 'In our country moral life is shaken to its foundations. Love of wealth and power has gained wide acceptance. Most of us live on the surface of life with no moral earnestness. There is hardly any corner of Indian life which has not been defiled by corruption'. Let us start with the temples. A colossal amount of gold and grain were donated to these. Some no doubt was used for maintaining the shrines, providing relief for the poor, assistance for pilgrims and paying the salaries of temple workers. But a good deal was systematically and cynically absorbed. The most outrageous incident was the 'disapperance' of 40,000 acres of land belonging to the Brihadesware temple in Thanjavur, Tamil Nadu. Both Hindu and Moslem religious endowments were eroded by corruption.

The rapid increase of corruption in India has given smugglers and the other criminal gangs a foothold in Indian society. Their illegally earned money is 'launched' into lawful use through legitimate business. They had set up a huge and powerful undertaking which paralleled the government in its area of operation. They had at their disposals fleets of vessels, a counter-intelligence companies and a banking system. But they could not have been carried out without the connivance of influential politicians and bureaucrats. The black marketeers also had an influence on Indian politics. They would join a political party, become office-bearers, and eventually control the party. They fund the parties which did not have independent sources of income. Once entrenched, they would seize any available opportunity to indulge in corrupt practices.

School principals usually favour children of parents who can dispense patronage or favours, as well as those who can pay. In some schools teachers squeeze out gifts from students. The good old practice of giving flowers to the teacher has been replaced by giving a watch, an imported pen, lipstick and even a sari. Admissions are not based on the results of a written test: questions are leaked to certain people the school wishes to oblige, or marks are falsified. The illegal, unreceipted fees vary from 2000 -12000 rupees, depending on the prestige of the school. The situation is no better in higher education. The same state prevails in the courts. According to one advocate's estimate, 95 per cent of the staff in the lower courts are corrupt. One way of bribing a judge is to sell him luxury goods cheaply. In the transportation and building industries corruption finds one of the most fertile soils. Bureaucratic positions favourable to corruption are called 'wet posts'. So, all the forms and manifestations of corruption are beyond description. Corruption is the largest single element to be found most in India. All roads, from maternity hospital to the crematorium, smell of corruption. No individual is free from it, no area can be found where corruption is not a ritual. Baba Virsa Singh stated that there are no leaders, no matter to which side they may belong, who can escape the blame of corruption. They put their energy into obtaining other's women and amassing other's wealth. They are misleading the public.

In a scathing attack on the state of polity Central Vigilance Commissioner N. Vittal in 2001 said, Democracy in India is run by corruption and the corrupt are taking shelter under interpretations of law and constitution. Corruption has taken politics, bureaucracy and business of the country in its grasp. It is a vicious cycle where everybody seems to conforms to the prevalent norms. We have more than Rs. 58000 crore of non-performing assets in the country (T. O. I., 2003). All this forced the President, A.P.J. Abdul Kalam to take an unusual step on the eve of Republic Day (2004) to administer an oath to Children that they will be honest and endeavour to make a corruption-free society.

CAUSES

Corruption took a drastic turn following independence (Alatas, S.H., 1990), mainly due to widespread corruption during the war period preceding the achievement of independence; a sudden increase in bureaucracy; a sudden increase in opportunities for corruption on a bigger and higher scale; the invasion of different levels of leadership by people of low moral integrity; inexperience of leaders fighting for independence in building an incorrupt and efficient government—some were indifferent and lacking in moral integrity; and manipulation and intrigues of foreign financial and business powers through means of corruption. There were also cumbersome and dilatory procedures and practices in the working of government offices which gave rise to 'speed money' corruption. In Asian countries following independence, the leadership was either corrupt or lenient towards corruption, the corrupt elements surface and consolidated their position. Nehru was often taken to task for his permissiveness. The best known instance concerned his friend Khrishna Menon, who committed several irregularities in the so-called Jeep scandal while he was the Indian High Commissioner in London. There are many other instances where Nehru had even been protective of the corrupt politicians. Another cause of corruption was the rapid increase in the number of civil servants, resulting in chronic low pay. This in turn made a second income necessary. The rapid extension of the power and opportunities of the bureaucracy, coupled with the weakness of supervision from top, and the influence of political parties, provided a fertile soil for corruption. Institutional reforms to combat corruption had been tried several times in the past but failure was usually due to the human factor. These factors are significant in understanding the extent and manifestation of the phenomenon, but they are not the terminal point of explanation. They are the starting- point. The terminal point is the nature of man. The 'modernization thesis' of corruption has been articulated among others by Huntington (1968), Myrdal (1968) and Scott (1969). According to Huntington (1968: 59-71), corruption is most prevalent during the most intense phases of modernization of a country and tends to decline with institutionalization of advanced democracy. Myrdal's idea of the soft state point to lacking in discipline which promotes corruption at all levels.

EFFECTS

The effects of corruption on society and the individual are so complex and varied that I shall focus attention only on some of the more conspicuous. Corruption does not only affect man in his economic and political life but also in his psychological and philosophical growth. Philosophically, corruption promotes nihilism and cynicism. It is also nurtured by them. Corruption creates composite problems such as the 'brain drain' of educated people for the developing societies. In such problems corruption is a major constituent and combines with others to form a composite whole. Administrative inefficiency and parasitism are other examples of a composite problem. The losses caused by corruption exceed by far the sum of individual profits derived from it, because graft distorts the whole economy. Important decisions are determined by ulterior motives regardless of consequences to the wider community.

Advancement up the academic career ladder is no longer influenced by research and publication, but by connections with the right people, sycophancy, administrative need, or the sheer ability to crawl up the ladder. Teachers show no interest in their subjects, no intellectual commitment to the cause of education, no inclination to keep abreast of the latest work in their field, no motivation to discuss their subject, no sense of self-esteem. Routine work only is done and with the minimum of effort.

Corruption generates overall inefficiency in the bureaucracy. It is a myth that corruption improves efficiency. The efficiency which is improved concerns the isolated cases of corrupt transactions. The gain accruing to the firm is a loss to the government. The cost of the commodity in question is always inflated. Negligence is caused by corruption also. It is deliberately fostered to serve the interests of corruption. Doctors and nurses in corrupt hospitals deliberately neglect their patients in order to extract bribes. Roads are deliberately neglected in order to increase repair works. Obstruction and neglect are the integral and instrumental components of corruption. So, the catalogue of the effects of corruption in all fields of activity is endless. Corruption affects the productivity of society as well as neglecting people's welfare. Its tendency is to generate further economic difficulty for the society. Myrdal (1968) reported that corruption is one of the forces that help to preserve the, 'soft state' with its low degree of social discipline. Besides being a most objectionable corrupt practice, this custom of speed money has become one of the most serious causes of delay and inefficiency. As a result of corruption, criminals are now even joining politics as they, probably, feel that there is no difference between them and politicians.

REMEDIES

N. Vittal (2001) rightly concluded that corruption cannot be eradicated without curbing political corruption as it starts from top and trickles down to the bottom. However, following suggestions will go a long way in curtailing corruption from our society.

1. Pay special attention to education, especially value education. How else will children learn to discern and discriminate? Getting into IITs and IIMs is fine, but what about making them better human beings? All schools should offer the humanities stream so that life in all its hues is imbibed.
2. Simplify rules and procedures. The more rules there are the more scope for corruption. Red tap has now been replaced by green tape. All kinds of environmental clearances are now needed—all the more scope for corruption.
3. Punish the corrupt. Why should law-breakers get away? The legal system has to get its act together. Discipline yourself, else the world will discipline you.
4. Nothing like a committed media to expose scams. Make the common man aware of the details of corruption to start a movement against it.
5. Dilute the powers of appointing and transferring offices. How about involving the public in selecting important officials. Also have an integrity pact in all government dealings.

6. Enact the Lokpal Bill and see the big fish get caught and brought within the purview of law.
7. The public outcry against corrtruption must be regarded as a constructive force. As those people who can benefit personally from corrupt practices are a tiny minority, the public outcry against corruption should support a government intent on serious reforms.

REFERENCES

1. Alatas, S.H. (1990) Corruption: *Its Nature, Causes and Functions*. Avebury, Hong Kong.
2. Azam, M.A. (1970) *The Anatomy of Corruption*. Dacca, Society for Pakistan Studies.
3. Report of the Committee on the Prevention of Corruption, Ministry of Home Affairs, Government of India, New Delhi, 1964, The Santhanam committee.
4. Myrdal, G. (1968) *Asian Drama–11*, Allen Lane the Penguin Press, London: 937-58.
5. Maholtra, I. Kohli, S. (ed) 1978. *Corruption in India*. Chetana Publications, New Delhi 43.
6. Narendra, K. Singhi, (1974) *Bureaucracy: Positions and Persons*. Abhinav Publications, New Delhi: 205.
7. Monteiro, Johan B. (1966) *Corruption*, Bombay, Manaktalas.
8. Ministry of Information and Broadcasting, Government of India, SADACHAR – Movement for Purity in National Life, New Delhi.
9. Scott, James C., (1972) *Comparative Political Corruption*, Englewood Cliffs, N.J., Prentice – Hall.
10. Pavarala, V. (1996) *Interpreting Corruption –Elite Perspective in India*. Sage Publications, New Delhi.
11. *Times of India* special Correspondent (2004) "Oath for Children by the President, A.P.J. Abdul Kalam on the eve of Republic Day".
12. Vittal, N. (2001) "Democracy by the corrupt, of the corrupt", *Hindustan Times*, New Delhi, August 10, 2001: 13.
13. Vittal, N. (2003) "Corruption Index: Who's Dirty, How Dirty?" *Sunday Times of India*, New Delhi, December 7, 2003: 7.
14. Virsa Singh (2004) "Appeal to Leaders", *Gobind Sadan Times*, New Delhi, January, 2004.

Part - 3

CORRUPTION IN INDIAN POLITICS, ADMINISTRATION AND PUBLIC LIFE

21

CHALLENGES TO EDUCATIONAL SYSTEM TO ELIMINATE CORRUPTION

H.D. Bist

[Ex-Professor and Emeritus Scientist (CSIR), IIT Kanpur],

INTRODUCTION

Education is a critical requisite and a primary weapon for overall economic and social developments of an individual (and hence of society). Education generates awareness of the rights and obligations of an individual towards him and the society. It creates self-confidence and self-respect. It improves opportunities for development of an individual and upgrades his quality of life. Exploitation of individuals or groups in a society is minimized or eliminated. The progress of a country wholly depends on the working capacity and efficiency of its people. Both of these virtues are enhanced by proper training and education. The seeds of appropriate education have to be shown in the very young age through procedures of an all-round development in the (a) Physical, (b) Mental (Intellectual), (c) Emotional and (d) Spiritual (i.e. socio-intellectual) domains. At the right time, these seeds, on receiving proper nourishment from family, friends and environment, have to produce branches, buds, leaves, flowers and fruits; lasting through the lifespan of the individual.

Education polishes an individual to his/her taste and makes him a good professional with optimum capabilities in the field (of this liking) to suit the time and the place. Education, emphasizes on gaining knowledge, skills and attitudes of a general nature. However, education is a wider term that goes beyond the boundaries of any profession or a job. For example, a well known Sanskrit saying is: *Sa Vidya Ya*

Vimuktaye; i.e., knowledge is that which gives liberation (from poverty and backwardness, ego and imperfection etc. leading to Moksha).

Likewise, another Sanskrit saying is:

> *Vidya dadati vinayam, vinayatdyati patratam, Patratwat dhanmapnoti, dhanat dharm tatah sukham;*

> "Knowledge generates humility in a person, which helps him to develop (highly valued, distinctive) personality; the acquired personality helps him to earn money (wealth). Money acquired guides him subsequently to perform 'dharma'; to lead a contented and joyful life."

The emphasis on 'dharma' (duties) may be personal choice. However, it points to the duties to himself, to his family—spouse, father, son, brother, other relatives; to his community and society near him; as a citizen to the village district, state and country; and as a human being to the global mankind. The overall perspective may be different to individuals; but could be identified with the ambient needs and expectations at a particular place and time, with his independent thinking, process and training. The duties towards self include keeping him fit physically using the age-old techniques of Yam, Niyam, Asan and Pranayam. Education throughout life is based on four pillars; (i) 'to know', (ii) 'to do', (iii) 'to live together' and (iv) 'to be'. This was also aimed in our ancient system of education. A balance of Dharm, Arth, Kam and Mokshya concept; with moral, democratic, secular, views was advised for the complete man. The present education system lacks it.

To-day the global value system has to guarantee quality and freedom of individuals on following their religion, training against exploitation, and for opportunities for education and cultural activities. The dissatisfaction of the people will be removed if the economic fruits are distributed uniformly for the human race in the world. The educational aspects have to be strengthened globally to make the persons aware of their rights.

CORRUPTION IN SOCIETY

Corruption in India has been from times immemorial; from Satayug, Treta, Dwapar through Kalayug. The strategy of SAM (love-affection); DAM (money, cost); DAND (punishment) and BHED (division) has been suggested for getting the work done (by any means) and it tells volumes about the corruption in ancient India. In the present day society, corruption has taken the front row and deep roots. It is trying to hinder the progress of humanity. In the words of Elliot and Merrill "Corruption is a willful failure to perform a specified duty in order to receive some direct or indirect personal gains." Alternatively, it could be defined as doing the duty after taking some illegal graft in the form of extra money/time etc.

If we go through the views expressed by various authors in this book/seminar; corruption has been identified with various facets of public activity. A few of the acts of corruption have been defined as: treason; subversion, illegal foreign transactions, smuggling; privatization or misappropriation of public funds; stealing; abuse and misuse of power; underserved pardon and remission; deceit and fraud; cheating and swindling; perversion of justice; false evidence; unlawful detention; non-performance of duties; desertion; cronyism; bribery and graft; extortion; illegal levies; kickbacks; tampering with elections; vote rigging, misuse of inside knowledge and confidential information, manipulation of regulations, purchase and supplies; bias and favoritism in decision-making; tax evasion; excessive profiteering; acceptance of improper gifts and entertainment; illegal surveillance; misuse of mails and telecommunications; improper use of electronics and computers etc. Corruptions have also been elaborated as: autogenic, extortive, coercive, collusive, nepotistic, supportive, etc. Examples have been cited from various historical facts for these types of corruptions. Corruption has penetrated all fields of human activities; e.g. political, educational, medical, religion, police, business, social relations etc. This seepage is observed all around, e.g. in the distinguished offices of Comptroller and Auditor General; Union Public Service Commission, Staff Selection Committee, State Public Service Commission, Attorney General of India etc. In day-to-day life, a Govt. Doctor's refusal to admit a patient unless he is paid extra money, storing away free medicines etc.; a Police Officials-denying to file a FIR unless paid a kick-back; and a teacher's engagement in tutoring at home, for a price, rather than teaching at school; are all examples of corruption in public life. Going through the details of even few the main scams since independence, on could also tell about the causes of corruption in India Few well known scams are: Jain Hawala, HDW submarine, Churhat lottery, Bihar fodder, Bituman, Anantang transport subsidy, JMM, Nagarwala, Sukhram telecom, Urea, Bofors, Tahalka etc. In the Bihar fodder scam: Rs. 253 crores (against a grant of 105 crores) were spent on the purchase of fodder for 959 sheep, 5664 pigs, 40504 hens, and 1577 goats! Two buffaloes were transported from Haryana to Bihar (1000 km) by a two wheeler scooter (as per the Registration Number of the vehicle) to explain the vast amount pilfered from the public exchequer.

Further, the root cause for the increase in the cases of corruption has been the Indian Politics. Present day politicians are surviving as the old system of social structure, based on sub-castes, communes, languages and region, etc exists even today in India. The individualism revamped with favouritism, a nexus among politicians (money, muscle and mafia), bureaucrats, criminals; and constitutional bodies (and even judiciary made for its eradication) to a certain extent have helped this process of seepage of corruption.

Continuing right education at right time could eliminate the menace of corruption from the social structure, in all countries and societies. Hence it should be a challenge, to devise such an educational system to eliminate corruption. Specifying the strict qualifications and training for every job and emphasizing on a religion of future without caste, color, or creed, are few of the suggestions to remove the presently prevalent corruption from public dealings.

TYPICAL CASES

(i) "India Corruption Study-2005" conducted by Transparency International

It has become a fashion to bribe the concerned functionaries (Speed Money) for getting a work done within a specified time. A national survey "India Corruption Study-2005" conducted by Transparency International in 20 states and 151 cities in India, with 14405 samples, was released on July 1, 2005. It saysz citizens pay over Rs 21000 crore a year (2004-5) as bribe. The report summarizes that Bihar emerges as the most corrupt; HP, Gujarat, AP, and Maharashtra as less corrupt; UP stands on 11th place and Kerala is the least corrupt! the corruption is on the rise with respect to 2003-4. The police, the lower courts, the land administration, the government hospitals, and the electricity services have been mentioned in decreasing order of corruption. The public distribution system and water supply figure at the lower end of the corruption chart. The reason for this malaise is the bureaucratic procedures laid down for a file to move, after it is given a shape in the (main) concerned office. A system lacking in efficiency, transparency, and decentralized governance has been made responsible for this state of affairs. We present below the two typical routes that a file is made to follow.

(ii) District Level Office (of DM, say)

In a typical case of getting the verification of the antecedents of an NGO by a district magistrate, an application has to be sent to the main office of the DM. After the DM's consent, and submitting necessary documents to the satisfaction of the PA/officer concerned for dealing the case for accepting the application, the "file" is prepared. The application has to be complete in all respects with requisite information on all the questions itemwise. If the DM agrees or has to do the job as per his duty, he refers the case to his personal assistant or the concerned officers. The next step is to issue the number of letters; as many as may be thought necessary in a case; in this particular case one to SDM of the place for verifying civil aspects and another to SSP for verifying the criminal aspects of the antecedents of the NGO. One has to spend speed-time (or speed-money!) at various tables of the office to (a) prepare the document for the two officers and (b) dispatch to them. The third factor will be (c) the offices of the next level officer's (SDM and SSP). The document has to be delivered to the offices of these next level officers by delivery machinery/mechanism if the machinery is functional on those days. This delivery part, some time, could be overcome by working as a peon of the first office to deliver the letters to the two lower offices (spend speed-time again). The fourth part is the offices of the lower officers, who may or may not receive the document. Even if they receive them, they may keep the documents in their table, unless again you spend speed-time/money to accelerate the process. The setup is such that one has to spend speed time to get the file backwards to the lower rank officers (Tahsildar/Naibtahsildar/Peshkar/Patwari), in that order, in SDM's territory. Likewise in the second (Police) stream, the hurdles of the local Officer's, City officers and offices in the lowest Police/Local Intelligence Unit etc have to be overcome. The verification may not take place unless the concerned person desirous to get the work done presents the documents to the verifying officers of both the streams. After the lowest of the officer prepares the report in each of the two streams, the two reports are independently forwarded via the same route to the highest officer. The final report is prepared in the office of the highest officer, taking cognizance of the two independent streams of verification, by a person conversant with the verification process and is forwarded to the office of the ADM of the place. After final verification of the requisite certificate along with the prepared forwarding letter, the DM may issue the certificate. His office may forward the document to the office of (say) State (Dehradoon) in UA or Central Govt. (New Delhi). If the file is followed at each step, it may take time from 2 weeks to six months! Sometimes it may be lost in one of the various offices visited by the file.

(iii) Central Govt. Office (Secretary for a particular task) at New Delhi

Another typical case could be cited for the file received in the receipt unit of a Central Govt. office from the office of a DM in one of the districts of Indian Union. Normally the letters addressed to a Secretary for a particular task are received by his office and then sent to the under-secretary of the Department, following a set route. The letters may not be opened for weeks or months for very genuine reasons provided to anybody concerned with the result. The office staff being one leave in various desks (or now computers being out of order), could be given as a very convincing reason. Another reason for not getting attention could be given as the office being moved from one location to another. Even if the letters have been opened, they may not get filed properly for further processing. After filing is completed, the path of greatest downward resistance is offered to the file through the desks of the Section Officer, dealing clerk and the like. The dealing clerk has to prepare a file and put it before the section officer. Now it takes the forward route, if it reaches the office/desk of the Under-Secretary. The Deputy Secretary in charge takes the decision and then it is signed by the Joint Secretary of the Department giving approval or otherwise! The final decision will be communicated to the concerned person (after it follows the downward path) through the Dy. Secretary or under-secretary as per decision of division of tasks in the office. The file needs speed-time or speed-money from the concerned person to get the job done in most of the offices. If the concerned officer in any desk is on leave, the file may not see the light of the day for any action. In this regard the office of the passport officers is now more efficient, as the time limit has been imposed for issuance of the document, after its receipt in the office.

The way out from this situation faced by the general public is to make the desk officer responsible to clear the file in a day or two and forward it to the next one. The transparency in the task will demand that each note by a desk is transmitted to the person concerned for his modification, if needed! The need of the speed money or time should vanish, if transparency and efficiency are maintained by each office and its desks. Additionally one does not need the long chain of offices and officers for dealing a problem. One dealing assistant should be responsible for one type of tasks to be done, and may take the help of the one office at the most.

The reason for combining time and money together is the experience that a right task will be done by the offices without charging any money, as is the experience of many persons. However the time has to be spent in every office, if one desires the task to be done with some speed. The time (86400 sec per day at the possession of every individual) is the most valuable (more than money) thing. "Yesterday is history, tomorrow is mystery and today is a gift and present it is called" is a citation that everybody has to be taught in govt. offices. One should get utmost benefit in health, success and wealth by investing the time of the present day. There should be no room for investing the valuable time (and money) in getting petty things done through the offices. Finally again, the onus of keeping delivery agencies on their toes, lies on the enlightened public.

(iv) Changing Scenario

Nine states have enacted right to information laws, which has culminated in the "Right to Information Act at the Center". The central law and the state laws prescribe punitive action against officers who fail to disclose information within a specified period. The law needs political and social processes to empower citizens and communities. Present scenario, where the Ministers are like "feudal Kings" and bureaucrats like their "Courtiers" has to change. Swindling of development budget by a nexus between them, without any development task performed, has to change. The education of the masses of their rights and obligations and limiting contracts (till the retirement age of 60/62 years) of Government employees, and fixing accountability at each desk and office, will go a long way after Politicians are also educated and punished for amassing wealth.

POLITICAL CONSTRAINTS AND SHORT TERM INDIVIDUALISM

Political corruption has affected all aspects of our life and systems. The state and central governments appoint pliable officers to important posts. Today a large number of civil servants and IAS officers are politicized. The bureaucratic corruption, results in lack of accountability, mis-governance, and inefficiency. Today, it is almost impossible for a civil servant to function outside the political system. Hence the political system should first be cleansed; the bureaucracy will follow suit.

In India the present day politics is governed by various short-sighted elements; Casteism and Communalism etc. Corruption is supported further by Linguism, Regionalism and Terrorism, and is fortified by desire of individuals for power; and attainment of quick unlimited wealth. Today, it seems that political domination has changed the social behaviour of the general residents of the 21st century; especially so in the developing third world countries. The politicians, who become MLA, MLC or MP, may have no qualification to work as law-makers of the country, but would like to be elected to these posts, by hook or by crook. For this they may have to spend a vast amount of money, gained through unethical means. Additionally, they may have to use unlawful force and methods to get elected. Some of these individuals of dubious character, are installed to the post of Ministers and Heads of states, under compelling circumstances. No wonder if they use unethical means to get elected/selected to these posts; and subsequently, continue to misuse their positions for personal benefits and amassing of personal wealth.

21st century is striving hard for the development of highest technological and informative skills. The entire world has become a global village. It is essential to impart right education to the world citizen, especially to those affecting the lives of the entire country (or even the world). Hence the political constraints and the short term individualism should be removed by imparting right type of education to these persons; emphasizing a blend of global, modern scientific temper and with human values and emotional-intellectual social components.

TOP HIERARCHY POLITICIANS AND PUBLIC SERVANTS

The youth and the public are the blood streams for health and survival of any society. It is evident that only few persons could be the public representatives of people at various levels. The entrance tests, subsequent training and evaluation processes are important for maintaining the quality in any social structure. The selection process of candidates for various posts in public life has to be categorized accordingly. The first category needs brilliant people possessing the fast track inherent exceptional capabilities of originality, creativity, innovation, integration, imagination and dreaming. This task has to be done by the country-level politicians and (bureaucrats). The second category consists of the hard working people, having above average potentiality, interest and dedication to do corresponding jobs at state level. The third category should be for handling most of the jobs needed by the contemporary society at the district level. The forth category people should be for the village level developmental tasks. Some infrastructure for training the bureaucrats exists in the country. It is high time that the country should create institutions also for training top class politicians. The grinding of the four categories of people in these institutions with high level of public consciousness and moral, ethical values may turn the table in public polity and governance.

PROFESSIONAL EDUCATION AND TRAINING OF TOP VIPs

Professional education is a personalized training of individuals by specialized methods to develop attitude, aptitude, talent, basic skills, knowledge and behavioral pattern to perform adequately a given job or task; both the theoretical knowledge and the practical training being an essential part of the exercise. Professional education is essential as it gives perfection in the trade. The doctors (medical); engineers (engineering branches), lawyers (law), businessman (commerce), scientists, IT personal etc, all need perfection; and hence proper training for the jobs. Its role in the learning society has been summarized by

M. Yorke[2] in the context of assuring quality and standards in global higher education. The term learning-society (which has capabilities to read, analyze, adapt-to, act on, and interact with the environment) has been borrowed from learning-organization. This term emphasizes the essential needs for a society, if it does not want to suffer a decline. Professional and higher education have to advance with time and continually adapt to the ever changing and galloping developments in scientific, technological and societal innovations.[2] All Institutions have to devise a system of education to imbibe honesty, integrity and ethics in the individuals.

It is sad that there is no qualification for being a public representative and law maker (i.e. for MLA's and MP's etc.) even today. It is strongly recommended that there should be basic qualifications of education and honesty and training for public position holders in the country. Additionally, there should be special institutions for continuous updating of the training of the top hierarchy politicians and bureaucrats in top ranking institutions established for the specific task. Moral education should be a part of this training, emphasizing the ultimate goal of life; as explained in the book edited by Gupta and Bist.[3] Acquisition of this type of Professional Education at the top hierarchy will definitely help in eradicating corruption.

ORIENTATION SEMINARS FOR TOP HIERARCHY

It should be amply clear that the Prime Minister, the President in the country and the Chief Ministers and Governors in the states in India (and the other Council of Ministers and the other administrative staff associated with them) have the most important roles to play in Elimination of Corruption (EoC) in the States and Union territories in India. For EoC under various situations, they should also undergo some sort of critical management program for facing issues, planning budget, human resource development with an effective leadership. The programs should be devised to help the top administration to increase their capabilities and to adapt them to the ever changing needs of the youth and society, by developing effective strategies within the marked areas of duties and responsibilities. In USA, the incumbent President and his team, works and prepares for ~6 months with the outgoing team-mates. The new team is to be familiarized with the weaknesses, strengths and opportunities lying for them; and threats that are likely to be faced by them in their new job. Thus the newly appointed Heads of various sectors will go well prepared and with confidence to discharge the responsibilities and mandate of their new office. The other officials of the top administration in the country should also undergo continuing training programs organized for them to pave their path for better management. These types of professional training programs on a continuous basis provide a mentoring and an insight for the better governance. They also offer opportunities to numerous people, having identical interests and sharing similar talents and dreams for close interaction. Peers guide each other through difficult decisions and quandaries. Most successful people from various fields should be invited as resource persons, to participate in these Seminars to share their experiences. The process of good hiring and evaluating practices for term work and commitments of the participating officers could also be discussed in these seminars. These measures will definitely help to curb the menace of corruption in the country.

THE GOVERNORS IN THE STATES

Recent incidences of governors decisions in Goa, Jharkhand and Bihar (in May 2005) have pointed out that the office of the Governor has been reduced to the level of an agency which is set up in the states to execute the will of the political bosses in New Delhi at any instant of time. The Governors are thus causing trouble and constitutional embarrassment; instead of "protecting and defending the Constitution and the law of the land." these posts should be without political interference and persons chosen with due procedure of selection should be of highest caliber and track record in their field of attainment. The governors are the first (top) persons in the state. They could contribute significantly for elimination of corruption in the state of Indian union.

ERADICATING CORRUPTION

The public is the ultimate customer in the developmental processes. Hence, the saying that "Beauty lies in the eyes of the beholder" could be translated as "Corruption lies in the eyes of the (public) customer". Likewise the saying "Yatha raja tatha Praja" has to be changed as "Yatha Praja tatha Raja". Hence the significance of general public to detect, evaluate, quantify and assess the corruption cases is a very important factor for judging the benefits of developmental efforts. Equally important factors are the law makers (MP's etc.), the government bureaucrats and other participants in the Governance. Preparation of politicians, administrators, and the general public in society through a superior educational system, bringing out excellence, to root out corruption, is essential.

COLLECTIVE CONCERN TO CHECK CORRUPTION

Serious efforts by both the government (by improving the existing acts continuously) and the general public by showing concern (without showing helplessness or apathy) have to be made, simultaneously. Teaching of morals and character-building in the children, youth and officers has already been emphasized. Electoral reforms deregulation and privatization, decentralized governance with transparency and accountability may help in reducing the corruption. Promotional aspects involve in giving an encouragement to respect and compliance of laws. Inculcating a culture of value-based politics and administration will be immensely helpful. Strengthen the laws for punitive steps and rules to quickly detect and pursue the cases would also be supportive for checking corruption. A deterrent for corruption would also be a harder punishment for corrupt practices of various kinds through good education.[5]

RELIGION FOR GLOBAL VILLAGE THROUGH A UNIVERSAL EDUCATIONAL SYSTEM

Noble laurate Albert Einstein has written regarding the future religion as follows: "The religion of the future will be cosmic religion-based on experience and free of dogma." It is becoming increasingly clear that strength lies in unity. The age-old dogmas of religion, region, caste, language etc. are so intertwoven with the human emotions, that it may be difficult to get these value systems out of the global societal structure. However, efforts could definitely be made through proper system of education to develop more broader views in the minds of young generation to leave the narrow sectarian views. A balanced blending of the social value system from different faiths, by generating a scientific temper in the young generation, through future educational system has to be essentially inculcated. An intellectual and emotional environment has to be developed in the complex heterogenous structure prevalent today. The common good teachings from all world religious groups—Hindus, Buddhist, Christians,

Muslims, Sikhs, Jains, Suphis, Jewish, etc. should be introduced in the (global village) education system and future religion of mankind. The narrow dogmas and small differences should be shelved permanently in the back drawer not to be opened in future. This will be the only way to develop the world society (and humanity) on sound ethical background.

In good old times in India, the Gurukuls taught equality of mankind as a whole with the aim to make a man; "Manurbhav". At that time it was taught that the world was like a vast family "Vasudhaiva Kutumbakam". This enlightenment and consciousness brought an attitudinal change in human thinking and feelings. The inner illumination (with profound knowledge and universal love) is for unfailing health, vitality, happiness; and the outer illumination automatically brings respectful prosperous life. In the words of poet Tulsidas:

"Jimi sarita sagar mamun Jahin, Jaddapi tahi kamana nahin Timisukh sampati binahi bolaye, Dharam-seel pahi jahi subhaye"

(Happiness and property flows to a developed and balanced personality; like the water from the rivers flows to ocean; even though the ocean does not aspire for it.)

QUOTABLE QUOTES

We will present few quotations on education and corruption in the text given below; as we think it will be instructive to have the views of the past and present luminaries of the world on significance of these topics:

On Education

"Democracy depends for its very life on a high standard of general, vocational and professional education."

— S Radhakrishnan.

"Man is neither mere intellect, nor gross animal body, nor the heart or the soul alone. A proper and harmonious combination of all the three is required for the making of the whole man and constitutes the true economics of education."

— Mahatma Gandhi

"While computers have IQ (Intelligence Quotient), and animals have EQ (Emotional Quotient), it is SQ (Spiritual quotient)

that sets humans apart. SQ isn't necessarily connected to religion, although it can be. It is about wholeness, flexibility, self awareness, compassion, creativity, the ability to ask why, and the like."

— D. Zohar and I. Marshal

"A university stands for humanism, for tolerance, for reason, for the adventure of ideas, and for the search of truth. It stands for the onward march of the human race toward higher objectives. Universities are places of ideals and idealism. If the universities discharge their duties adequately, then, it is well with the nation and the people."

— Jawaharlal Nehru

"The past is our foundation, the present our material, the future our aim and summit. Each must have its due and natural place in a national system of education".

— Sri Aurobindo

"The highest education is that which does not merely give us information but makes our life in harmony with all existence."

— Rabindra Nath Tagore

"The deepest sources of all calamities in history is ignorance, for where we do not understand, we can never be just."

— Rabindra Nath Tagore

"When the lights are gone in the universities, they are not likely to burn long in churches, in industry, press or state,"

— Peter H Odegard

"If you are planning for one year, plant rice;

If you are planning for 5 years; plant trees,

If you are planning for future; educate your children."

— An old Chinese saying

On Corruption

"Just as it is impossible not to taste honey or poison that finds itself at the tip of the tongue, so also it is impossible for a government servant not to eat up at least a bit of the government

revenue. A fish moving under water cannot possibly be found out whether drinking water or not. Likewise, government servants cannot be found out [while] taking money [for themselves]. It is possible to mark the movements of birds flying high up in the sky; but it is impossible to ascertain the movement of Government servants for his hidden purpose."

— Arthashastra of Chanakya

"It is essential that the three pillars of democracy—legislature, executive and judiciary—are strong in structure, pure in form and uncorrupted and unblemished in conduct."

— APJ Abdul Kalam,

"For every rupee spent by government for poverty alleviation, only fifteen paise is reaching the beneficiary, another forty paise may be spent on administrative overheads and the remaining forty five paise lost in corruption."

— Rajiv Gandhi

"Corruption is a behavior which deviates from the formal duties, of a public role because of private, (personal, close family, private clique) pecuniary or status gain."

— Huntington

"It is an illegal payment to a public agent to obtain a benefit that may or may not be deserved in the absence of pay-offs."

— Susan Rose-Ackerman

"Corruption occurs when a function, whether official or private, requires the allocation of benefits or the provision of good or service. In all cases, a position of trust is being exploited to realize private gains beyond what the position holder is entitled to."

— World Bank

"Corruption = Monopoly + ***Discretion*** *— Accountability"*

— Robert Klitgoard

REFERENCES

1 M. Yorke; Assuring quality and standards in globalised higher education, *Quality Assurance in Higher Education*, 7, 14-24, 1999.

2. H.D. Bist and S. Bhargava; *Lasers and Their Applications—The Indian Spectrum for 2001 AD*; Tata MC Graw-Hill Publishing Company Ltd, New Delhi, (1996).

3. R.K. Gupta and H.D. Bist, *Higher Education, Challenges for the Future*, Anamika Publishers, New Delhi, 2005.

4. A Stella and A Gnanam, *Assessment and Accreditation in Indian Higher Education: Issues of Policy and Prospects*; Books Plus Pub. New Delhi (2001).

22

CORRUPTION IN INDIAN POLITICS: AN OVERVIEW

Jagbir S. Narwal and Ranbir S. Gulia

Deptt. of Public Administration, M.D. University, Rohtak

&

Deptt. of Political Science, M.D. University, Rohtak

There are many challenges to Indian politics such as communalism, regionalism, casteism, terrorism, corruption, linguism etc. putting over the democracy at stake. Corruption is the most serious threat riding into the rank and file of our system. The canker of corruption is eating into the vitals of our polity and spreading like cancer in the body politics, making its defence mechanism hollow. It is a cause of immense concern not only for the intellectuals and the media, but also for the high officials of the country.

The gravity of problem can be understood from the speeches of the President and Prime Minister delivered on the various occasions to fight the demon of corruption. While addressing a conference of Governor's Mr. K.R. Narayanan the former President of India indicated the rising nexus among politicians, bureaucrats and criminals and advised them to use their constitutional power and influence against it. His views were fully endorsed by the Vohra Committee report. At the time of golden jubilee of the Election Commission on January 17, 2001, he further expressed deep concern about increasing role of money, muscle and mafia in our election.[1]

Corruption exists in various forms in different parts of governmental machinery. It has tightened its grip not only on legislature and bureaucracy, but also has taken judiciary into its clutches. Even the constitutional body like Comptroller and Auditor General, Union Public

Service Commission, Staff Selection Commission, State Public Service Commissions, Attorney General etc. cannot claim to be above board. Corruption is not a new phenomenon, way back in 200 B.C. Kautilya meticulously described forty (40) different types of corruption in the *Arthashastra*. He has highly remarked:

"Just as it is impossible not to taste honey or poison when it is at the tip of the tongue, so also it is impossible for a minister or a government servant not to eat up a bit of government revenue. And just as it cannot be found out whether a fish swimming through water drinks or not, so also government servants cannot be found out while taking money for themselves."[2]

CONCEPTUAL FRAMEWORK

Like all other social phenomena "Corruption" is too complex to be defined. The *Oxford Advanced Learners Dictionary* defines it as being immoral, dishonest or depraved.[3] In everyday life, it stands for the misuse of authority by a civil servant to obtain an extra income from the public.[4] Broadly speaking, corruption refers to perversion of power, or the violation of a country's legal system,[5] the destruction or perversion of the integrity or fidelity of a person in his discharge of public duties. Thus corruption can be defined as moral depravity, misuse of one's official position for his personal gain or for the benefit of his nears and dears, etc. at the cost of the public. But the term 'Political Corruption' is a narrower one and refers to misuse of public power by political office holders for private profit.[6] Interference of wealth in the political arena for protecting and promoting personal interests of political power wielder, begets deviant behaviour. When such behaviour deviates from the normal duties of a public role and influenced by a particular motive, namely that of private gain at the cost of public interest, political corruption tends to develop. To be very concrete, it refers to 'official misconduct'[7] of the politicians, a kind of behaviour which deviates from the norms actually prevailing or believed to prevail in a given context, such as political.

In general, it is illegal or improper use of political power for securing pecuniary or other advantages directly or indirectly for oneself or for those in whom one is interested. To put it more tersely, it is trade of public interest for private gain. In countries like India, Pakistan, Indonesia, Bangladesh, Philippines, Yugoslavia and other third world countries corruption affects every walk of life. In the entire developing region of Asia, Singapore is the only government that is more or less free from corruption. China has curbed it with heavy hand, while the daily holds of the public can still be obtained without bribery in Malaysia. But it has become rampant in India and reached disconcerting levels, particularly after independence. It flourishes as luxuriantly as the bush and weeds which take away the goodness from the soil and suffocate the growth of plants which have been carefully and expensively bred and tended.[8]

FORMS OF CORRUPTION

The forms and dimension of corruption are constantly changing with the exposure of new deals in corrupt practices day by day. Bribe, patronage, nepotism, favouritism, misappropriation, transfers and appointments of officials at lucrative posts, procuring goods or services at rates higher than those prevailing in market with a view to getting commission, forming baseless and unprincipled conditions, trying to get cheap popularity at the cost of State exchequer including, installing statues of their political mentors enmasses and forming trust on their names and getting forcible donation of real estate to it, misuse of governmental machinery, not paying dues of IAF aircraft and illegal occupation of government accommodations etc. are some of the manifested form of corruption. Broadly it can be divided into six types—transactive, extortive, defensive, inventive, nepotistic and facilitative.

1. Transactive type infers to the mutual arrangement between donor and recipient to the advantage of and actively pursued by both parties at the public cost. It normally involves businessmen and government. This can be in the form of granting licences, permit, quotas etc.
2. Extortive type is the kind where the donor is compelled to bribe in order to avoid norm being inflicted upon his person, his interest, or upon those persons or things dear to him.
3. Defensive corruption is the behaviour of the victim of extortive corruption. His corruption is in self defence.
4. Investive corruption involves the offer of goods or services without any direct link to a particular favour but in anticipation

of future occasions when the favour will be required. This system of patronage has become an integral part of Indian politics.

5. Nepotistic corruption is the unjustified appointment of relatives or friends on public office, or according them favoured treatment, in pecuniary or other forms, violating the norms and rule of the organisation.
6. Facilitative or speed money corruption originates where procedures and practices in public office are cumbersome and dilatory. Here the bribe giver does not want to get anything unlawful, but wants to speed up the process of decision-making.

CORRUPTION: A RELOOK

Corruption is an age-old phenomenon, a deep-rooted evil and a universal malady. According to Ralsh Braibanti, government corruption is found in all bureaucracy, in all periods of political development though it varies in degree.[9] It is more common in some societies than in others and at one time than others in the evolution of a society. It was wide spread in western countries in ancient and medieval times. Though India was not an exception, but the extent of evil was certainly for less than what it is today.

The corruption in India in its present form, is a legacy of British rule or a progeny of colonialism. It became active in Indian Polity with the implementation of provincial autonomy in 1937. That's why Mahatma Gandhi expressed disappointment on the moral decline of Congressmen and stated that it seems that we have become too weak internally. I will not hesitate to bury the whole Congress organisation but not ready to live with corruption.[10] The Second World War provided a hope for freedom on one side and gave opportunity for flourishing corruption on the other. Corruption become a lucrative business in post-World War situations and developed as an institution of contractualism among middle and lower level leaders, zamindars and fueds. Corruption breeds corruption. When it sets in, it grows like weeds. It penetrated and overpowered the higher ranks of administration even before Independence. That's why Dr. S. Radha Krishanan warned Jawahar Lal Nehru against this evil and Nehru publically announced that people found indulging in corrupt practices will be hanged to electric poles.[11]

As far as Nehru was concerned he was particularly keen to keep his hands clean in money matters, but he did not object to others dirtying their hands to raise funds for the Congress party or causes in which he was interested. That's why he not only ignored but also helped the politicians who were very close to him in matters of financial improprieties. Whether the case may be of T. Prakash who formed a Ministry in Madras in 1946 and was charged of collecting a lot of money and proved by the investigating committee consisting of Nehru, Patel and Rajender Prasad, but was exonerated on the ground that persons concerned were no longer ministers.[12] Within a short period another case of corruption cropped up in 1948. It was V.K. Krishna Menon, the then High Commissioner in London, involved in many financial irregularities including the Jeep scandal. Though, in the beginning, Nehru defended him saying that 'the only thing scandalous about the Jeep scandal is the use of the word scandal, yet when the inquiry was made by a Parliamentary Committee (1951)[13], he was found guilty and therefore, a judicial enquiry was recommended. But the Prime Minister was very keen to protect him, hence all the charges of corruption against Menon were dropped and further appointed him a minister without portfolio on February 3, 1956.[14] After sometimes he was made the Defence Minister.

T.T. Krishnamachari, the then Financial Minister was found to have indulged in corruption by Chagla Commission of Inquiry in Mundhra affairs. As a result, T.T.K. had to resign in 1958, but after a brief political exile, he was again inducted in the Union Cabinet by Nehru in 1962.[15] As Nehru had to eat a humble pie in TTK case, hence when charges of corruption were levelled against K.D. Malaviya, Minister for Mines and Fuel, the matter was referred to C.K. Daphtary, the then Attorney General instead of appointing a Commission of Inquiry. Ultimately Malaviya had to resign on adverse remarks from Justice Das, yet Nehru said, "I am not personally convinced that Malaviya has done anything which casts a reflection on his impartiality and integrity."[16] He also refused to make the report public and Malaviya was appointed minister after a short exile. Similar was the case of Partap Singh Kairon, Chief Minister of Punjab (1958-65) when charges of corruption were levelled against him and member of his family for amassing wealth. This was acknowledged by Shriman Narayan, General Secretary of Congress Party in his enquiry but Kairon was exonerated from the charges of corruption. Nehru in a Press

Conference in June, 1958 called these charges as 'fantastic, frivolous and absured as there was no evidence at all, not the faintest and slightest shadow of it. Kairon is a leader of masses, living simple life and dedicated to the service of the people.[17] Meanwhile the Supreme Court passed strictures against Kairon in Pratap Singh case on September 2, 1963. Nehru tried to minimize the gravity of charges and after great reluctance, had to appoint Das Commission of Inquiry on November 1, 1963. The Commission found Kairon to have indulged in corruption but this happened after the death of Nehru. Thus Nehru though himself absolutely honest, tried often to shield his trusted lieutenants and hence corruption started crawling from top to bottom.

The approach of Lal Bahadur Shastri towards political corruption was not very different from that of Nehru. He also shielded corruption in the interest of party. In Kairon case, he was reluctant to make the report of Das Commission public and did so only when Kairon refused to resign on the basis of report, to force him to resign. Similarly in the case of Biren Mitra, the then Chief Minister of Orissa and Biju Patnaik, Ex-Chief Minister Shastriji referred the matter to a sub-committee of Union Cabinet, instead of appointing a regular Commission of Inquiry. Even after the approval of allegations, the matter was hushed up by Shastriji under the pressure of the Syndicate on the ground that Chief Minister has resigned.[18] However, it is noteworthy that Khanna Commission of Inquiry appointed by Singh Deo, the then Chief Minister of Orissa, on October 26, 1967 indicated Biju Patnaik, Biren Mitra, S. Tripatha, all ex-Chief Ministers and Nitamani Routray, ex-Deputy Chief Minister for indulging in corruption. Similar attitude was adopted by Shastriji in case of K.B. Sahay, the then Chief Minister of Bihar and his colleagues' case in 1965, when the matter of corruption charges were given to a Sub-Committee of party, which gave them a clean chit. But latter on, they were indicted by Aiyer Commission of Inquiry.[19] Shastriji again shielded corruption in case of T.T. Krishnamachari in 1965 when no Commission of Inquiry was appointed and the matter was hushed up on his resignation. Corruption got an up-boost and recognition when Shastriji stated that 'Congress is a large party and it has to field its candidates throughout the country for election. It requires a lot of money, which they have to take from various firms in the form of donation. Santnan Committee (1964) also noted that corruption has spread in those levels of administration, where its influence was not observed earlier.[20]

Mrs. Indira Gandhi not only followed the footsteps of her predecessors but also established new record of corruption during her tenures from 1966-77 and 1980-84. Charges of corruption were levelled against L.N. Mishra[21] in the Pondicherry Licence Scandal Case, Sanjay Gandhi, Devraj Urs[22]; Vengal Rao, D.P. Mishra, Parkash Singh Badal, M. Karunanidhi, the then Chief Ministers of Karnataka, Andhra Pradesh, Madhya Pradesh, Punjab and Tamil Nadu, in that order. Except Badal and Karunanidhi all other belonged to the Congress Party, hence she refused to appoint any Commission of Inquiry against them. But she was quick in appointing such commissions whenever a non-Congress Chief Minister was involved i.e. in case of Prakash Singh Badal[23] and M. Karunanidhi.[24] In both the cases, the Commission found the charges of corruption as substantially true; same was the fate of Congress Chief Ministers and above mentioned leaders except Vengal Rao, when Commission of Inquiries were appointed against them by the United Front (1967-71) and the Janata Party Government (1977-79).[25] Gupta Commission indicted Sanjay Gandhi on the Maruti Project for his various acts of omission and commission. The Commission also indicted Bansi Lal, N.D. Tiwari, Herdio Joshi, S.C. Shukla and Giani Zail Singh, the then Chief Ministers of Haryana, U.P., Rajasthan, Madhya Pradesh and Punjab respectively.[26] Similar was the attitude of Smt. Gandhi in A.R. Antulay and Gundu Rao case both Congress Chief Ministers of Maharashtra and Karnataka respectively. She defended corruption by saying that it is worldwide phenomena. However, in the Spirit scandal in which some of the non-Congress Minister of Tamil Nadu and Kerala were involved; she immediately appointed a Commission by the State Government.[27] It is interesting to note that the report of Shah Commission which indicted Mrs. Gandhi for declaring emergency and committing excesses therein and also of Gupta Commission which exposed the irregularities committed by Sanjay Gandhi in Maruti Project, were rejected by the Cabinet headed by Mrs. Gandhi.[28]

The approach of Morarji Desai towards political corruption was not much different from that of Mrs. Gandhi. He too was very quick in appointing various Commission of Inquiry against Congressmen but was reluctant to appoint against Kanti Desai, his son, Padma Desai, his daughter-in-law and Mrs. Gayatri Devi, wife of Charan Singh, the then Home Minister when allegation of corruption were levelled against them. He resisted to appoint the commission even after passing a resolution by Rajya Sabha by 164 votes to 78 in its favour. When the Congress Party blocked the proceedings in Rajya Sabha, Desai agreed to appoint justice C.A. Vaidyalingam for finding out whether there was a prima facie case or not.[29] When the Commission held that there was a prima facie case for proper inquiry, he described the report as cock and bull story.[30] However, Charan Singh asked the government to send the case of his wife to the special court. Thus, all the Prime Ministers except Charan Singh dragged their feet behind in appointing Commission of Inquiry when their own kith and kin or lieutenants were involved.

SECOND PHASE

In the second phase, the charges of corruption were levelled against Prime Minister themselves besides various Chief Ministers and ministers. Rajiv Gandhi, who was considered Mr. Clean, was alleged to be involved in the Bofors Gun and Submarine deals and appointment of fair fax against FERA violations. Similarly the involvement of Ram Lal's sons in Tanta timber smuggling, J.B. Patnaik in the mustardrid deal, P.C. Sethi in the Kua oil deal, J.N. Mishra in Patna Co-operative bank scandal, Moti Lal Vohra in Raipur Land deal, indictment of N.T. Rama Rao by Andhra Pradesh High Court in respect of certain charges of corruption and filing of F.I.R. against Hiteshwar Sakia, dismissal of Nerbahadur Bhandari by Governor were some of the notable incident of corruption committed by then Chief Ministers of various states.[31] The cases of corruption against ministers and legislators were countless. The terrible face of corruption reflected in Rajiv Gandhi's statement, "Only 15 paise out of 1 rupee granted, reach to the actually headed and 85 paise will remain in bottleneck". But no concrete step was taken by him to counter it except making some emotional speeches.

Corruption touches new heights in the regime of P.V. Narsimha Rao (1991-96). Securities scam by Harshad Mehta (1993), JMM bribery case (1993) and horse-trading of MPs to save Rao's minority government, St. Kitts forgery case (1993) etc. was among the major scandals in which the Prime Minister himself was found indulged.[32] Even in the former two cases, Rao was punished by the CBI designate court in its historical decision in September, 2000. It was the first incident of this type in which a former Prime Minister was sentenced.

The other politicians involved in JMM bribery case were Buta Singh, Satish Sharma, Bhajan Lal. R.K. Dhawan, Ajit Singh, V.C. Shukla etc. The Chief Ministers alleged to be involved in corruption during this period were J. Jayalalitha, the C.M. of Tamil Nadu. Tansi Land Scandal, Coal import case, Pleasant Stay Hotel Case, Sari Scam and amassing wealth by impropriation and Laloo Prasad Yadav, the then Chief Minister in Fodder Scam. In Urea Scam (1994), involvement of Prabhakar Rao son of former Prime Minister Narsimha Rao and Hawala Scandal (1996) in which eminent leaders of all political parties including L.K. Advani, Arjun Singh, Motil Lal Vohra, Sharad Yadav, Balram Jakhar, Jagan Nath Mishra, Madan Lal Khurana, Madhav Rao Scindia etc. were alleged to be involved.

Keeping in consideration the rising trends of corruption, the Central Government directed the Central Vigilance Commission (CVC) to probe into the allegations of the involvement of middlemen in all identified major defence deals of more than Rs. 75 crore since 1985. The CVC N. Vittal admitted the existence of middlemen in most of the above stated deals.[33] Ajit Jogi, former Chief Minister of Chattisgarh, alleged the involvement of Prime Minister Office and Arun Shoorie former, Disinvestments Minister in Rs. 100 crore bribery while setting 51 per cent of the shares of Bharat Aluminium Corporation 'BALCO' to a private company 'Sterlite' of Anil Aggarwal in mere Rs. 551.5 crore, though it was giving profit regularly.[34] Defence scandal is the latest in this series exposed by 'Tehlaka.com' in which Bangaru Laxman, the then President of BJP, Mrs. Jaya Jaitly, President of Samata Party, top official of Prime Minister Office and Defence Ministry were shown taking bribe in videotapes from West End International a non-existent London based firm for facilitating defence deals.[35] The issue rocked into the Parliament and opposition demanded resignation of government. There was a split in NDA when Mamta Banerjee and her party minister Ajit Panja resigned in protest against Defence Minister George Fernandes still holding the office, which ultimately resulted in his resignation.[36] The government appointed a Commission of Inquiry to investigate into the matter headed by Justice K. Venkataswamy, who later resigned in protest. Now Justice S.N. Phuken is heading this commission. Meanwhile, George Fernandes was reinstated in Union Cabinet. Thus the number and gravity of corruption is touching the highest level day by day.

CAUSES OF CORRUPTION

It is not difficult to locate the causes of corruption. Corruption breeds at the top and gradually filters down to the lower levels. Gone are the days when people who joined politics were imbued with the spirit of serving the nation. Expensive election, degeneration of moral values, unemployment, poverty, illiteracy, lack of political will to eradicate it, prolonged and loose trial system to punish corrupt persons, recognition of corruption of higher levels, lack of Ombudsman like institution etc. are the major causes of ever rising evil of corruption. Public Service Commissions and other recruiting bodies in most of the states have become the dens of corruption. Being on constitutional posts and enjoying immunities, majority of the members and Chairman of Public Service Commissions, can not preserve their fidelity. They play in the hands of politicians and try to appease their political bosses. There are so many incidents of paper leakage and misappropriation with answer-sheets in competitive examinations. Hardly any appointment is made on purely merit basis, it has not only confined to the matters of appointments but also has crept into case of admissions in professional courses. Undeserving persons appointed at Lucrative posts cannot assert and they surrender before their political bosses.

Withdrawal of corruption cases lying in different courts and lack of strong movement against corruption as launched by Jai Prakash Narayana and Vinoba Bhave in the seventies, have also promoted the evil. The trend of hung Parliament, multi-party system and politics of opportunism have made the situation even worse. Instability, defection, horse trading of MLAs and MPs, formulating of baseless coalitions just to barter and capture power, rising role of regional and local parties in national politics have added to the score of corruption. Uncertainty in politics and increasing role of money, muscle and mafia in election have provocated corruption. Rising of H.D. Dev Gowda and Inder Kumar Gujaral as Prime Ministers, Mayawati, Rabri Devi, Jayalalitha etc. as Chief Ministers have filled up each politicians with unending passion of power, as they were not the forefront leaders. It has been proved time and again that some politicians who were considered politically dead or remained in long political exile, rebounced in active politics on the basis of their money power which encouraged them to amass as much as wealth as they could. Recognition of corruption at higher level has made it an integral part of our political, economic and social system. Some people have chosen politics as an occupation to become rich. The control, permits and licence system has opened new vistas for corruption.

IMPACT OF CORRUPTION

Power tends to corrupt and absolute power tends to corrupt absolutely. This has become true with the present politicians of India. It has become the cause of political instability and defection, eroded the moral values, lessened the credibility of our political system and leaders. Criminalisation of politics and rigging of polls, baseless political coalitions and rise of opportunism in politics has threatened the authority of state and alienation in citizen. It has resulted in unrest among people and created an environment of violence and anarchy all round and has spoiled our political life. People are frustrated as nervous as they have no clear cut alternative. Honest and genuine persons cannot dare to contest elections. Corruption has increased the role of mafia in politics and has acknowledged the significance of extra constitutional sources of power which encourage cheap popularity in politics.

As far as economic implications are concerned, corruption has created a parallel market of black-money which is responsible for loss in revenue collection, centralization of capital, hoarding, adulteration, artificial deficiency of essential commodities rise in prices, inflation etc. The wealth collected through corrupt means is used in anti-national movements or activities to encourage instability and disintegrating forces. It has brought a bad name for India abroad and put at stakes her credit and dignity in international arena. A direct impact of corruption can be seen on share market, foreign investment, trade and commerce, even the economy of the nation as a whole.

Inferences of corruption can be seen even in the social system. It is getting recognition and acceptance even in those sections of society as an opportunity to rise who earlier criticized and noted it as an evil. It has become a value of our society. People whose ancestors have amassed wealth and got political designation by corrupt means, are enjoying respect and status in the society. Honesty has become a bane now a days. One, who has not innumerable wealth, can not seek better relations in the society. A lot of money is spent on social ceremonies. If an honest man does not want to indulge in corrupt practices, it has become a general perception that he did not get opportunity for it, if he gets the same, he will not remain far behind. On the one hand, a corrupt person is designated as active and advance, on the other, it is becoming highly inconvenient for honest people to fulfil their social obligations and social ceremonies. Even an honest person is not getting the desired respect in his own family and pressurised from all corners to get more.

REMEDIAL STEPS

There are, however, many legal provisions to deal with corruption in politics, but most of them have, in practice, become impertinent because of procedural defects or other obstacles. Under articles 102 and 171 of the Indian Constitution, the Election Commission acts as a permanent statutory tribunal to inquire into complaints of some type of misconduct by the member of Parliament and Legislative Assemblies. On the adverse report of the Commission, the President of India or the Governor of the State, as the case may be, can dismiss the MP or MLA concerned. Moreover, a recurring fine of Rs. 5000 per day of attendance in the Parliament or the Assembly can be imposed under section 104 or 93. Besides, the Election Commission, the higher judiciary can also inquire into cases relating to corrupt and fraudulent practices adopted by candidates during elections. However, in most of the cases, the findings of the commission and even the judiciary remained in-operative, as the cancellation of Indira Gandhi's election by Allahabad High Court in 1975 for adopting corrupt means resulted into emergency in the country. In some cases the decisions were delivered too late that they have no virtual significance by them. Similarly section 163 of the Indian Penal Code covers a wide range of cases of nepotism, but this too becomes in-operative in most of the cases, as section 197 of the Code of Criminal Procedure requires prior sanction of the concerned government before prosecuting any public servant or minister which again is a matter of discretion and provides protection to them against their purported acts.

The most popular device to inquire into the misconduct of the ministers is an Inquiry Commission appointed under the Commission of Inquiry Act, 1952, to deal with inquiries into 'definite matters of public importance' various commissions have been appointed so far, but the pity of these commissions is that their reports have been thrown into the dustbins or treated as mere scraps of paper due to lack of political will to implement these reports or withdrawal of criminal cases from the court of law. Therefore, the recommendations of commission of inquiry should be mandatory for government and a strong political will to root out corruption is need of hour. Institutions like Lokpal and Lokayukts need to be strengthened. Central Bureau of Intelligence, Central Vigilance Commission, State Vigilance Department or Bureaus are also not proving much effective against corruption due to political interference and various other reasons. The legal procedure to deal corruption cases should be straight forward and quick so that charged persons can be indicted and punished quickly.

As corruption has developed as an industry, in which all except some are involved from top to bottom, therefore, various laws and provisions made to counter it are proving futile, hence needed new thought on the topic. A strong movement against corruption needs to be launched on the same line as done by Jai Prakash Narayan in 1974. More vigilant, and free and fair mass media is required to expose people indulged in corrupt practices and to make public opinion against them. Moral code of conduct needs to be implemented properly during elections. Candidates and political parties should be asked to maintain their complete and transparent record of election expenditure. Persons with criminal background or charged in criminal cases should be banned from contesting elections. It may be possible that unsubstantial allegations may be levelled against persons on high rank and file of government, but Ceaser's wife should be above board. Our educational system needs to be reviewed. Recruitment process should be made objective and transparent. Competent persons should be given due weightage. The intellectuals have to come out of their confinement in workshop or research papers in closed rooms and to play a significance role to guide anti-corruption movement in practice.

Though the problem is undoubtedly grave, yet once the government is determined to fight corruption and it has time to do so, it is not difficult to change the situation gradually but steadily. The planning has to be very sound. Merely a flash of publicity will not work. A strong motivated leadership is the first requirement to eradicate corruption.

REFERENCES

1. *Dainik Bhaskar*, March 1, 2001.
2. Venktappih, B., "Misuse of Office", David L. Shills (ed). *International Encyclopaedia of Social Science*, Vol. II U.S.A.: The MacMillan Company and The Free Press, p. 272.
3. *Oxford Advanced Learners Dictionary*, Delhi: Oxford University Press, 1974, p. 193.
4. Kalaveren, Jacob Van, "The Concept of Corruption", Arnold J. Heidenheimev (ed.), *Political Corruption: Reading in Comparative Analysis*, N.Y. Holt, Rinchart and Winston Inco, 1970, p. 38.
5. Scott, James C, *Comparative Political Corruption*, New Jersey: Prentice Hall: 1972, p. 4.
6. Sentuna, Joseph J., "Political Corruption", R.A. Edwin Salingem, et al. (ed.), *Encyclopaedia of Social Science*, Vol. III and IV, London, 1931, p. 448.
7. Myrdal, Gunnar, *The Asian Dramma: An Inquiry into the Poverty of Nations*, Great Britain, Allen Lane, 1968, p. 837.
8. Wraith, Ronald and Simpxins, Edger, *Corruption in Developing Countries*, London, George Allen and Unwin, 1963, pp. 12-13.
9. Braibants, Ralph, "Reflections on Bureaucratic Corruption", *Public Administration* London: Winter, 1962, p. 357.
10. *Op. cit.*
11. Mathai, John, *Reminiscences of the Nehru Age,* Delhi: Vikas, 1978, p. 116.
12. Chaudhary, G. Rudrayya, Prakasan: *A Political Study*, New Delhi: Orient Longman, 1971, p. 148.
13. Privedy, S.N. and Bhargava, G.S., *Political Corruption in India*, New Delhi: Popular, 1967, pp. 43-62.
14. *Op. cit.*
15. Siwach, J.R. *Dynamics of Indian Government and Politics*, New Delhi: Sterling Publication, 1990, pp. 763-64; Nehru, J.L. Lok Sabha Debate, Vol. VIII, 3rd Series, Col. 14211, April 25, 1963, May 07.
16. Noorani, A.G. Parkasam: *A Political Study*, New Delhi: Orient Longman, 1971, p. 131.
17. Ibid.
18. Ibid.
19. Ibid., pp. 102-128.
20. *Op. cit.*
21. *The Times of India*, July 21, 1981.
22. *The Tribune*, May 11, 1979.
23. *The Statesman*, July 29, 1975.
24. *The Times of India*, May 13, 1978.

25. Ibid., July 29, 1981.
26. *The Tribune*, September 13, 1979.
27. *The Tribune*, June 18, 1981.
28. *The Times of India*, July 29, 1981.
29. Ibid., May 1, 1979.
30. *Indian Express*, Feb. 6, 1980.
31. *Op. cit.*
32. *India Today*, October 11, 2000, p. 32.
33. *Hindustan Times*, March 16, 2001.
34. *Amar Ujala*, March 4, 2001.
35. *The Times of India*, March 14, 2001.
36. *The Hindustan Times*, March 16, 2001.

23

CORRUPTION IN INDIA: SOME OBSERVATIONS ON POLITICAL CORRUPTION

Manoj Dixit

Dept. of Public Administration,
Lucknow University, Lucknow

Corruption is a universal phenomenon. It is not something new either. Corruption in one form or another existed since time immemorial. A review of penal codes utilized in various ancient civilizations clearly demonstrate that bribery was a serious problem among the Jews, the Chinese, the Japanese, the Greeks, the Romans as well as the Aztees of the New World (Thakur, 1979:7).

PRESENT CONCERN WITH CORRUPTION

"If corruption has been an age-old phenomenon, deep-rooted evil and an universal malady afflicting each and every society in one form or another at one time or another" (Padhay, 1986:1). then why there is so much concern at the present time with corruption. The reasons are obvious. Pope of Transparency International provides the *raison d'etre* for this concern.

"Corruption at the highest levels distorts competition so denying the public access to the competitive market place. It induces wrong decisions resulting in wrong projects, wrong prices, wrong contractors, substandard delivery to recoup overpricing, promotes corruption at lower levels and erodes public confidence in leaders. At lower levels, petty corruptions are damaging because they add to transaction costs, exclude those who cannot pay, foster contempt for public servants amongst public and erode capacity for revenue collection".

Still other reasons as to why now corruption is receiving serious attention could be:

1. Widespread perception that the level and pervasiveness of corruption is not only much greater but may well be increasing (Harris-White, 1996:1).
2. Developments in the 1980s and 1990s against the backdrop of increasing economic liberalization, third wave of democratisation and floating of good governance agenda have heightened expectations that an effective and root-and-branch cure of corruption may be found (Harris-White and White, 1992:2).
3. The coming into prominence of such concepts as decentralization, accountability and transparency, human rights, rule of law and sustainable development have considerably influenced efforts to minimize political and administrative corruption in many countries.

DEFINING CORRUPTION

Defining corruption is also important in the context of global efforts to reduce its influence in public life. But that is not an easy task. Corruption is a social, legal, economic and political concept enmeshed in ambiguity and consequently encouraging controversy.

The moralists view "corruption as an immoral and unethical phenomenon that contains a set of moral aberrations from moral standards of society, causing loss of respect for and confidence in duly constituted authority".

The functionalists usually look at corruption in terms of the actual function that it plays in socio-economic development. Claims are made by functionalists that corruption flourishes as a substitute for the market system; offers an acceptable alternative to violence; increases public participation in public policy.

In view of the multitude of approaches and views on corruption it is not easy to agree on a unanimous definition of the term. Two definitions of corruption can prove handy. The shorter definition of corruption includes "abuse of authority, bribery, favoritism, extortion, fraud, patronage, theft, deceit, malfeasance and illegality" (Caiden, 1991a).

The broader definition of corruption refers to "use of one's official position for personal and group gain and that includes unethical actions like bribery, nepotism, patronage, conflict of interest, divided loyalty, influence peddling, moonlighting, misuse of government property, selling of favours, receiving kickbacks, embezzlement, fraud, extortion, misappropriation, under or over-invoicing, court tempering, phony travel and administrative documents and use of regulation as bureaucratic capital (AAPAM, 1991).

In conformity with these two definitions of corruption the following definitions of political corruption and administrative corruption are adopted here. **Political corruption** is "the behaviour of (elected) public officials which diverges from the formal components—the duties and powers, rights and obligations—of a public role to seek private gain." **Administrative corruption** is defined as "the institutionalized personal abuse of public resources by civil servants" (Gould, 1991). In both cases public officials (elected and appointed) can convert public office into private gain in many ways or stealing.

Some of the major reasons as to why people "collude in different ways, rationalize corrupt practices and tolerate corruption in a large scale" are because of the presence of a number of factors. These are: governments act as monopolies in many respects, discretion that government and its monopolistic public agencies enjoy in their decision-making and allocative role, lack of effective accountability in government except in the normal sense of presenting annual audited accounts and reports to parliament or answering questions in the Parliament, citizens have limited information about the rules of the game and the standards of service they can expect from public agencies and exposure of the average citizen to corruption in the public sector tend to be episodic.

Corruption has been differentiated into three types—collusive, coercive and non-conjunctive (Arora, 1993). In collusive corruption the corruptees themselves are willing and active participants in the process and use of corruption as an instrument for inducing wrong action or inaction on the part of authorities, deriving benefit greater than the costs of corruption on their part. Corruption is forced upon the corruptee by those in the position of power and authority in coercive corruption. In non-conjunctive corruption benefits are obtained at someone else's cost and victims are unaware of their victimization.

Five major strategies—mystification, distancing, folklore, colonisation and pacification—have been used by beneficiaries to protect, promote and sustain corruption in diverse contexts (Arora, 1993).

POLITICAL CORRUPTION IN INDIA

"*I would go to the length of giving the whole congress a decent burial, rather than put up with the corruption that is rampant.*" — ***Mahatma Gandhi, May 1939***"

This was the outburst of Mahatma Gandhi against rampant corruption in Congress ministries formed under 1935 Act in six states in the year 1937. The disciples of Gandhi however, ignored his concern over corruption in post-Independence India, when they came to power. Over fifty years of democratic rule has made the people so immune to corruption that they have learnt how to live with the system even though the cancerous growth of this malady may finally kill it. The recent Tehelka episode surcharged the political atmosphere of the country but it hardly exposed anything, that was unknown to the people of this biggest democratic polity.

Politicians are fully aware of the corruption and nepotism as the main reasons behind the fall of Roman empire, the French Revolution, October Revolution in Russia, fall of Chiang Kai-Shek Government on the mainland of China and even the defeat of the mighty Congress party in India. But they are not ready to take any lesson from the pages of history.

The history of corruption in post-Independence India starts with the Jeep scandal in 1948, when a transaction concerning purchase of jeeps for the army needed for Kashmir operation was entered into by V.K. Krishna Menon, the then High Commissioner for India in London with a foreign firm without observing normal procedure. Contrary to the demand of the opposition for judicial inquiry as suggested by the Inquiry Committee led by Ananthsayanam Ayyangar, the then Government announced on September 30, 1955 that the Jeep scandal case was closed. Union Minister G.B. Pant declared "that as far as Government was concerned it has made up its mind to close the matter. If the opposition was not satisfied they can make it an election issue." Soon after on February 3, 1956 Krishna Menon was inducted into the Nehru cabinet as minister without portfolio.

In 1950, A.D. Gorwala, an eminent civil servant was asked by Government of India to recommend improvements in the system of governance. In his report submitted in 1951 he made two observations: "One, quite a few of Nehru's ministers were corrupt and this was common knowledge. Two, even a highly responsible civil servant in an official report as early as 1951 maintained that the Government went out of its way to shield its ministers" (*Report on Public Administration*, Planning Commission, Government of India 1951).

Corruption charges in cases like Mudgal case (1951), Mundra deals (1957-58), Malaviya-Sirajuddin scandal (1963), and Pratap Singh Kairon case (1963) were levelled against the Congress ministers and Chief Ministers but no Prime Minister resigned.

The Santhanam Committee, which was appointed by the Government in 1962 to examine the issue of corruption in its report submitted in 1964 observed: "There is widespread impression that failure of integrity is not uncommon among ministers and that some ministers, who have held office during the last sixteen years have enriched themselves illegitimately, obtained good jobs for their sons and relatives through nepotism and have reaped other advantages inconsistent with any notion of purity in public life."

The following comments of Nehru on the memorandum of charges against Pratap Singh Kairon submitted to the President of India by the non-Communist opposition in Punjab suggest his approach on corruption — "The question thus arises as to whether the chief minister is compelled to resign because of adverse findings on some questions of fact by Supreme Court. The ministers are collectively responsible to the legislature. Therefore, the matter was one, which concerned the assembly. As a rule therefore, the question of removing a minister would not arise unless the legislature expressed its wish by a majority vote." (*Pathology of Corruption* by S.S. Gill).

Thus, we find that while Nehru's tolerance of corruption among his ministers legitimized this malady, his daughter Indira Gandhi institutionalized it by holding both the posts of the Prime Minister and party President. By doing so she was herself controlling the party funds, which gave birth to the money power in politics. The famous V.P. Malhotra (Chief Cashier of State Bank of India) case in which he got a telephone call believing from Indira Gandhi to pay Rs. 60 lakhs to one Nagarwal remained a mystery. Corruption cases like Fairfax,

HBJ Pipeline, and HDW Submarine deal came up since then. The famous Bofor's deal is well known. Narsimha Rao was the first Prime Minister being prosecuted in corruption charges. Cases like Rs. 2500 crore—Airbus A-320 deal with France involving kickback (1990), Harshad Mehta security scam (1992), Gold Star Steel and Alloys controversy (1992), JMM bribery case, Hawala scam of Rs. 65 crore and Urea scam (1996) also came up during the period of Narsimha Rao government.

Criminalisation of politics is another facet of corruption. N.N. Vohra, Union Home Secretary in his report (1995) on this issue observed: "A network of mafias is virtually running a parallel Government pushing the state apparatus into irrelevance." Quoting some 'DIB' sources, he added, "...there has been a rapid spread and growth of criminal gangs, armed senas, drug mafias, smuggling gangs and economic lobbies in the country, which have over the years developed an intensive network of contacts with bureaucrats, government functionaries at local level, politicians, media persons and strategically located individuals in non-state sector. Some of these syndicates have also international linkages including the foreign agencies."

Against the above discussed historical background of corruption during last fifty years, the only contribution of Tehelka is that the exposure has forfeited the right of the BJP to claim itself to be a party with difference. So long the BJP was in opposition, it was by and large known as a party with moral integrity, but when it aligned with the political leaders with shady background for the sake of power, the malady of corruption infected this party too. Once the moral integrity is compromised it opens the door of corruption. Perhaps the BJP leadership deliberately went for ideological compromise for capturing power at centre. L.K. Advani put the responsibility on middle class when he reacted to a suggestion by an important ex-National Executive member of the party against the "dubious coalition politics". Advani reportedly said: "The middle class does not like compromises and tends to be idealistic. At the same time, it is unhappy if we lose power. It wants power as well as ideological integrity. This is the dilemma of the party". (Inside BJP by Dr. Jay Dubashi published in *Times of India* dated March 22, 2001). Advani might have philosophised the situation but he cannot escape from the responsibility for the ideological compromise the BJP made for the sake of power.

Corruption is an abstract term. According to World Bank report 1997 abuse of public power for private gains is described as corruption. But this appears to be too simplistic explanation of corruption. In fact, it is a multi-faceted evil, which gradually kills a system. A basic conflict between the ethos and system has weakened the Indian polity. The feudal outlook of the ruling class polluted the people's mindset, which judge the status of an individual on his capability to flout the law to favour them. This is the reason why corruption is no more viewed by people with abhorrence in Indian society. Leaders like Laloo, Jayalalitha, Sukhram and others, who are facing corruption charges, continue to have wide range of people's support. Transparency, responsiveness, accountability, probity in public life and good governance are now only slogans. The legislature has failed to make the judiciary, executive and even media sensitive to the cause of the common people. The failure of the political leadership to take a principled stand against corruption has clouded the system to the extent that it is now difficult to understand whether the system is alive or dead.

In the present context corruption is so much linked with power that our politicians have adopted a cynical attitude toward political morality. Maneuvering the anti-defection law for electoral politics with the help of both money and muscle power and other unfair means for the sake of power have affected the political morality of all the political parties and as such none of them can claim themselves to be faithful to nation in true sense. It was pathetic to see an excellent orator of Congress struggling to brush away the past of the Congress in the recent "Big fight" programme on Star TV.

The collapse of the Janata Party Government (1977-80), fall of V.P. Singh and Chandrashekhar Government (1990-91), turning his minority Government into majority by Narsimha Rao, split in Telugu Desam Party (1994), defection of Ajit Singh with his supporters to Congress (1993), defection of S.S. Vaghela from BJP, maneuvering defection by Kalyan Singh to keep the BJP led Government in power in UP are some of examples to prove that a sizeable number of our politicians are not immune to corruption.

With Tehelka exposure, we may like to refer to our ancient law book, which said, "That monarch, whose subjects are carried from his kingdom by ruffians, while they call aloud for protection, and he barely looks on them with his ministers, is a dead, and not a living king." (*Manusmriti* VII/143). Tehelka is simply an addition to thousands of past and present eruptions in the cancerous body polity of the country.

Manu may not be relevant to the present century, but as human nature more or less remains same and states either in monarchy or democracy are governed by the same human beings, he is still relevant. License to govern does not mean license to be corrupt. Mahatma Gandhi believed in the need for creating a social climate against corruption, which meant creation of an atmosphere in which the corrupt could not thrive. The need of the hour therefore, is to wipe off the tormenting system, which could be possible only after its thorough overhaul. For this our national leadership is expected to devise a political mechanism to create a social atmosphere by empowering of people. The ongoing war cry against corruption, which is nothing but a mad fight to replace one corrupt system by another is not going to transform the beleaguered nation to a sustainable social order.

Checking corruption is no easy task. Still no one denies the need to check corruption effectively. It may not be possible to eradicate corruption completely but then vigorous and determined actions will go a long way to minimize it. The measures suggested are too many and defy any easy characterization. To contain and minimize corruption a number of measures have been recommended. These include: driving out corruption by means of usually one-off purges of campaigns, setting up of anti-corruption boards, commissions and the like, campaign for moral regeneration or moral re-armament, strengthening of checks on abuse of power and the enhancement of accountability of powerful as well as public officials, ensuring transparency and openness in governmental activities, develop positive social attitudes, enforcing a code of public ethics, supporting the role of media, improving educational procedures (Theobald, 1990; UN, 1990).

To reduce corruption drastically, a number of fundamental changes must be brought about. These include: reducing the opportunities for corrupt transactions by cutting back the state's activities; emergence of new centres of power outside the bureaucracy; development of competitive party politics; ascendance of universalistic norms; effectuation of far-reaching administrative reform measures affecting policy, institutional and process levels, strengthening of preventive structures and tightening of prosecuting techniques (Theobald, 1990; UN, 1990).

Corruption is a complex multifaceted social phenomenon with innumerable manifestations. It takes place as an outcome of deficiencies in the existing public administration apparatuses and systems as well as cultural, economic, political and social factors. Differences of opinion still exist as to the meaning of the term corruption. This is primarily because individuals look at corruption from their own vantage points influenced by surrounding environment. But what is heartening is that in recent years corruption is viewed from a much broader perspective rather than looking at it from moral and functional angles only.

24

ADMINISTRATIVE CORRUPTION IN INDIA: THE NEED FOR SCANDINAVIAN MODEL OF MECHANISM TO COMBAT CORRUPTION

S. Balamurugan and S. Suchitra Varma

Deptt. of Political Science & Public Administration, DDE, Annamalai University, Annamalai.

Indian citizens are proud of the democratic system of governance, but one cannot ignore the fact that a vast majority of the people particularly the under-privileged and less-privileged feel that a system of non-governance characterized by rampant corruption exists in Public Administration.

In the governmental set-up, the critical task of public administration is entrusted to the popularly elected politicians called Ministers and officially appointed personnel called Bureaucrats. Good conduct and ethical practices are two cardinal principles of public administration. The expectations of the people for fairness and justice in public administration are the same everywhere irrespective of their race, culture and the structure of the Government.

The responsibility of the Government has increased leaps and bounds with the growth of the concept of Welfare State. It has been perceived many a times that there is a tendency of the ruling class to protect the interests of the "haves" and ignore those of the "have-nots." Therefore, it is essential that people should have faith and confidence in the administrative elite and at the same time be assured that any action taken by them is for the overall development of the nation and its people. If the public servants do not resort to arbitrary, capricious, discriminatory and fanciful actions, there could be good rapport between the people and the Government and consequently the greatest good for the largest number of the people could be achieved. Transparent and clear public administration is a "must" for any Government of the time and public accountability is the core and conscience of the public administration.

It is unfortunate that with the passage of time corruption in India has substantially increased. A non-governmental organization Transparency International based in Berlin has come with the corruption perception index. It ranks countries according to the level of corruption. This year (2004) out of 102 most corrupted countries India occupies the 33rd position. For a developing country like India corruption is a scourge. It is anti-national. It seriously retards country's economic development.

The World Bank has defined corruption as the use of "Public Office for Private Profit." Corrupt acts include bribery, embezzlement, etc. International anti-corruption convention of the United Nations defines corruption as "... promise or giving of any advantage to another person as undue consideration for performing or refraining from the performance of that person's duty, or the soliciting or accepting of any advantage as undue considerations for performing or refraining from the performance of one's duty."

The Administrative Reforms Commission was appointed on January 5, 1966 by the President of India. While dealing with one of the terms of reference, namely, "to consider the problems of citizens' grievances", it unanimously recommended that the Ombudsman type of machinery be set up in India. The Commission recommended two types of Ombudsmen i.e., Lokpal at the Central level and Lokayukta at the State level to inquire into allegations of corruptions against public functionaries and for investigation of authorities in certain cases and for matters connected therewith. The commission had felt the urgent need for such institutions in view of the inadequacies in the existing system and for introduction of supplementing the already existing agencies like the Courts and Tribunals which were not always within the reach of the common people because of various factors including cumbersome procedures, long delays, litigation costs etc. In addition, the Commission found that there was a vast area of cases arising out of the unjust exercise of executive power for which no remedy was available. Again, in the context of the off-expressed public opinion against the prevalence of corruption and for ensuring the highest standards of efficiency and integrity in the public administration and for making administrative wing accountable and transparent, the commission had underscored the need to set up 'Ombudsman' type of institutions throughout the country.

The basic idea of the Lokpal is borrowed from the office of Ombudsman, which has played an effective role in checking corruption and wrongdoing in Scandinavian and other nations. In a climate where, to use the former Prime Minister's Vajpayee's own words, "corruption has bred contempt for the law an additional mechanism which takes note of public grievances and can take cognizance of wrong doing in public life deserves to be welcomed". Just how effective the Lokpal legislation will be in checking corruption in high places has been a matter of longstanding and inconclusive debate. The Lokpal is no substitute for judicial action and by itself the institution is unlikely to magically transform the manner in which the administration works. But, as conceived in some earlier draft Bills, the scope and jurisdiction of the Lokpal is reasonably wide and the very existence of an institution which can bring public figures to book could act as an important check on the misuse of power. Given that virtually every major party has routinely supported the setting up of a Lokpal in their manifestos, the Bill will not fail because of the lack of political support. All it requires now—just as all it had required before—is the requisite political commitment to see the proposed legislation through Parliament.

The Government of India introduced the Lokpal Bills in the Parliament in 1968, 1971, 1977, 1985, 1989, 1996, 1998 and 2001. It had been referred three times to joint select committees of both the Houses and as many times to the Parliamentary Standing Committee on Home affairs. They had also submitted their reports. Thus, up to now, there is no national Ombudsman in India.

The bill has failed to get Parliament's approval several times in the past due to lack of consensus among lawmakers about the exact functions of the Lokpal (Ombudsman) and whether to include the office of the Prime Minister in the definition of public servant.

The UNDP Report on Human Development in South Asia, says that if corruption levels in India were reduced to those of the Scandinavian countries, the investments in the country could increase annually by 10 per cent and GDP growth by almost 1.5 per cent each year. One recent study shows that investing in relatively corrupt country compared to a relatively honest one is equivalent to additional 15 per cent profit on investment.

WORKING OF OMBUDSMAN IN SCANDINAVIAN COUNTRIES

The office of Ombudsman is a Scandinavian institution that has received much attention in recent years. New Zealand and Canada and several state in the U.S. and some of the new countries of Africa have adopted the idea, and the name at least has been applied to officials in business concerns and on college campuses. The concept of an Ombudsman originated in its present form with the Swedish Constitution of 1809, and it has been adopted and even extended in the other Scandinavian countries such as Finland (1919), Denmark (1953), and Norway (1962).

Bureaucracy sometimes rides brutally over the rights of the individuals, either because of careless disregard, or because regulations cannot cover exceptional cases, or for other reasons having to do with the fallibility of laws or officials. Any society that seeks justice must provide channels for appeal and correction of mistakes, but too often the procedures of complaint go through the same governmental structure as the thing objected to. Therefore, the Swedes provided for a judicial agent, the Judicial Ombudsman (JO), acting under the authority of Parliament to be a watchdog over administrative officials and acts.

The JO is a person respected in the community, with salary and position comparable to that of a Supreme Court Judge. He or she has the right to see all relevant documents and access to whomever he wishes to consult. The press checks with the JO each day, so the power of publicity is at the JO's disposal. The constitution of each country empowers the JO not only to accept complaints from individuals but also to initiate proceedings whenever he or she senses there may be injustice. Occasionally the JO makes inspection trips, visiting courts, hospitals, schools, smelling out little and big cases of wrongdoing, suggesting remedies.

The JO also makes an annual report to Parliament but is never ordered by Parliament to undertake a case or to desist from prosecution. Thus, the JO is free agent, appointed for a several-year period and frequently reappointed. The JO has a deputy and staff of lawyers but still has difficulty handling the workload. The office of JO gives people confidence that there's someone concerned not only with the welfare of society as a whole but with their own rights as individuals. More recently, Ombudsman offices are being created in the former socialist countries of Eastern Europe (Poland, Hungary, Slovenia, Albania, Bosnia-Herzegovina, Macedonia) as well as in the Russian Federation.

During the last decade, Latin America has witnessed a process in favour of a more democratic rule compared to the tradition of authoritarianism long developed in the area. As a consequence, many countries began to include the figure of Ombudsman with different names: Defensor del Peublo, Procurador de los Derechos Humanos, Defensor de los Habitantes, Comisionado Nacional deDerechos Humanos. Until then, just Peurto Rico (from 1977) and Gautemala (1985) had institutions like this. From 1990 on, it was created in Mexico, El Salvador, Colombia, Costa Rica, Paraguay, Honduras, Peru, Argentina, Bolivia, Nicaragua, Panama, Ecuador and Venezuela. It is also in agenda for Chile and Uruguay. All the Latin American Ombudsman are integrated in the Federation lberoamericana del Ombudsman to give their efforts an international support.

Regardless the name of the office, all Ombudsman institutions respond in essence to the basic pattern of an independent investigator capable of receiving complaints from the public to make the state administration accountable for wrongdoings and facilitate redress to the victims of maladministration or violations of human rights.

Not all the Ombudsman are however, equal since traditionally the Scandinavian and European Ombudsman has been responsible only for cases of maladministration or administrative injustice. Lately under the influence of the Spanish Constitution of 1978 a so-called hybrid model has been developed to include within the Ombudsman jurisdiction the responsibility for human rights violations. In some cases, the enlarged mandate has gone even further as to include the protection of the environment, freedom of the press and supervision of elections.

The Scandinavian countries and especially Finland have been regarded quite highly in many international ratings of anti-corruption. What are the reasons for this fine situation? It is useful to look at some Finnish experience of combating corruption.

There have been times in Scandinavian history, too, when corruption has filled the front pages of the tabloids. Every now and then cases do emerge when an individual, a lower or a high-ranking public official, is caught red-handed committing some criminal offence. In most cases this has led to the resignation or dismissal of the person and, depending on the case also to a criminal prosecution. Yet ordinary Finns do not come across corruption in their daily lives. Recently, there was a survey done on the citizens' perceptions of public institutions. The police scored the top rating for honesty.

As noted, in international ratings of corruption Finland has enjoyed high esteem for a number of years. The corruption index by Transparency International has had Finland ranked number one as the least corrupted country for many years. A few possible explanations for this phenomenon.

The model of the present-day Finnish welfare society is widely known. It is, however, useful to point out some background facts as to its origins. In Finland, democracy and the rule of law were consolidated in the beginning of the twentieth century. In those days, good education was seen as one of the most powerful social tools. Being a nation of 5 to 6 million people, they know that everybody's skills were needed in building welfare and prosperity. Education became compulsory for everyone.

The Finnish legal norms on corruption have been basically the same for the past 100 years. They are for administrative principles of good governance effective in Finland, are (1) the principle of equality, (2) the principle of objectivity, (3) the principle of proportionality and (4) the principle that any action must be appropriate in view of its purpose. The main idea of the Finnish anti-corruption legislation is that it is never considered as a separate phenomenon, with separate laws or separate supervisory bodies. Instead, corruption is seen as part of criminality and as part of bad governance and/or politics. The prevention of corruption also involves creating and observing ethical norms of behaviour, increasing transparency and preventing procedures.

Both in state administration and in local administration, a so-called employment instruction system is being applied to new officeholders. This is a form of introduction training. If there is a great risk of corruption in the field in question, matters related to corruption shall naturally be emphasized during the introductory training. New officeholders are also given examples of some typical situations where the risk of bribery may arise. Management training, as well as other kinds of staff training in public administration are moreover planned so that they include sections on values and ethics.

According to the Finnish Constitution, some of the most important guarantees of good governance for the citizens are the right to be heard, the right to hear the grounds for decisions, and the right of appeal.

TRANSPARENCY AND OPENNESS

The transparency of public decision-making promotes anti-corruption work. Open access to public records makes it possible to apply transparency and good information practices in public activities. It also makes it possible for individuals and associations to control the exercise of official authority and the use of public finances, freely to form their opinion, to influence the exercise of official authority, and to assert their rights and safeguard their interests.

Transparency in public administration is enhanced by the obligation of the highest officials to declare their commitments, and by restrictions on secondary occupations. Training, leadership and publications increase the consciousness among civil servants of values and ethically sound proceedings in public administration. Informing partners in the private sector of the requirements of civil service ethics is a factor for promoting transparency. In local administration, a clear definition of the eligibility for office for members of a municipal executive board and other institutions promotes transparency and reduces corruption.

Finland was one of the first countries to allocate state funds for political parties. The elimination of conflicting interests and liabilities and thus corruption is also pursued through the publicity of election financing.

LESSONS LEARNED FROM THE FINNISH EXPERIENCE

The key contacts that can be distilled from the Finnish experience and other Scandinavian countries are 1. Access to education for all; 2. Well functioning democracy both at national and local level; 3. Civil service based on meritocracy; 4. Openness in public administration; 5. Low hierarchical structures; 6. Devolution of decision-making powers to civil servants in their respective fields of responsibility; 7. Non-politicisation of key civil service posts, and above all, 8. The effort to defend the values of an open society.

In India it is proposed to create one national Ombudsman with general responsibilities, which will combine the characteristics of the classical Scandinavian Ombudsman model with some of the new features of its modern versions existing in the European countries, and with some adjustments according to condition in India. The most essential function of the Ombudsman institution will be to guarantee more efficiently the rights and freedoms of private persons. If the former are abused by the public authorities, the Ombudsman shall be entitled to propose measures for terminating the acts of abuse, compensating the incurred damages and creating conditions for the smooth and efficient exercise of their rights in the future.

More specifically, the Ombudsman must have the authority to monitor and control the exercise of administrative power, the organization and regulation of the judicial system's administration, as well as any other exercise of public authority. However, the subject and scope of the Ombudsman's activities must not include certain institutions, such as the Parliament, the President, and the Judiciary.

It can be proposed that the Ombudsman be elected by a simple majority directly by the Parliament. It has been suggested that the Ombudsman's mandate should be longer than the mandate of the Parliament—five or more years. The number of the Ombudsman's mandates will be limited to no more than two. At the same time, he will enjoy immunity similar to that of the members of Parliament.

Because of its Parliamentary origin, the Ombudsman will report to the Parliament once a year, which would secure a high level of publicity and transparency for its activities and the results thereof. This effect will have a positive influence on those public institutions, which do not fully respect the rights and freedoms of private persons.

TYPES OF RESPONSIBILITIES AND AUTHORITY

In general, the responsibilities and authority of the Ombudsman are:

- To review petitions in any form from private persons—individuals and legal entities, whether local and/or foreign, as well as from individuals with no citizenship;
- To conduct investigations and examinations when a particular case has been referred to him;
- To make proposals and recommendations to all observed institutions with public powers or functions regarding their respect for human rights and freedoms, and to recommend possible remedies for the infringement of certain rights and

freedoms and the reasons for that infringement, notwithstanding whether the ombudsman acts at somebody's request or his own initiative;

- To extend recommendations and give advice to petitioners;
- To act as an intermediary between private persons and public entities in order to overcome the existing infringements on private rights and freedoms;
- To request and receive timely, complete and precise information from all observed institutions;
- To have direct access to the observed institutions, including their meetings, discussions and other forums;
- To give and announce publicly his opinions on cases he has been approached with or on issues on which he makes summaries and conclusions at his own discretion;
- To approach the prosecution bodies when, as a result of his observations and investigations, the Ombudsman has obtained information on a committed crime;
- To prepare and present an annual report to the Parliament;
- To prepare special reports, if necessary and to inform the Parliament incidentally about particularly serious cases of disrespect and abuse of rights.

CONCLUSION

In the modern world especially after globalization in India the influence and range of activity of the administration at all levels is increasing. More and more central or local governmental authorities with their actions, visible or invisible, affect the private persons—individuals and legal entities—on a daily basis. The existing mechanisms are not always in a position to secure a quick, timely, efficient and easily accessible protection of the parties affected by the actions of the administration. This creates the need for a new mechanism Ombudsman, which will not duplicate the functions of the existing mechanisms but, rather, will operate parallel to them, add to their work, initiate directly or indirectly their interference, and under some circumstances, be their alternative. With few modifications, as mentioned in this paper, this system will be highly suitable to the Indian condition.

25

PROPOSED LOKPAL BILL 2001: A CRITICAL ANALYSIS

S.S. Chahar and Rajesh Kundu

Department of Public Administration,
M.D. University, Rohtak (Haryana)

INTRODUCTION

The Scandinavian Office of Ombudsman[1] as an agency for redressing of citizens' grievances, has in recent years attracted the attention of many countries. Now it operates in over 40 countries[2] both developed and developing. Interestingly, it has emerged distinctly in developed countries which are adhering to the original Swedish model of the 'grievance man'. But the developing countries have perceived it essentially as an instrument of investigating the allegations of corruption or misconduct by ministers and other public officials.

In so far as India, is concerned the demand for the establishment of Ombudsman has been raised from time to time by individual scholars[3] and other bodies.[4] Having realized the relevance of this institution in India as well, the Administrative Reforms Commission[5] (ARC), 1966 headed by Morarji Desai recommended in its interim report on "Problems of Redress of Citizens' Grievances" to set up the institution of Lokpal on the general pattern of Ombudsman in Scandinavian countries. Since our country is quite a big one in comparison to any other country which has adopted the institution of Ombudsman, the ARC provided for two separate authorities designated as Lokpal and Lokayukta, the former to deal with the complaints against ministers and secretaries to government and later with complaints against other public officials. But today practically, Lokpal is meant for central affairs whereas Lokayukta is for state affairs. In pursuant to ARC recommendations, the Lokpal and Lokayukta Bill[6] was moved in Lok Sabha on May 9, 1969. The Bill provided for the appointment of one Lokpal and one or more Lokayuktas to inquire into the allegations of corruption and maladministration against the Central ministers and secretaries to the Union government. The Bill was referred to a Joint Committee of Parliament. It was passed by the Lok Sabha but lapsed on its dissolution at the end of December 1970 while it was pending in the Rajya Sabha. Thereafter, it was moved in the Parliament many times[7] but could not get through. Lastly, it was presented in the Lok Sabha in 2001.

MAIN FEATURES OF THE LOKPAL BILL 2001[8]

The bill provides for the establishment of the institution of Lokpal to inquire into allegations of corruption against public functionaries including the Prime Minister, provided the offence committed is within ten years from the day the complaint is lodged. The Lokpal shall consist of a chairperson who is or has been a Chief Justice or a Judge of the Supreme Court and two members who are or have been the Judges of the Supreme Court or the Chief Justices of the High Court. The chairperson and members shall be appointed by the President of India on the recommendation of a committee headed by the Vice-President of India and comprising the Prime Minister, the Lok Sabha Speaker, the Home Minister, the leader of the opposition in both the Lok Sabha and the Rajya Sabha. The bill provides for a fixed tenure of three years for the chairperson and the members. The bill ensures that the Lokpal is able to act independently and discharge its functions without fear or favour. For this, it provides that the chairperson or a Member of the Lokpal shall not be removed from office, except by an order made by the President on the ground of proved misbehaviour or incapacity. He can issue the removal order after an inquiry by a committee consisting of the Chief Justice of India and two other Judges of the Supreme Court (next to the Chief Justice in seniority). The Lokpal will inquire into complaints alleging that a public functionary has committed an offence punishable under the Prevention of Corruption Act, 1988. The expression 'public functionary' covers all the three categories of union ministers including the Prime Minister and the Members of Parliament. The constitutional functionaries such as Judge of the Supreme Court, the Election Commission have been kept out of the purview of the Lokpal. The allegations against the Prime Minister related to his functions in the areas of national security and maintenance of public order have been kept out of the purview of the Lokpal. To enable the Lokpal to function effectively and in a quasi-judicial manner, it has been vested with the powers of a Civil Court in respect of summoning and enforcing the attendance of any person and examining him on oath. The bill provides for an open court or if the Lokpal wishes in-camera proceedings. The proceedings have to be completed within six months, with a provision for extension of six more months. The Lokpal is vested with penal powers to discourage frivolous complaints. For such complaints, the fine could be an imprisonment from one to three years including a fine upto Rs. 50,000.

APPOINTMENT PROCESS[9] — A CRITIQUE

For appointment of Chairman and Members, a Committee is provided under Clause 4(1) to recommend names for consideration of the President. This is no doubt a welcome provision and an advancement over the recommendation of the ARC. This Committee recommended it to comprise seven persons, including the Prime Minister and Minister-in-charge of Ministry of Home Affairs are members of the Committee. In our view the Prime Minister and these ministers should not be associated with the appointment process as their offices fall within the purview of the Lokpal institution and as such it will not be good on grounds of impartiality and fairness. Under clause 4(2) of the Bill, there is a need to mention the requirement of quorum of at least three members, including Chairman.

JURISDICTION[10] OF THE LOKPAL

The Lokpal is empowered to entertain a complaint alleging that a person who holds or has held the office of Prime Minister, Cabinet Minister, Minister of State, Deputy Minister, Chief Parliamentary Secretary or Parliamentary Secretary of the State and any other public servant has committed any offence punishable under Chapter IX of the Indian Penal Code, 1860 or the Prevention of Corruption Act, 1988 or under any law for the time being in the force for prevention of corruption. Further, he may on receipt of a reference from the government or *suo-moto* proceed to inquire into the allegations and grievances made against a public servant. He may also inquire into any act or conduct of any person other than a public servant in so far as he considers it necessary to do so for the purpose of his inquiry into any such allegation of misconduct against a public servant.

FILING OF COMPLAINT[11]

Any person other than a public servant[12] may make a complaint under this Act to the Lokpal. The complaint shall be in the prescribed form and shall set forth particulars of the offence alleged and shall be accompanied by fees prescribed, if any, an affidavit in support of such particulars and a certificate of deposit furnished under sub-section (3) or, if the complainant is unable to make the deposit, an application for exemption from the requirement as to such deposit. The complainant shall deposit such sum of money in such manner and with such authority or agency as may be prescribed and the certificate for such deposit shall be furnished in the prescribed form. Notwithstanding anything contained in the foregoing sub-sections, any letter written to the Lokpal or, as the case may be, to the appropriate authority, by a person in any jail or other place of custody or in any asylum or other place for insane persons may, if the Lokpal, or as the case may be, the appropriate authority is satisfied that it is necessary so to do, be treated as a complaint made in accordance with the provisions of this section. Notwithstanding anything contained in any other enactment, it shall be the duty of a police officer or other person incharge of any jail or other place of custody or of any asylum or other place for insane persons to forward, without opening, any letter addressed to the Lokpal or to the appropriate authority by a person imprisoned or detained in such jail, place of custody, asylum or other place, to the Lokpal or the appropriate authority, as the case may be, without delay.

MACHINERY AND PROCEDURE FOR INQUIRIES[13]

The Lokpal can appoint in consultation with the Government such officers and staff as he may consider appropriate for the discharge of function under this Act. He can also utilize the services of any officer or investigating agency of the state government for the purpose of conducting any inquiry or investigation under the Act. The Lokpal institution should be armed with a core investigating agency, entirely at its own disposal, in addition to the power to secure the services of any officer or employee or investigating agency of the Central Government or State Government with the concurrence of that Government or the services of any other persons or agency. In this regard, Karnataka and Madhya Pradesh Lokayukta models might be adopted. The Lokpal should be given *suo moto* power of investigation to protect community and collective rights of the depressed, deprived and downtrodden members of the society. It should also be given power to review and revise its own decisions/recommendations under appropriate circumstances. If, after the consideration and verification in respect of a complaint, the Lokpal proposes to conduct any inquiry, it shall forthwith forward a copy of the complaint to the competent authority; it may make such orders as to the safe custody of documents relevant to the inquiry as it deems fit; and it shall, at such time as it considers appropriate, forward a copy of the complaint to the public functionary concerned and afford him an opportunity to represent his case. Every inquiry shall be conducted by the Chairperson and the Members sitting jointly and the place in which such inquiry is conducted shall be deemed to be an open court to which the public generally may have access so far as the same can conveniently contain them, provided that in exceptional circumstances and for reasons to be recorded in writing, such inquiry may be conducted in camera. The Lokpal shall hold every such inquiry as expeditiously as possible and in any case complete the inquiry within a period of six months from the date of receipt of the complaint, provided that the Lokpal may, for reasons to be recorded in writing, complete the inquiry within a further period of six months. Save as aforesaid, the procedure for conducing any such inquiry shall be such as the Lokpal considers appropriate in the circumstances of the case.

REPORT OF THE LOKPAL AND ACTION TAKEN[14]

After the conclusion of inquiry, the Lokpal shall determine whether all or any of the offences alleged in the complaint have or has been proved to its satisfaction and by report in writing shall communicate its findings to the complainant, the public functionary and the competent authority. The Speaker, in the case of the Prime Minister or a member of the House of the People, and the Chairman of the Council of States, in the case of a member of that Council shall, as soon as may be after the receipt of report under sub-section (1), cause the same to be laid before the House of the People or the Council of States, as the case may be while it is in session, and if the House of the People or the Council of States, as the case may be, is not in session, within a period of one week from the reassembly of the said house or the council, as the case may be. The competent authority shall examine the report forwarded to it under sub-section (1) and communicate to the Lokpal, within a period of ninety days[15] from the date of receipt of report, the action taken or proposed to be taken on the basis of the report. The Lokpal shall present annually to the President a consolidated report on the administration of this Act and the President shall, as soon as may be after and in any case not later than ninety days from the receipt of such report, cause the same, together with an explanatory memorandum, to be laid before each House of Parliament.

SHORTCOMINGS OF LOKPAL BILL, 2001

The Lokpal Bill of 2001, no doubt, had wide ranging provisions to empower the institution in a bid to fight corruption but it did not focus on redressal of people's grievances. So Bill reveals some specific shortcomings which are discussed below:

- The Indian model does not match with the original Swedish model of 'grievance man' where the Lokpal is treated as an agency of investigation. Thus, it provides no relief to common man from administrative failure and injuries.
- The proposed Bill barred the Lokpal from taking *suo-moto* cognizance. For initiating any case, a complaint has to be filed along with the fee and full responsibility is to be taken by the person have leveled the allegations.
- The provision of punishment to complainants is widely feared that this might act as a dampener on attempts to expose the corrupt deals where hard evidence is not produced.
- The Lokpal has not been given wide powers of inquiry and officers conducting such inquiries are not kept independent of the government agencies. So, there is no point in having a Lokpal if he has to depend only on other agencies to investigate complaints. In case of no cooperation from them, the investigation can be held up. Moreover, the use of government agencies for investigation cannot be free from corrupt practices.

- The provision of "in-camera proceedings" by the Lokpal corroborated the principle that in theory every person is equal but practically some persons (the public functionaries, i.e., M.Ps., Ministers and Prime Minister) are more equal than others.
- The first bill of 1968 talks about to curb maladministration but this Bill considers it as the mechanism to stop corruption. So it deviates the institution from being a grievance redressal machinery.
- The 'competent authority', is under no obligation to accept the recommendations of the Lokpal. This clearly defeats the very purpose for which the institution is proposed to be set up.

CONCLUSIONS AND SUGGESTIONS

The institution of Lokpal will certainly be an improvement over the existing system. It is the need of the hour in the light of a large number of political scandals. The Bill has certainly provided a wide jurisdiction of inquiry to the Lokpal. The complainants are also allowed to approach him to file their complaints without depositing any fee. However, the Lokpal has not been treated as 'grievance man' but an investigating agency. The pattern of investigation resembles to those of civil courts which is not prompt and simple. He is heavily dependant on the government for his investigations and implementation of his recommendations. The Bill has not been framed while avoiding the flaws existing in the Acts of other states.

So for making the institutions of Lokpal an effective one, following suggestions may be given:

- If he is to function as a formally independent institution, the method of his appointment should be above board. He can be directly selected on the pattern of New Zealand.
- In order to insulate him against political pressures, he should be appointed for life.
- He should have his own independent investigating agencies having its own small secretariat.
- Proceedings should be held in open to expose the corrupt public servant in the society. There should be freedom of information on the pattern of USA so that assets owned by government employees can be revealed.

- It should have two wings: one attending to allegations, the other to grievances.
- Enquiry should not be conducted only under the Prevention of Corruption Act but also under the Criminal Procedure Code.
- The Lokpal need not depend on the decision of the competent authority for the implementation of his verdicts but he should have powers to prosecute the corrupt public servants himself.

REFERENCES

1. Ombudsman refers to a person who acts as a spokesman or the representative of another person.
2. The work of hearing the grievances of the people is performed by different institutions in different countries, e.g. Parliamentary Commissioner. For Administration in Britain, the Mediator in France, Lonobayan in the Phillippines. Wifaque Mohtaseb in Pakistan, Director of Public Prosecutions in Guyana, Investigator in Zambia, Inspector General of Government in Uganda, Permanent Commission of Inquiry in Tanzania, Chief Complaints Commissioner in Nigeria, Lokayukta in Indian states, See Subhash C. Kashyap (ed.), *Judicial Activitism and Lokpal*, New Delhi: Uppal, 1997, pp. 93, 108.
3. In 1950, for the first time after independence, an academic duo-Professor Karve and Bodh Raj Sharma suggested the institution of Ombudsman for India. Similarly, in 1951 A.D. Corwala, in his Report on Public Administration had mentioned certain machinery for the improvement of the integrity or moral standards of, as well as efficiency in the administration. He had recommended a Tribunal of Enquiry for ministers and high government officials. Further, in 1957 C.D. Deshmukh, while delivering his Lecture in Madras University has suggested a high level impartial Standing Judicial Tribunal. In 1958, K.M. Munshi also demanded for sub-institution. In 1960, a group of Members of Parliament raised the demand of an Ombudsman there. See Subhash C. Kashyap, (ed.), *Judicial Activism and Lokpal*, New Delhi, Uppal, 1997, pp. 107-08.
4. The Santhanam Committee, 1962 recommended that specific allegation of corruption on the part of a minister at the Centre or a State should be investigated by an agency whose findings will command respect. For this purpose, the Committee suggested to constitute a 'National Panel' of eminent persons, *Ibid*., pp. 81-82.
5. See, Administrative Reforms Commission, Government of India, Interim Report on Problems of Redress of Citizens Grievances, 1966.
6. See, P.K. Tripathi, '*Lokpal: The Proposed Indian Ombudsman*', 1967; MP Jain, *Lokpal: Indian Ombudsman*, 1970, S.K. Aggarwal, *The Proposed Indian Ombudsman*, 1971, Donald C. Rawat (ed.). *The Ombudsman: Citizens Defender*, 1968; D.R. Saxena, *Ombudsman (Lokpal): Redress of Citizens' Grievances in India*, 1987.

7. Since then, it has been introduced in Parliament in 1971, 1977, 1985, 1989, 1996, 1998 and 2001 but could not be adopted for various reasons including a controversy over the jurisdiction of Lokpal.
8. *Lokpal Bill*, 2001, pp. 12-13.
9. *Ibid.*, Clause 4(1) and (2), p. 2.
10. *Ibid.*, Clause 10, p. 4.
11. *Ibid.*, Clause 12, p. 5.
12. Public servants means any person who is a member of a defence service or of a civil service of the Union or a State or of an all-India service or holds any post connected with defence or any civil post under the Union or a State; any person in the service or pay of a local authority, a corporation established by or under a Central, Provincial or State Act or a Government company, as defined in section 617 of the Companies Act, 1956; any person in the service of any other institution, concern or undertaking which is established by or under a Central, Provincial or State Act or which is controlled, or financed wholly or substantially by funds provided, directly or indirectly, by the Central Government or a State Government.
13. *Ibid.*, Clause 14 and 15, p. 6.
14. *Ibid.*, Clause 17, p. 7.
15. In computing the period of ninety days referred to in this sub-section, any period during which Parliament or, as the case may be, either House of Parliament, is not in session, shall be excluded.

26

CORRUPTION IN INDIA: ORIGIN, CAUSES AND SOLUTIONS FOR CORRUPTION IN PUBLIC LIFE

Vibhuti Gupta
Department of Public Administration,
University of Lucknow, Lucknow.

"*Corruption is not less than terrorism but we can say that it is 'Financial Terrorism', which shows wide impact in our society, politics, and economy and in other spheres of life.*"

Former CVC of India

Etymologically, the word "corruption" comes from Latin word "corruptus" (to break). It literally means broken object. The thing that is broken might be a moral, a social norm or an administrative rule.

Corruption can be of various types—Bribery, Nepotism, Tax Evasion, Abuse of Power, Illegitimate Profit, Mismanagement of Public Funds, extortion, Linency, Descrimination, Non Transparent behaviour, Illegal tendering of contracts etc.

According to K. Santhanam, Chairman of the committee on Prevention of Corruption —

"*Any action or failure to take action in the performance of duty by government servant for some advantage is corruption.*"

Section 161 of Indian Penal Code defines corruption as such —

"*Whoever being or expecting to be a public servant, accepts or obtains or agrees to accept or attempts to obtain from any person for himself or for any other person any gratification whatever other than legal remuneration as a motive or reward for doing or for bearing to do any official act or for sharing or to show in the exercise of his official functions favour or disfavour to any person or for rendering or attempting to render any service or disservice to any person with the central or any state government or Parliament or Legislature of any state or with any public servant as such, shall be punished with imprisonment of either description for a term which may extend to three years or with fine or with both.*"

Corruption can be both **need based** and **greed based**. Need based is that which forces a person for corruption keeping aside ethical values whereas greed based is unending and infinite lust and appetite for more money. Both are widely prevalent in India. At present India is ranked 73rd most corrupt country out of 102 countries for the year 2002 by a German NGO called Transparency International located in Berlin, West Germany. According to it, Finland is the least corrupt whereas Bangladesh the most. The malaise of corruption is so pervasive in the government apparatus that the then Prime Minister Mrs. Indira Gandhi, while inaugurating a conference of the officers of the CBI in 1981, with the authority of her great office and with all the information available to her, said that *the increasing corruption at all levels, not only bureaucracy and of political life, but also in trade and commerce was a matter of major concern, and there was a feeling among the people that persons known to be corrupt escape the clutches of law because of their power and influence while the small fry are caught in the net.*

Bofors, Tehelka, Fodder, Stamp Duty scam etc are just a few examples to introduce Indian Polity.

"*Our dreams to root out corruption have been shattered so far.*"

The Home Minister of India while addressing the IAS officers, in 1978.

Ever noticed why a cancer patient dies? Because cancer is incurable. But what makes it incurable? The cells in the affected area starts multiplying abnormally affecting that particular area or organ, destroying it forever. Slowly the tentacles of cancer cover the entire body, leading to the death of patient. Corruption is much more fatal than cancer.

Today the condition is such that no area is left corruption free. Previously where corruption existed was when somebody had to get some illegal work done. But now the condition has so deteriorated and worsened that even to get simplest and legal work done bribe is a must, and that is pathetic. *The Times of India,* dated, Feb. 25th, 1972, noted that "*It has been found that every department of the government has become a den of corruption*". People have lost faith in Public Administration due to rampant corruption. It has entered even those area from where it was absent in the past, like cancerous cells. Romain Rolland said on the fall of France, "*French fell because there was corruption without indignation.*"

CORRUPTION IN INDIA IS OMNIPOTENT

What will be the future of India is a matter of grave concern.

Causes of Corruption

Though the government provides enough pay and additional facilities, but we know "*Man is a perpetually wanting animal*" and so whatever he gets is less for him as one satisfied need gives birth to another Abraham Maslow said. But Maslow expressed it in terms of pyramid:

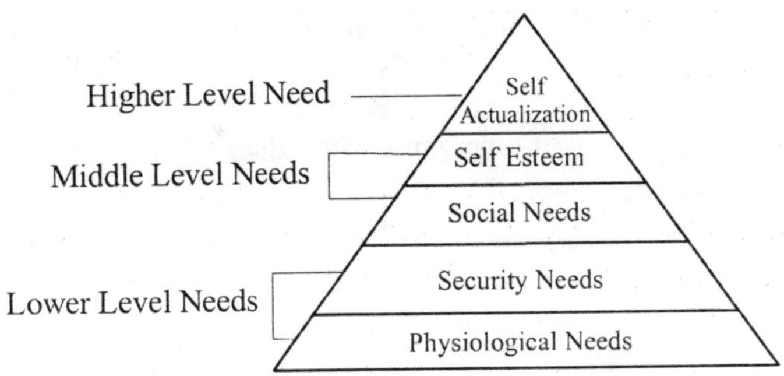

Meaning thereby one need satisfied, move to higher order needs in the hierarchy. And finally according to Maslow, man reaches at the position of Self Actualisation, i.e. excellence in chosen field. But is it really so today?

Today where men is focusing most in lower order needs, i.e. Best Clothing (Multinational Brands, obviously expensive), best build huge villas with marble and granite, eating in costliest food joints (Pizza Hut, Dominos, Barista, Cafe Coffee Day, etc.) They are status symbol now.

Globalization has also increased corruption. Unlimited needs and variety of choices in the market is motivating people for corruption. The consumer today have so many products in the market that to avail all these modern goods/gadgets he compromises with his moral values, keeping aside what has been taught since the childhood or through training.

The process is something like —

Variety of goods in the market

↓

Increased wants

↓

Increased Demand

↓

Limited Income

↓

Lust to have all or more

↓

Compromise with values

↓

Corruption

Once compromised, the spirit is crushed forever, and then sky is the only limit.

Need Based Corruption

- Inflation is yet another cause of corruption. It has forced people to be corrupt, though, not justified, but it can be termed as need based corruption. According to the latest issue of *India Today* inflation is at 8.17%, for the week ending August 18th, highest in the last four years.
- Poverty is one major cause which forces one honest person to be dishonest.

Political cause

- Millions of rupees are funneled to the election funds of the political parties by major industrial houses. This results in higher prices of goods used by general public.
- Political leaders who believe in self preservation rather than nation building.
- Politicians, Bureaucrats and Businessmen — *a fatal triangle... The Rich and Mighty* — they manipulate the system according to their whims and fancies, where poor people are busy in earning square meals for the day.

According to Narayan Hazare

"*Corruption owes its origin to important political causes. Though at the top people preach integrity, more often then not, they lack the virtue of example... Corruption like sacrifice starts at the top and percolating down, colours the whole society.*"

Statutory Cause

- Immunity of officers from action. Either they are not caught, if so, they are suspended for few months or so and then reinstated with full pay etc.
- Due to slow proceedings and cumbersome procedures single file (even the legal ones) take long time to reach to the destination that is why people have very comfortably adjusted to the situation that "*Pay and get your work done.*"

Legal cause

- Inadequate legislation and loopholes in laws.

Modernized mindset — End not means is important

- A feeling is prevalent in the society that one who is rich is respectful. One who lives in palace like houses, moves in a Mercedes or Sonata (costing anything between 25-45 lacs) is much more respected than one who moves in a Maruti 800 or a Two wheeler, immaterial of how he managed to maintain it.

Costliest Mobile handsets are available in the market everyday. To afford all these is an uphill task and corruption is the simplest/ easiest way out.

Constitutional cause

- Article 311 of the Constitution of India is a protection shield for the civil servants, which obviously should be there, keeping in view the prestige and authority attached with the office, but sometimes it acts as a negative shield.

Kautilya in his *Arthashastra* identifies forty types of corruption whereas modern CVC of India has identified thirty types of corruption. "*Corruption was always there but now it has become loot*" said the Editor of a leading National daily in an article on Independence Day, 1982.

Since 1982 till today, corruption has advanced a lot. Stringent Laws are the need of the hour, those Laws that are not only for books, but action is also taken; to check corruption Prime importance should be given to make an aware citizenry, who should know their rights and also Claim them. They should be aware enough not to get exploited anymore.

Moreover, laws and their sub-laws, should also be simplified, so that the educated and not so educated may clearly understand them. The anti-corruption bureau and vigilance organization must be strengthened.

The message to the citizens should be

Know Your Rights and Claim Them

Knowledge is Power and Ignorance is Bliss

Bliss not for the ignorant, but for those who manipulate the ignorant.

27

CORRUPTION IN PUBLIC LIFE: STRATEGIES AND MEASURES

Rajesh Kundu and Suman Lata

Department of Public Administration,
M.D. University, Rohtak (Haryana)

It is not an exaggeration to talk about corruption in terms of a crisis or a cancer endangering India's society, polity and economy. There has been a distinct increase in transactions in Central and State Governments where the presence of corruption in higher bureaucracy and elected political functionaries, often in collusion or in nexus with criminal elements.[1] Lord Acton's insightful remark, "Power corrupts and absolute power tends to corrupt absolutely" appears to have universal validity. It is a hydra-headed monster with no Hercules in sight to slay it.[2] So corruption is a complex phenomenon which is prevalent in all forms of government and for which various factors—sociological, economic, administrative and justice are responsible. Kautilya, the author of "*Arthashastra*" refers in cynical mood to its various forms, and even its inevitability.[3] He remarked "Just as it is impossible not to taste honey or poison when it is at the tip of the tongue so it is impossible for a government servant not to eat up a bit of revenue. And just as it cannot be found out whether a fish swimming through water drinks or not, so government servants cannot be found out while taking money for themselves." Thus, the problem is of a serious nature.[4]

In primitive and medieval days the scope of public administration was minimum. As a result the scope for corruption was also diminished. The outbreak of war unleaded forces of corruption. The unscrupulous officials got golden opportunity to grab wealth. According to the Bengal

Administration Enquiry Committee (1944-45). "The Second World War... breeds conditions which make money making easy... The possession of a license became a thing of high value and dishonest and unscrupulous persons did not hesitate to after bribes in order to secure the license to trade in the commodities effected... War conditions thus, provided the opportunity, and it cannot be denied that it became all too easy for dishonest men to seize the opportunity of illicit gain by reason of two things, namely, (i) ill advised administrative action. (ii) defects in the Law which make detection of offences difficult and which provide inadequate penalties for convicted offenders.

After independence and especially in the last three decades, there is not a day, when you find a newspaper without any news of corruption. Some examples are Mundra Scam 1957, Nagarwala Scam 1971, Tullu Mohan Rao Scam 1974, Cement Scam 1982, Chorhat Lottery Scam 1982, HDW Submarine Scam 1987, Bofors Scam 1987, Chec Pistol Scam 1987, Keo Oil Scam 1988, Air Bus Scam 1991, Security Scam 1992, Sugar Scam 1994, Ms Shoe Scam 1994, Jain Hawala Scam 1995, Telecom Scam 1995, Reliance Scam 1995, Urea Scam 1995, JMM Bribery Scam 1996, Fodder Scam 1996, Indian Bank Scam 1996, ITC Scam 1996, Petrol Pump Scam 1996, Stock Scam 2001, UTI Fisco 2001, Tehelka.Com 2001, Petrol Pump Allotment Scam 2002.[6] Besides, individual cases of corruption are unlimited.

MEANING OF CORRUPTION

Corruption has a variety of meanings. The World Bank has defined as the "Use of public office of private profit". Section 161 of the Indian Penal Code defines "Corruption" in legal terms as under "Whoever being or expecting to be public servant accepts or obtains or agrees to accept or attempt to obtain from any person for himself or for any other person any gratification whatever other than legal remuneration as a motive or reward for doing or for bearing to do any official act or for showing or to show in the exercise of his official function favour or disfavor to any person, or for rendering or attempting to render any service or disservice to any person with the central or any state government or parliament or legislature of any state or with any public servant as such shall be punished with imprisonment of either description for a term which may extend to three years, or with fine, or with both"[8]. In the view of Jacob Van Kalveren, "Corruption means that a civil servant abuses his authority in order to obtain an extra income from the public."[9] As defined by Robert C. Brooks "corruption is the intentional mis-performance or neglect of a recognized duty, or the unwarranted advantage more or less directly personal." According to David H. Bailey. "Corruption is a general term covering misuse of authority as a result of considerations of personal gain which need not be monetary.[11]

ANTI-CORRUPTION STRATEGIES AND MEASURES

There has been several legislative and administrative reports to combat menace of corruption in India. The Prevention of Corruption Act, 1947, which was later amended in 1988 and section 5 of this Act identifies five characteristics of corruption. These are (i) habitual acceptance of gratification, (ii) obtaining valuable items for a kind consideration, (iii) abuse of position to obtain advantage, (iv) possessing property disproportionate to ones income and (v) misappropriation. Former Prime Minister Lal Bahadur Shastri in 1964, set up the Santhanam Committee to review the problem of corruption and give suggestions to make existing measures and machinery more effective. It recommended to set up Central Vigilance Commission (CVC) in 1964. After the Supreme Court stopped into revive in December, 1997 and entrusted it with superintendence over the functioning of the Central Bureau of Investigation (CBI).[12] So the existing machinery and agencies through which corruption is being sought to be eliminated are:

The Special Police Establishment (SPE)

The Special Police Establishment was created by the Government of India under an executive order in 1941 to investigate cases of bribery and corruption in the War and Supply Department as the Defence department was then known. Later, the jurisdiction of the Special Police Establishment extended over the entire governmental machinery of the nation. In 1953, an enforcement wing was added to the Special Police Establishment to deal with offences relating to export and import regulations. With the establishment of the Central Bureau of Investigation (CBI) in 1963, the Special Police Establishment become a part and parcel of the CBI.[13]

Central Bureau of Investigation

The CBI was set up in 1963 by a resolution of the Ministry of Home Affairs. Presently it is under the Ministry of Personnel and enjoys the status of an attached office. It is the main investigating agency of the Central Government and plays an important role in preventing corruption and maintaining integrity in administration. It also provides assistance to the Central Vigilance Commission. Like this every State and Union Territory there are anti-corruption bureaus looking after the anti-corruption work in those states. The Ministry of Home Affairs resolution provided for the following divisions within the Central Bureau of Investigation.

— Investigation and Anti-Corruption Division
— Technical Division
— Crime Records and Statistics Division
— Research Division
— Administrative Division

Presently the CBI deals with the following three broad categories of criminal cases:

(i) Crimes of corruption,
(ii) Economic crimes including frauds,
(iii) Special crimes such as terrorism, bomb blasts etc.

The work load on the CBI is of late increasing. Being the premier investigating agency in corruption cases, it must be made autonomous and be staffed with competent and honest officers.

Central and State Vigilance Commissions (CVCs & SVCs)

The CVC was established in 1964 on the recommendation of the Santhanam Committee on Prevention of Corruption. It was set up by an executive resolution of the Union Government. As such, originally it was neither a constitutional nor a statutory body.

Before August 1998, the CVC was a one-member commission headed by the Central Vigilance Commissioner appointed by the President of India for a term of 6 years, subject to the upper age limit of 65 years. In August 1998, the Central Government promulgated an ordinance conferring statutory status on CVC. The ordinance provides for the constitution of a multi-member commission headed by a Central Vigilance Commissioner and assisted by not more than three vigilance commissioners. They shall appointed by the President of India on the recommendations of a high powered committee under the chairmanship of the Prime Minister, with the Home Minister and leader of opposition in the Lok Sabha as members. The Central Vigilance Commissioner shall have a fixed tenure of 4 years while the vigilance commissioners shall have a fixed tenure of 3 years subject to the upper age limit of 65 years. This ordinance has given the CVC wide ranging powers to supervise the functioning of investigation agencies like the CBI and Enforcement Directorate, and recommend appointment of their heads.[14]

The jurisdiction and powers of the commission covers all the employees of the central government, all the employees of public undertakings, corporate bodies, all the employees of the Delhi Metropolitan Council and the New Delhi Municipal Committee. However, its present jurisdiction is limited to the gazetted officers and officers of equivalent status only. It advises on individual vigilance cases relating to higher civil servants only. It has no power to probe into the cases of political corruption.

The commission receives complaints against corruption and malpractices directly from the aggrieved citizens. It can also gather information about the same from press reports, audit reports, various departments/enterprises concerned, allegation made by member of Parliament reports of Parliamentary Committees. The Commission submit its annual report on its activities to the Personnel Ministry which then lays it before both the Houses of Parliament.

Various States have also on the pattern of CVC, established State Vigilance Commissions in 1964, with similar functions as the CVC.

The CVC is troubled by two factors, e.g. its dependency on the CBI, which leads to avoidable delays and effects the equality of investigation, and the second factor has been the appointment of outgoing commissioner to other government posts, such a practice on the part of the executive does detract from the independence and autonomy of the CVC.[15]

Lokpal and Lokayukta

Citizens in a democratic society should not feel that they are under the governance of the rule of man. The role of the Ombudsman is to establish and promote the governance of the rule of law. An Ombudsman is the Scandinavian institution for the redressal of public grievances, first established in Sweden in 1809. The ombudsman institution is based on the principle of administrative accountability to parliament.

The Administrative Reforms Commission of 1966 headed by Morarji Desai, recommended the creation of two special authorities designated as Lokpal and Lokayukta. The Lokpal was intended to deal with complaints against administrative acts of ministers and secretaries to the government at the Central and State level and the Lokayukta in every state.

A damnsquib for the legislature to table the Lokpal Bill eight times in a row starting from 1968, 1971, 1977, 1985, 1989, 1996, 1998 and 2001 all went in vain. These bills lapsed due to either the dissolution of Lok Sabha or withdrawn by the government. This has happened largely because, there is no political will to eradicate the corruption.[16]

The salient features of the 2001 Lokpal Bill are as follows[17]:

- The bill provides for the establishment of the institution of Lokpal to inquire into allegations of corruption against public functionaries including the Prime Minister, provided the offence committed is within ten years from the day the complaint is lodged.
- The Lokpal shall consist of a chairperson who is or has been a Chief Justice or a Judge of the Supreme Court and two members who are or have been the Judges of the Supreme Court or the Chief Justices of the High Court.
- The chairperson and members shall be appointed by the President of India on the recommendation of a committee headed by the Vice-President of India and comprising the Prime Minister, the Lok Sabha Speaker, the Home Minister, the leader of the House other than the House in which the Prime Minister is a member and leaders of the opposition in both the Lok Sabha and the Rajya Sabha.
- The bill provides for a fixed tenure of three years for the chairperson and the members.
- The bill ensures that the Lokpal is able to act independently and discharge its functions without fear or favour. For this, it provides that the chairperson or a Member of the Lokpal shall not be removed from office, except by an order made by the President on the ground of proved misbehaviour or incapacity.

He can issue the removal order after an inquiry by a committee consisting of the Chief Justice of India and two other Judges of the Supreme Court (next to the Chief Justice in seniority).

- The Lokpal will inquire into complaints alleging that a public functionary has committed an offence punishable under the Prevention of Corruption Act, 1988. The expression 'public functionary' covers all the three categories of union ministers including the Prime Minister and the Members of parliament. The constitutional functionaries such as Judges of the Supreme Court, the Election Commission have been kept out of the purview of the Lokpal.
- The allegations against the Prime Minister related to his functions in the areas of national security and maintenance of public order have been kept out of the purview of the Lokpal.
- To enable the Lokpal to function effectively and in a quasi-judicial manner, it has been vested with the powers of a Civil Court in respect of summoning and enforcing the attendance of any person and examining him on oath.
- The bill provides for an open court or if the Lokpal wishes in-camera proceedings. The proceedings have to be completed within six months, with a provision for extension of six more months.
- The Lokpal is vested with penal powers to discourage frivolous complaints. For such complaints, the fine could be an imprisonment from one to three years including a fine upto Rs. 50,000.

Though the Central Government is still debating the establishment of the institution of Lokpal, many states have already set up the institution of Lokayuktas like Maharashtra, Rajasthan, Bihar, Uttar Pradesh, Madhya Pradesh, Andhra Pradesh, Himachal Pradesh, Orissa, Karnataka, Gujarat and Haryana on the lines suggested by the Administrative Reforms Commission, to deal with the problems of maladministration and administrative injustice.[18] But the Haryana Governor on the advice of Cabinet in September , 1999, repealed the Haryana Lokayukta Act, 1997.[19] Now the Haryana Government has started the process for re-establishment of the institution of Lokayukta after amendment in 2002 but the case is still pending due to the writ laid down by the former Haryana Lokayukta I.P. Vasishth before Uttar Pradesh High Court, Lucknow.[20]

Public Interest Litigation (PIL)

Public Interest Litigation is an innovative strategy that was essentially devised to enable an aggrieved individual to cut through the cumbersome and labourious legal procedures. The credit for the introduction of the PIL goes to the learned judges of the Supreme Court like P.N. Bhagwati and V.R. Krishna Iyer in the late 1970s and it flourished further under many other judges like Venkatachaliah, J.S. Verma and Kuldip Singh.[21]

Public Interest Litigation covers cases filed by any bona fide citizen or their organizations in the courts, to prevent anything like breach of law, or in the matter of awarding public contracts, failure of concerned authorities to enforce laws, or unfair distribution of public resources. The provisions of the civil procedure code are applicable usually in cases of corruption. The court can summon, after examining the related records and orders, the arguments for and against. The accused can defend themselves by filing an affidavit. This does not amount to trial and punishment under the criminal law. The findings are hence not enforceable.[22]

Anti-Corruption Measures

It is not possible in any short treatise to dwell upon all the possible strategies for combating corruption, since a holistic analysis would demand a focus on socio-cultural, economic, political, administrative, legal, judicial and even technological aspects of reforms in the governance system. So the country has not yet reached the point of no return. A set of measures which can be of help are:

- There is a need of Constitutional status to Ombudsman and the Central Vigilance Commission to prevent misuse of discretion and corruption by politicians as well as administrators. In January, 2001 in a national meet of Lokayuktas held in New Delhi, inaugurated by the former Prime Minister Atal Bihari Vajpai, a resolution was adopted to have a common and effective legislation for all State Lokayuktas. The draft legislation was ready in June, 2001 and is yet to be adopted. However, these bodies and the proposed national Lokpal will have genuine legitimacy only if these are made integral components of the Indian Constitution. There is little doubt that with Constitutional teeth, CVC, Lokpal and Lokayuktas will prove to be efficacious.

- Corruption will flourish until the general mass of people resists it with determination and strength. Most of all, the elimination of corruption requires widespread and stead fast opposition to it, coupled with the courage to act against it. There can be no doubt that the people of India can get rid of corruption. So there should be a healthy public opinion against corruption.
- The fountain head of corruption in India, is in the form of election funds. It has to be made less expensive and more rational (Donations to political parties should be made more transparent and laws governing political parties should be made stricter. So election system needs reforms).
- There are the sets of conduct rules for Government servants like All India Services (Conduct) Rules, 1954; Central Civil Services (Conduct) Rules, 1955; Railway Services (Conduct) Rules, 1956. Apart from these there are several rules and instructions dealing with public servants.) In this regard Justice H.R. Khanna has observed "The present condition of rules of conduct or declaration of assets cannot assure rectitude among ministers and other members in the public life. What is needed is a climate of strong public opinion wherein none may dare to deviate from the path of rectitude. The ramparts of a clean and healthy administration are within the hearts of people; laws can only punish occasional lapses."[23] (So effective implementation of conduct Rules is required).
- The root cause of corruption seems to be the complicated procedures of the governmental offices. Delays must be prevented and officials made fully responsive to the needs of all people. These procedures of working need to be evaluated and simplified.
- A system of performance appraisal of public servants and rewards appropriate to their performance may help reduce illegal money transactions. The present system of automatic promotion, annual increments and the like, based on seniority, should undergo changes to ensure efficiency, discipline, honesty and integrity.
- Most corruption is an upshot of secrecy and avowed confidentiality in the conduct of government affairs. Laws relating to official secrecy in India particularly the Official Secrets Act of 1923, have resulted into inaccessibility of information

about and knowledge of government policies, rules, regulations, decisions, accounts and discretionary acts.[24] So most citizens are unable to obtain justice at the hands of manipulative and intelligent bureaucrats. Recently, legislative measures adopted by several States such as Tamil Nadu, Maharashtra, Goa, Rajasthan, Karnataka and Delhi as well as the Central Right to Information Act, 2003 have paved the way for enforcing transparency in the administrative system. There is an inverse correlation between transparency and corruption and therefore, there is a hope that people's control over the governance system will be augmented and in this process, corruption will be mitigated.

- Rules and legal provisions should be amended to enable immediate and exemplary prosecution and removal of corrupt officials without recourse to any political protection.
- Wives of corrupt officials can stop them to become a corrupt person. For instance, the wife of a Food Corporation of India official had been on indefinite fast in the part of city of Visakhapatnam since September 15, 2004 with the avowed intention of weaning away her husband from corruption and she said that her fast was as much against her husband as against the corrupt system and she would continue her agitation till this systematic corruption was dealt with.[25]
- While the complicated and confusing laws should give way to foolproof legislations, least likely to be misused by the culprits, the judicial system must become active to prevent the further erosion of national ethos and ethics. The Indian Prime Minister, Manmohan Singh expressed concern over growing incidents of corruption in judiciary and said judiciary should bring accountability and transparency in its functioning, on inauguration of the Third Conference of Chief Justices and the Chief Ministers at Vigyan Bhawan. Chief Justice of India R.C. Lahoti declared the year 2005 as the "Year of Excellence in Judiciary" and said there will be no place for any corrupt or indolent in the system.[26]
- Elimination of corruption in public services should address preventive, surveillance and deterrent punishment, and deal ruthlessly with the nexus of officials with criminal elements and venal political functionaries.

- Objective and transparent criteria for the transfer and promotion of officials in order to insulate them from political influence in action taken according to law and in public interest.
- Encouraging adoption of code of ethics not only by civil servants but also all public functionaries, media, professionals, and the corporate sector based on constitutional principle and moral values.
- Strengthening role and powers of audit in the identification of financial and procedural irregularities to be followed by investigation for possible corruption.

Mentioned above are a few measures that can be helpful in containing corruption in public life in India. Though a holistic approach will be ideal in tackling the menace of corruption, one cannot wait for all the strategies to synchronize simultaneously. Therefore, incremental and segmented approaches may have to be taken recourse to but even these ought to be consistent and continuous.

CONCLUSION

In essence, the nexus between corrupt individuals and parties to appropriate the State, explains the crisis of Indian governance. In India those who govern the nation are supremely impervious to curb corruption, because the hands of many of them are not clean. The real remedy for the evil of corrupt practices lies in creating a clean and healthy atmosphere in which every person holding a prominent position in the political, social, religious even educational spheres shall follow a certain standard of conduct, a life of austerity and simplicity, and imbibe the good values of our country.[27]

In the end, while moral indignation and political actions are necessary to limit the phenomenon of corruption which grows and distracts the dynamism of the body politics. It is the social fabric of India makes arms length relations difficult to maintain, there is only one way that corruption can be reduced significantly by reducing the role of the government or minimizing government interest in the economy because the role of the government should be facilitator or promoter not as distributor or doer.

REFERENCES

1. Aftab Alam, *Crisis of Governance*, New Delhi: Raj Publications 2003, p. 245.

2. R.K. Arora, "Challenging Corruption in the Indian Public Service" in *Public Governance and Decentralization*, ed. By. S.N. Mishra, A.D. Mishra and Sweta Mishra, New Delhi: Mittal Publications 2003, p. 105.
3. Binayak Prasad, "Corruption at Public Places' New Delhi: *Civil Service Chronicle*, October, 2001, p. 36.
4. S.L. Goel, *Advanced Public Administration*, New Delhi : Deep & Deep 2003, p. 536.
5. *Ibid.*
6. Shariq Mashhadi, "CVC's Attempt to Cleanse the System," New Delhi: *Civil Service Chronicle*, April, 2000, p. 35.
7. *Ibid*, p. 34.
8. Binayak Prasad, *op. cit.*, p. 36.
9. Jacob Van Klaveren, "The Concept of Corruption" in *Political Corruption*, ed. by Arlond J. Heiden heimer, New York: Holt Rinehart and Winston, Inc., 1970, p. 38.
10. *Ibid.*
11. *Ibid.*
12. Shariq Mashhadi, *op. cit.*, p. 34.
13. P. Sri Latha, "Governance in India: The Issue of corruption", in *Governance for Development*, ed., by Pradeep Sahni and Uma Medury, New Delhi: Prentice Hall of India, 2003, p. 89.
14. M. Laxmi Kanth, "*Public Administration*", New Delhi: Tata McGraw Hill, 2003, p. 214.
15. Binayak Prasad, *op. cit.*, p. 37.
16. M. Laxmikanth, *op. cit.*, p. 216.
17. Lok Pal Bill 2001.
18. M. Laxmikanth, *op. cit.*, p. 216.
19. *Hindustan Times*, September 19, 1999.
20. *Dainik Bhaskar*, August 17, 2004, p. 5.
21. P. Srilatha, *op. cit.*, p. 92.
22. *Ibid.*
23. S.L. Goel, *op. cit.*, p. 468.
24. R.K. Arora, *op. cit.*, p. 127.
25. *Hindustan Times*, September 16, 2004, p. 1.
26. *Hindustan Times*, September 18, 2004, p. 8.
27. S.L. Goel, *op. cit.*, p. 474.

28

CORRUPTION IN PUBLIC LIFE: CAUSES AND SOLUTIONS

Sudha Kumari

Department of Education, Aligarh Muslim University, Aligarh, U.P.

The wealth through pious means flourishes;
Those who earn through dishonest means destroyed. — ***Atharva Veda***

Corruption is the enemy within us and around us
Behind every corrupt man there is a greedy family
The honest have value; the corrupt have a price
The corrupt have wealth, the honest have worth
Bright future awaits the honest; shady past haunts the corrupts
The war against corruption is the mother of all wars
If you think you are too small an entity to play any role in the fight
against corruption, think of the potential of an atom!
Just kick start the anti-corruption movement and
it will get momentum!

Corruption is anti-national, anti-economic development and anti-poor. Everyday we read some scams or other cases of corruption in the newspaper headlines. Unfortunately the impact of corruption is all-pervasive that the nation has become immune to the adverse impact of corruption. Corruption is a road block for national prosperity. We must be able to do something about it. We must put into practice the advice of the *Taitreya Upnishad* to resolve our problem. In fact, corruption has become a common part of life. Mainly corruption depends upon three factors:

(a) The first is the set of individual sense of values.

(b) Second is the set of social values which are accepted by the society as a whole.

(c) The system of governance or administration.

Broadly speaking there are two broad factors which determine the extent of corruption.

(i) The social roots of corruption.

(ii) The system of governance.

(i) 1. **Hindu Philosophy:** The social roots of corruption: From a sociological point of view the family is the basis of our society. In the present time the joint family system has been changed into nuclear family, especially in the rural area, but caste still prevails in our society. The bases of entire politics is based on casteism. Jawahar Lal Nehru was speaking about building India into a casteless and classless society. The classless society could never evolve. In the present time caste defines the basis of politics. Hinduism preaches the concept of tolerance. In my opinion, none of the social roots of corruption in India can be traced to basic philosophy of Hindu ethos. We have eternal message of tolerance the sense of forgiveness, the hope held for sinners to come to right path. As many examples are given in *Purans* where a sinner can get redemption by taking the name of Lord Narayan in his last moments.

2. **Family relations:** The root of corruption perhaps arises from the extreme attachment of people to their families. A man who is working in an office thinks that he should earn enough not only for himself but also for his children and his grand-children and for his many generations. Perhaps this is the basic motivation for the accumulation of wealth by the corrupt in our society today.

3. **Power:** Power is misused in our society. The people earn wealth by corruption when they are in power. Society tolerates and does not question how this money is accumulated by them.

4. **Dowry:** Another cause that promotes corruption is the

dowry system in our country. Most people want that their daughters are married off well. In this way people want to earn more and more money. Dowry system is definitely one of the social roots of corruption in our country. The people, who had a clean life in the beginning of their career become vulnerable to corruption in the end because they had to marry their daughters and to see them happy.

5. **Admissions in Public Schools and in Self-Financing Colleges:** The parents right from the preparatory stages want to give their children best education in public or English medium schools, where there is pressure of competition. These schools and colleges charge a lot of donation money and capitation fees which is collected in black.
6. **Public Life:** Corruption which a common man faces at every stage in his day-to-day life is more widespread. There is corruption at higher levels where massive deals or even policies are modified taking into interest one or the other group. Indian voter knows that our entire politics is based on the corruption. Every political party needs funds and this is collected in cash. The voter thinks that all parties are corrupt, there may be some difference in the parties, some are less corrupt and some are more corrupt.
7. **Speed money:** In our country we have red tapism leading to delays, which can be speeded by money. This makes the common man consider paying a bribe as speed money is a part of the system. The common man thinks that the bribe given as speed money as an additional tax by which his work is done. In the public offices, fighting against corruption leads to more harassment to him.

(ii) The system of governance: The second element responsible for corruption in our country is system of governance. Our system of democracy is based on corruption. Why? Because all the political parties have to collect funds in cash, which is black money. The political parties have to oblige the people from whom they collect this black money. We have a scenical view of people living with corruption. The people are accustomed with the view of corruption.

Corruption due to Globalization

Corruption is lack of integrity. Fighting corruption has become a global issue. It is good thing, the globalization process itself has lead to a focus on corruption. In Globalization four elements of economy move across the borders. They are:

(i) Physical capital in terms of plants and machinery.

(ii) Financial capital in terms of money, invested in the capital markets and FDI.

(iii) Labour.

(iv) Technology.

The World Bank defines corruption as the abuse of public office for private gain. While this definition does not include totally private sector corruption. Some of the examples are bribery in purchasing government contracts, benefits, licenses, judiciary decisions, evading custom duties, taxes, or misappropriating budgetary funds.

The present state of India is as a corrupt country is really pathetic. Transparency International, Berlin based NGO published corruption perception index CPI countries from least corrupt to the most corrupt. India ranks 73 out of 102 countries.

SOLUTIONS

1. **Motivate the younger generation for certain values:** Younger generation are to be motivated for certain values like integrity, patriotism, commitment to work, commitment to excellence and so on. The transmission of values happens through a process of emotional or psychological osmosis. The question arises how younger generation is to be motivated? The answer is through role modals. The next question is who are the role modals available in the society? In India politicians and sportsmen play dominant role in shaping values. The values imbibed by the youth today therefore are negative. There is an issue "who will shape the future of our country? Who will motivate younger generation?" The answer is educational

institutes play a very significant role in the plastic years of an individual's life. (Early five years, according to Freud). There is a need for strict discipline. It has been well said that one cannot be a good leader unless one is a good follower. There is a big responsibility of educational institutes in this respect. Mobilization of the youth is very important if we have to fight against corruption. We must systematically inculcate the right values in our youth so that at least in the next 20 years we can bring the basic change in the social perception about corruption.

2. **There is a need for value based education:** NCERT has already prepared a modal syllabus taking this aspect into consideration. Fighting corruption should also be one of the subjects included so that students in the secondary schools and colleges about fighting corruption. The educational institutions should not only focus on imparting the skills but also on values. The institutions will be successful because they will be acting on the advice of the shlokas of *Bhagvad Gita*. The shlokas bring out the facts that where there is vision an action, there is wealth, justice and success.
3. **There should be judicial control of corruption:** The degree of corruption depends upon three factors. The first is the individual values cherished by a person. This depends upon religious background, family background and the culture in which he is brought up. The second factor that affects the level of corruption is the social values. In Indian society we take a very tolerant view of corruption. The third factor that affects the level of corruption is the system of governance, that is the legal framework and the institutions that form the basic structure of government. Corruption in our system flourishes because of the following factors:
   (a) Scarcity of goods and services.
   (b) Red tape and delay
   (c) Lack of transparency
   (d) Cushions of safety which have been created by the legal system on the principal that everybody is innocent till proved guilty. The legal provisions and procedures are effectively exploited by the corrupt to escape punishment.

If we have to think of legally preventing corruption we will have to see whether we can frame laws in such a way that the basic factors which promote corruption, at least in the Indian context can be checked. In the Indian context there are four major players in corruption. These are—the corrupt politicians, the corrupt officials, the corrupt businessmen and the criminals. In so far as the Indian context is concerned our laws do not seem to have been effective so far. Absolute laws can be very conducive for corruption therefore there is a need for introducing a "sunset principal" so that the obsolete and obscure laws do not become an instrument of corrupt public servants to exploit the public. Equally important is the need for transparency. Greater transparency and empowering of public is the second major method using law to prevent corruption. An increasingly aware public can be an effective support to the concerned legal authority in checking corruption. If we want to use the law of checking corruption we should look at the basic motivation of the corruption. It is the greed.

The effectiveness of judiciary can be enhanced if we can find a method by which the entire legal process can be expedited. The challenge before us in India is what can be done to improve the legal system so that the quick punishment is meted out to the corrupt. The major weakness is the delays inherent in the legal system, the lack of adequate number of judges and courts and so on. We have to tackle this issue effectively if we want to see judicial control in India. It is not the laws that matters but the extent to which they are implemented.

1. **Need for accountability in every sphere.** Accountability means responsibility for performance. In our country we find that we have the best articulated policies and programs. But when it comes to information we generally find that
   (i) Policies are not implemented at all.
   (ii) If they are implemented they show counter-productive results.
   (iii) If and when they are implemented there is great inefficiency and lack of grace in implementation. Examples of implementations of policies may be seen in the many antipoverty programs launched by the government with the great vigour. But the result is that only a small fraction of the benefit in these programs reaches to the target population. Rajeev Gandhi observed that for every rupees

meant for the poor, hardly 15 paisa reached the poor and out of remaining 85 paisa, 40 paisa may be spent on administration overheads, but 45 paisa definitely is corruption.

The first factor that comes in the way of effective implementation of the policies is the failure of the system of checks and balances which our Constitution provides. The judiciary, executive and the legislature have their role to play. If the agencies which are designed to play their respective roles do not function effectively. The issue of political interference in administration has been raised by many as one of the reasons why implementation of policies do not take place. Benjamin Franklin said "nothing is more certain in life than death and taxes." For a civil servant nothing is more certain than death, taxes, transfer, retirement.

The politicization is one of the important feature of the administration today. After nearly 5 decades of independence, the relationship between the political leadership and beauracracy therefore is a very important factor when it comes to implementation of policies and better governance. Accountability can be induced if there is a fair assessment of performance; and performance which is outstanding is rewarded and the performance which is below par is punished.

2. There is a need for the inclusion of the new fundamental right like the right to corruption-free service. It sends the signal throughout the country that there is a national consensus recognizing the problem of corruption as a social evil and has conferred the right on the citizens to enable him to take on the corrupt public servants. There should be awareness about the inclusion of a new fundamental right among new generation of the students. Which will modify social behaviour?

I would like to conclude unless there is a plan of action, mere sentiments or unguided action will not bring results. It is very important to sensitize and empower every Indian citizen who want to fight corruption. What is needed is a new, well thought out programs for national regeneration on the basis of shared ethical values and ideals of transparent integrity in governmental administration as well as in all aspects of political and public life. The vision of corruption-free society has to be translated into action. The watch word must be: act, do not wait for the act.

REFERENCES

Vittal, N., *Corruption in India*. Academic foundation, New Delhi, 2003.

29

CORRUPTION IN PUBLIC LIFE

Mritunjay K. Misra
Department of Political Science,
Govt. P.G. College, Lohaghat

Corruption in politics and public life is not a new phenomenon. As early as 1000 B.C. the laws of Manu stated that corrupt officials who receive bribes from villagers are to be banished and their property should be seized. This speaks not only of the prevalence of corruption but the condemnation of such practices. Throughout history common people, officialdom and others such as foreign observers have remarked upon and condemned Corruption, bribery, greed and the coveting of another's property. Ibn Batuta, an Arab visitor to the court of Mohammad-Bin-Tughlaq and later the Qazi of Delhi for sometime (in the 14th century) wrote about the fondness of the Sultan for giving and receiving gifts. This practice was actively encouraged by the merchant community which would advance sums of money to people desirous of audience with the Sultan. These merchants would then get back their dues from the gifts given by the Sultan to his visitors in return for theirs! Edward Gibbon in his introduction to the Decline and Fall of the Roman Empire calls Corruption "the most infallible symptom of constitutional liberty". Lord Acton in his Historical Essays and Studies said these words which are oft quoted now: "Power tends to corrupt, and absolute power corrupts absolutely. Great men are almost always bad men".

The word corruption according to the Chamber's Dictionary means rottenness; impurity; bribery. But in the broad understanding of people Corruption is associated with bribery. If we look closely for a moment we will realise that it is an impurity or rottenness in the moral fibre that then manifests itself in the taking of bribes. These connotations are actually related to each other in this context. In recent times we have heard about large, public scandals related to the stock market and defense purchases. None of these facts can reconcile us to the reality that barely five decades after independence corruption has established itself firmly in our country. Functionaries expect to get bribes in order to do work for which they are paid by the government to do but which they have neglected deliberately in their exepectation.

People now believe that no work however small or routine can be done without paying "something" to "someone" in government offices, educational institutions and even in legal matters. One may call it a douceur (a sweetener), "speed money" (that which speeds up work), or "palm-grease" (to smoothen the working of the palm) or other such euphemistic terms to make the facts of bribery acceptable. The fact remains that there is no aspect of life that corruption has not touched. We can explain that the rising population has added to the numbers everywhere, to the number of applications and increased the requirement of college seats and work positions and scarcity of resources. In other words, the supply has not kept up with the demand. Hence, in order to avoid wasting time over red tape and official procedures we prefer to advance our case or our place in the queue by offering bribes which we know will get the work done. We can further explain it by saying that inflation erodes the salaries of employees who then expect to supplement their incomes by taking bribes, and hence the employee or functionary is not to blame but his circumstances. Here his circumstances corrupt him in two ways. In order to get the bribe he holds up or slows down the work which is his duty to do. He develops a frame of mind which is conditioned to the taking of bribes. Henceforth, he will do nothing without being offered the "incentive" to work. He not only corrupts himself but he also corrupts the work ethic. This contributes to the tardy functioning of government departments and to the expenditure of government machinery. We see that corruption as the taking of bribes is connected to corruption as a fall in human values.

The causes of corruption are many and complex. Any situation where there are large government expenses, a climate of shortage, an increase in bureaucracy and the functions of government, numerous controls and licences and a weak-willed or inexperienced government unable to check corrupt practices is conducive to the growth of corruption. Post-independence India with its democracy in its infancy, its teething problems, its rising population, and its vast sub-continent has had the ideal conditions for the growth of corruption. This situation has been compounded by the influx into different levels of leadership by leaders of low moral integrity. The first line of leaders during the independence struggle were giants who gave way to others who did not measure up to them. Gradually, the vision faltered and nepotism set in, bringing in its wake the distribution of favours and disbursement of largesse which could then be passed on to others with less influence in exchange of favours or money.

Western sociologists and writers often attribute the prevalence of corruption in eastern countries to their cultural and traditional mores. The solidarity of kinship has been seen as the cause of nepotism. Traditional loyalties to the family or clan than to the society and nation at large are said to contribute to the lack of clear perception between private gains and public good. However, eastern sociologists feel that there is an over simplification of the case and it may even be erroneous to an extent in its conclusion. Corruption is human in its wide prevalence and its causes are general and historical as people down the times and of different cultures have experienced the same type of corruption. We may safely say that cultural practices like the giving of gifts or kinship are avenues to corruption, rather than cause of it. People use these opportunities to serve their own ends.

It has been observed that along with high inflation rates which create the need for an extra income, readymade situations available within a system for corruption such as shortages and controls, and the weakness of a government's anti-corruption machinery, it is also the easy social acceptance of people who are known to have become rich on corruption that encourages an atmosphere conducive to corrupt practices. Although it is true that no society condones the taking of bribes or encourages corrupt practices, it is also true that individuals envy the amassed wealth and grand lifestyles of others and do not ask questions about the sources of their wealth. It is a sad fact that there is a dilution of moral values and not many voices are raised in protest when others and not they are victims of the greed of the system. It may be remembered that Mr. Khairnar created a brief stir when he took up a crusade against Mr. Sharad Pawar, the then Chief Minister of Maharashtra. People were impressed by the sincerity of

Mr. Khairnar's voice and the implications of his voice, but not for long, the power of office is such that a few dissenting voices can not harm it.

Popular magazines carry articles on particular cases of corruption, and interviews with key figures and the largely unquestioning and sensation-hungry public laps it up, seeing it only as a distant issue and often not aware of the deeper implications. People have become insensitive due to their inability to visualize a change in the system.

Arguments and justification such as "Politicians are known to be corrupt", when the rival party was in power, the corruption was more", "There is corruption everywhere, all over the world", "Our leaders are also human, and anyway what is a few hundred crores for such a large country as ours?" are all heard too often and are the indications of the fall of inhuman expectations and values. People are willing to accept a lowering of standards in their rulers and consequently in themselves. India is a country where people like cults and exalt cult-figures. We follow the examples set by our leaders.

The leaders of the country have become apologists for the prevalence of corruption today. The freedom struggle saw the appearance of political leaders who were men of vision. They led and the people followed unquestioningly, because they could see noble qualities in their leaders. Unselfish devotion for the common cause and personal sacrifice were the order of the day. What we find today is exactly the opposite of what was then. Our politicians are so many sores and cancerous growths in the body politic. They are motivated only by selfish interests for personal gains, utterly unconcerned by the sacrifice of national welfare at the alter of their greed, plundering and amassing wealth in order to make sure of a luxurious existence of their families and dependents. Politicians in office and out of it have been accused of hiding their ill-gotten wealth in foreign banks. There is a general atmosphere of chaotic unrest, lowered morale, an up-for-grabs philosophy at work, while the poor people become more and more abject in their misery. We may draw the conclusion that people deserve the government they get as it is they who elect such leaders. But like many other truisms this is only half true. Politicians forget the promises they made before the election as soon as they elected to office. Politics is a business in our country just like any other commercial ventures. It is the most successful and lucrative business. That is why elections are so important. That explains the vast sums spent on wooing the voters, on conducting elections and on winning or being re-elected. The electorate is a veritable cornucopia, the horn of plenty or even the mythical Kamdhenu which can be milked endlessly. The business of getting rich at the expense of the electorate and the country is conducted by the most important leader right from the top to the smallest politician at the bottom. It is open, very much in the public eye, as can be seen in the collection of party funds and the lavish expenditure on mammoth rallies. Such activities receive the blessing of even Prime Minister.

The whole election process is nothing but a corruption of all the moral values of a human being. In order to buy votes and ensure victory all manner of corrupt practices are followed. They can range from simple gifts of money, to advance distribution of licences and franchises in return for votes and vote-banks. Providing exemption from following the laws of the land and protection from prosecution by the law are further instances. The poor voter who places his trust in the election process and in the candidates for office is betrayed. He becomes pessimistic and fatalistic and utters such platitudes as "What do I care as long as I get my daily bread', "Somebody has to govern and it does not matter who; one is as bad as the other". But in the case of the millions living below the poverty line this can not be considered a mere mouthing of platitudes because they see all around them honest labour is rewarded with suffering without hope, whereas corrupt practices flourish from day to day. This is why anybody with a little money can tempt them to break social and moral laws. A number of people take to party work at the time of elections hoping to enhance their income with the handouts made then in order to swell the numbers or the following of any party or candidate. Due to such situations greed, selfishness, insensitivity, escape from justice, contempt for law and a burgeoning lawlessness contribute to the fall in human standards. People simply accept it as a part of everyday life, exercise a little stoic calm set aside additional allocation of expenditure when they need anything done. They have lost faith in straightforward dealings and thinks in terms of going to politicians to beg for favours, or buying the services of anti-social elements to settle disputes.

It may seem doubtful in the present circumstances to think of remedial measures. However, though the root has spread everywhere, there are certain steps which can be taken in order to set the process of cleaning up in motion. It is tantamount to Hercules' task of cleaning the Augean stables; but, it can be done with a concerted effort between determined leaders and a determined public. As with all other reform measures it must begin at home; that is, people should first exercise self-control in order to decide for themselves that they will put the country above self. They have to give up selfish interests and self-gain in the larger interests involved. They have to be sensitive to the exploitation around them and resist it wherever they see it. They have to help others to resist it also. They have to watch for accountability in the leaders they elect and press for the right to recall elected representatives if they see them becoming indifferent to the electorate.

A lot of the effort to stop corrupt practices has to come from the top, from a leadership which has the will to fight corruption and dismiss corrupt officials. Politicians should however, have reduced powers so that they do not interfere unnecessarily in the functioning of the different government departments. Issues and problems should be solved without allowing them to become politicised. The advice of professionals and professional bodies of a non-parliamentary type should be sought in tackling the problems before the country. The administration has to be streamlined in order to eliminate the possibility of corrupt practices. Economic policies which will ensure a moderate standard of living for the people will also discourage the need to ask and receive bribes. Moral and ethical considerations do not dominate the strata of society which does not receive even two meals a day. So instead of looking for mere moral upliftment, the road could be made easier by economic reforms and education. Above all else, we need leaders who by personal example and selflessness will set the ball rolling and allow the influence to permeate to the lower levels of politicians and functionaries.

REFERENCES

1. *Third Concept.*
2. *Mainstream.*
3. *Economic and Political Weekly.*
4. *The Hindu.*
5. *India Today.*

30

"POWER CORRUPTS...": A STUDY OF POWER PURCHASE AGREEMENTS IN ANDHRA PRADESH

M.V.S. Koteswara Rao & B.P.C. Bose

Department of Political Science and Public Administration, Archarya Nagarjuna University, Nagarjuna Nagar, Guntur, A.P.

"Corrupt influence is itself the perennial spring of all prodigality and of all disorder; it leads us with more than millions of debts; takes vigour from our arms, wisdom from our councils, and every shadow of authority and credit from the most venerable parts of the constitution."

Edmund Burke

We start the discussion by understanding corruption as a behaviour which deviates from the formal duties of public role because of private regarding, pecuniary or status gains; or violation of rules against the exercise of certain types of private regarding influence. This includes such behaviour as bribery, nepotism and misappropriation (Nye: 2000, 47)

The purpose of this paper is two-fold. One, to present the growth of Andhra Pradesh State Electricity Board, which is spectacular, and serves as a model, and two, to discuss the rationality of the Power Purchase Agreements, which ultimately turned out to be anti-people, benefiting the private companies at the cost of public money. This paper is divided into three parts. The first part presents the growth and contribution of the Andhra Pradesh State Electricity Board (APSEB), the second part discusses the Power Purchase Agreements and the last part bears some conclusions.

I

The Andhra Pradesh State Electricity Board (APSEB) was established in 1959 to take charge of generation and distribution.[1] At that time power was a comfort of the elite. Only a few families in a town used to enjoy this luxury. Most of the villages around the cities and all remote villages did not have the facility of electrification. In short, power was the costliest commodity, available to those few rich families in the society. The total power installation was a paltry 213 MW, against a population of almost four crores. Since then, the growth of APSEB was spectacular and sound like a folklore story.

Growth in the Services of the APSEB: The installation capacity rose to 5612 MW in 1999 from 213 MW in 1959. In addition, it gets

Table 1. The Details of Power Sector in Andhra Pradesh by 31-11-1999

S.No.		
1.	Maximum needs fulfilled	6.480 MW
2.	Production in 1998	4796 MW
3.	Electricity Purchase—Import (1998-99)	13.569 MW
4.	Units Handled by the System	38.788 MW
5.	Sold, Utilized Units total	26.168 MW
6.	Utilization per head	475 KWH
7.	Transformers Distribution	1,67,908 Numbers
8.	Electrified Cities	264 Numbers (100%)
9.	Electrified Villages	26,565 Numbers (100%)
10.	Electrified Satellite Villages	21,450 Numbers (65.34%)
11.	Electrified S.C. and S.T. Colonies	39,874 Numbers (92.52%)
12.	Electrified Minority Colonies	12,955 Numbers
13.	Agricultural Pumpsets (including Rescos)	18,84,678 Numbers
14.	Consumers total (including Rescos)	1,09,69,615 Numbers
15.	Total Employees	74,980 Numbers
16.	Earnings	4,824.68 crores
17.	Investment	1,832.28 crores

Source: 1. Computed from the tables provided by APSEB, 1998.
2. APSEB, 97 : 105

897 MW as its share from the Central sector and 273 MW from the Joint sector. So, the installed capacity of the State was 6782 MW— a

rise by 34 times. Its capacity to meet the peak demand rose from 146 MW in 1959 to 6480 MW in 1999—a rise by 44 times. The number of service connections rose from 2.7 lakhs in 1959 to one crore and ten lakhs by 1959—a rise by 36.7 times. The number of agricultural connections rose from 18,000 in 1959 to 18.85 lakhs in 1999—a phenomenal rise by 100 times. In 1959, 686 million units of power was supplied by APSEB. The supply rose to 40,574 million units in 1999—a rise by 59 times. The length of the transmission and distribution lines was 6,08,000 km in 1999. The total number of consumers was about eleven millions of which 1.8 millions were agricultural consumers (Government of Andhra Pradesh, 2002 and APSEB, 1998)[2]. The following table shows the spectacular growth of APSEB and its service to the society, particularly to backward sections.

The operational side of the Board was governed by the 1948 Electricity (Supply) Act. Section 59 of the Act stipulates that the power generation and distribution shall be so managed that the Boards must earn 3 per cent of profit on net assets value. The state governments are responsible for deciding the tariff. If any state government is not in a position to fix the tariff to ensure the 3 per cent profit, it shall meet that amount as subsidy to the Electricity Boards. Thus it is mandatory on the part of State Governments to ensure 3 per cent profit per year. In terms of Plant Load Factor, which reflects upon the efficiency of power generating units in utilising the installed capacity, the APSEB units showed an extraordinary performance.[3]

The following Table shows the details of power generation and the PLF of the APSEB (GENCO since 1999) from 1992 to 2001-2002.

However, the active persuasion of Rural Electrical Programme (REP) from early 1970s onwards started straining the resources of APSEB.[4] The importance rural of electrification in the socio-economic development of a country with a predominant rural area and agriculture oriented economy is unanimously accepted. But the problem lies in extending the network to remote areas located thousands of kilometers away from cities. Rural electrification means extending the power lines, establishing a number of substations, transformers and employing additional staff. To quote the Indian Institute of Public Enterprises report, "the transmission problem which India faces is that of rapidly electrifying vast rural areas. In fact, every MW of installed capacity in India has over 4 km of transmission lines with voltages of 66 KU

Table 2. Details of Power Generation and the PLF

Year	Plant Load Factor		Rank among SEBs
	APGENCO	All India Average	
1992-1993	64.9	57.1	III
1993-1994	68.7	61.0	III
1994-1995	70.1	60.0	II
1995-1996	78.2	63.0	I
1996-1997	78.1	64.4	I
1997-1998	82.3	64.7	I
1998-1999	77.6	64.6	III
1999-2000	83.2	67.3	II
2000-2001	85.1	69.0	I
2001-2002	86.3*	69.9	I

*Highest PLF achieved by APGENOC, APSEB till 1998.

Source: APGENCO, A Decade of performance (1992-2002), p. 3

and above. This may be contrasted with the situation in U.K. which has about 0.3 KM of HV lines per MW of installed capacity; U.S.A. which adds 0.6 HV lines for each added MW of capacity; and 1.5 KM/KW of added capacity in Canada. In Andhra Pradesh the total length of the power lines in terms of circuit Kms reached a figure of 1,55,877 by 1978" (IPE, 1982, 131).

Since, the rural India is very poor, the decision to extend the electrical facility implied the subsidised supply to agricultural sector. The average cost of delivering one unit of low Tension Power was paise 27.60 and paise 33.90 and the return from these sectors was paise 15.20 and paise 13.55 in '70-71 and '72-73 respectively. The power supply to agricultural consumers has become a perpetual source of vast losses for APSEB. So is the case with all Power Boards of South India. To quote from Institute of Public Enterprises (1982: 181) "... the power supply to agricultural consumers has become a perpetual source of vast losses for the four SEB's, since the profits earned on account of the supply to the rest of the consumers do not balance out when compared with the losses incurred in supplying this sector. The State Electricity Boards are finally left with marginal profits and many times pushed deep into the red. This, however, is in line with the Indian position in this context". As Dayal (1980: 252-53) rightly said: "Howsoever efficiently an electricity board may function organisationally, and howsoever economically its affairs may be managed and howsoever cost-conscious it may be and cost-oriented its rate structure may be for the non-rural sector consumers, as long as it is expected to assume the expanding obligations of rural electrification with the inevitable concomitant implication of a subsidised or concessional tariff structure for rural consumers, the Board cannot avoid incurring losses, mounting arrears of interest charges and continued inability to build up the various prescribed reserves, the receding prospects of its being able to repay the principal amounts borrowed from State governments or of generating any worthwhile internal surpluses to finance expansion plans.

The losses incurred by APSEB because of the Rural Electrification Programme were very high. In 1976-77 APSEB lost 1170 lakhs. Though it earned 1066 lakhs from other sectors, its year end balance was on the negative side with 104 lakhs loss, before subsidy. The trend was an all India one. Because of Rural Electrification programme, there was a sudden spurt in the consumption in the agrarian sector. The electricity consumption was only 6.0 per cent of the total Electricity consumption in India. The figure jumped up to 10.2 per cent in 1970-71, 14.4 per cent in 1975-76 and reached 31.2 per cent in 1998-99 (Economic Survey, 2000-2001, Govt. of India).

Further the rising prices in coal and Railway tariff also put burden on the finances of APSEB. In fact there was a 100 per cent increase in the prices (see Murthy, 2001: 42). Even under these highly adverse circumstances the APSEB never faced unmanageable financial crisis. It not only regularly met its debt servicing commitments with manageable loss. For the first time the APSEB faced a financial loss of 1134 crores in 1997-98. This was prior to subsidy component calculation. After the mandatory subsidy from the state government, the loss would have been covered and a minimum of 3 per cent profit would have recorded by the APSEB.

The State Government which is bound by the 1948 Act to give subsidy to ensure 3 per cent profit, if the State Electricity Board does not earn this amount on its own, never bothered to meet this obligation.[5] For example, the net assets of the APSEB were 2547 crore during

1985-1990 (APSEB 98: 8). The net profit after expenditure including debt servicing must be 76.5 crore. But the state government never bothered to keep the profit rate of 76.5 crores. The following table gives the details of profit of APSEB and the subsidy given by the state government during 1985-90.

Table 3. Net Loss faced by the APSEB because of Government's Failure to meet the Statutory Obligation.

Details	*1987-88*	*1991-92*	*1994-95*
Income/loss of APSEB	+ 29.23	+ 14.9	-836
Actual subsidy paid by the government	0.00	69.54	944.11
Mandatory subsidy to be paid by the government, i.e. 3% of net assets including the losses incurred	76.5[1]-29.23 =47.2 crores	105[2]-14.9 = 90.1 crores	186[3]+836 = 1022 crores
Due from the government or net loss to the APSEB	47.2 crores	90.1 crores	1022 crores

Source: APSEB, 97 : 105 and 98 : 105

Income: Sale of Power + miscellaneous - Revenue expenditure, Depreciation and interest charges.

Net Loss: Net Income + subsidy $\pm$ 3% assets.

(1) 3% profit on 2547 crores of assets of the APSEB.
(2) 3% profit on 3500 crores of net assets of the APSEB.
(3) 3% profit on 6190 crores of net assets of the APSEB.

II

It is in this background that the State Government decided to reform or privatize the Power Sector. The reasons like bridging the gap between demand and supply, need to improvise the financial performance of the APSEB, to control the commercial losses[6] etc., were offered as the immediate reasons for privatization (www.andhrapradesh.com. /07/16/2002 and also see Government of

Andhra Pradesh, 2001, IBRD, 1999, TRANSCO, 2000, World Bank 1997 and 1999).

The practical side of the reforms was rude shock including to those who saw privatization as a panacea. Each and every imagined and propagated advantage was evaporated within no time. Instead of free competition, both Government and consumers became captive in the hands of promoters. Government was forced/gratified to sign on the doted lines. Normally private sector means competition among producers and choice to the consumers to select the goods that are efficient and cheap. But what ultimately turned out to be an anti-thesis. Not only that the private power projects violated all formal conditions set in the PPAs but were also allowed to pocket hundreds of crores of public money at their will.

The *modus operandi* was unbelievably simple. Establishment of a power project was made lucrative. The promoters have to invest only 30 per cent of the project cost. The rest can be raised from lending institutions. If the promoters are shrewd enough, they can appreciate the cost of the project, get more loan and save their 30 per cent of investment. Even the interest paid to the bankers and the income tax on the earnings of the promoters will be paid by the TRANSCO. In fact there was a strong argument that the promoters over quoted the project costs to avoid investment.[7] The TRANSCO and the state government stood as guarantees on behalf of private promoters. In case the promoters fail to repay the money, the TRANSCO and the state government will have to pay. As per the provisions of the PPAs, every promoter has to complete the project within certain period or pay heavy liquidity damages. When the promoters failed to complete projects, the TRANSCO failed to impose the damages and lost hundreds of rupees of income. For example, just in case of two projects Lanco Kondapalli and Spectrum—the TRANSCO lost 150 crores.[8]

The power from the private power projects was purchased at prohibitive cost compared to the cost paid to public sector and Joint Sector power projects. For example the cost of the power generated by 100 Mega Watt (MW) Simhadri Thermal Power Station of NTPC was fixed at Rs. 4.18 crore per MW and the cost of the power generated by 420 MW Rayalaseema Thermal Power Project of APGENCO was fixed at Rs. 3.57 crore per MW. But in case of private sector power projects it was between 4.75 crores to 5.25 crores per Mega Watt. Converted into unit cost, the payment is as follows (Table 4).

Table 4. The Unit Cost Paid to Different Power Projects

Name of the project (gas based)	*Charge paid for a unit*	*Projected unit charge in case of appreciation in the cost of gas**
GVK unit II	1.84	2.55
GVK unit I	2.24	2.94
Konaseema Okwell Pvt. Ltd.	1.84	2.55
Gowtami Power Project	1.84	2.25
Vemagiri Power Generation Limited	1.84	2.25
Lanco Kondapalli	2.31	2.94
APGPCL (Public Sector)	1.60	2.00
Average cost of power generated by all public sector projects	1.43	

Source: APREC orders: www.ercap.org/.

Order No. 105/2003 in op 402/2002

Order No. 106/2603 in op 2/2002

Order No. 107/2603 in op 3/2002

Order No. 108/2003 in op 4/2002

Order No. 109/2003 in op 5/2003

Order No. 94/2003 in op 392/2001

Also see, www.cea.nic.in/data

Andhra Jyoti (vernacular daily) 14.7.2004 to 21.4.2004, Praja Sakti (Vernacular daily) 7.8.2002 to 9.8.2004.

On average the TRANSCO buys 1500 million units of power from each project. The difference of unit charges between public sector and private sector power projects works out to around 600 crores a year (average cost difference of 0.60 paise × 1500 million units each from six power plants in the private sector).

The Rate of Return (RoR) on fixed cost of the private power project was fixed at 16 per cent. Implication being all the power projects were allowed to regain their investment within a short period of six years (16% × 6 years = 96%). Surprisingly, the TRANSCO agreed to pay the RoR for the entire period covered by the PPA (the minimum period covered by the PPA is 15 years). If the PPA is for 15 years, then the private power projects get 16 per cent RoR for 15 years. Yet, another surprising clause of the PPAs is, the yearly payments are not deducted to decide the 16 per cent RoR on subsequent payments. If the cost of a project is assumed as 100 crores and it starts production in 2001, the TRANSCO pays 16 per cent RoR (i.e., 16 lakhs) in 2002. In 2003 it pays 16 per cent RoR not on 99.84 crores (100 crores — 16 lakhs paid in 2002) but on 100 crores. Therefore, an agreement on 100 crores fixed cost that is valid for 15 years fetches the promoter a whooping 200.40 crores. Besides, the variable cost of the project-fuel salaries, interest paid, income tax etc.—is also born by the TRANSCO. This ridiculous agreements are bound to cause heaviest damages to the public exchequer. The amounts paid and to be paid to the agreement period to various private power projects are given below:

Table 5. Amount Earned by the Private Power Projects on Their Fixed Cost

Name of the Project	*Installed capacity*	*Project cost*	*Payment made*	*Payment due for the remaining period*
GVK II	216 MW	816 crores	1540 crores	790 crores
Spectrum	208 MW	748 crores	1130 crores	1020 crores
Lanco Kondapally	351 MW	1380 crores	1288 crores	2256 crores
BSES	220 MW	850 crores	225 MW	1650 crores

Source: Individual power purchasing agreements between TRANSCO and promoters, as mentioned in APERC orders (see, www.ercap.org/)

Andhra Jyoti, Vernacular daily, 16th and 17th July, 2004.

The integrity of the government had become doubtful in the light of its failure to pay the 3 per cent RoR to the Andhra Pradesh Electricity

Board before the reforms. Had the state government respected the mandate of 1948 Act and duely paid 3 per cent return, the APSEB would have accumulated hundreds of crores as reserve fund.

As we have seen already the Thermal Projects in Andhra Pradesh consistently turned out 75 per cent and above PLF. But in case of IPPs, the PLF is fixed around 68 per cent (65 to 68 per cent). The surrender to the IPPs is such that, the Government accepted to pay 0.525 per cent on equity to the private power projects as incentive for every 1 per cent of PLF over 68 per cent. This works out to be Rs. 82 crores for every one per cent raise in the PLF. If the same 'affection' had showered on APSEB units, thousands of crores of rupees would have been earned by them every year, thereby permanently avoiding the poisonous bytes of the private projects.

More mysterious is the clause that the APTRANSCO shall buy the power generated by the IPPs, whether it needs it or not. Even if TRANSCO does not draw any power from IPPs it has to pay the fixed cost of the projects. The APTRANSCO did not buy a single unit of power from LVS Project and yet paid 37 crores each in 2003 and 2004 in the form of fixed cost and still has to pay the same amount for the next 13 years (see, Srinivasa Rao, Government gives into Reliance on PPAs. *Deccan Chronical*, 8th August, 2004) What happens if Hydel Centres start generation with full capacity and APGENCO meets the demand by itself? The Government is too busy to think about these sundry details (For a critical review of PPAs see, 1. K. Sreenu, M. Thimma Reddy, N. Sree Kumar, and D. Narasimha Reddy, www.prayasa pune.org/; Nair, PNV, 2002, Srihari, V. 1997; Peoples Monitoring Group on Electricity Regulation, 2001; Raghu, 2001 and Raghu and Satyanarayana, 2001).

III

Thus we have seen that the power purchasing agreements between APTRANSCO and private power promoters are highly mysterious. These agreements were entered by the APTRANSCO in the name of gap between increasing demand for power and available power. The report of the then House Committee of the Andhra Pradesh Legislative Assembly on Power Situation in the State in 1999, which estimated that the available power was more than enough to meet the demand (see, Rao, Koteswara, 2004) was ignored by the then government.

Even the observations of the Comptroller and Auditor General of India were not cared and the signing spree was continued (see Appendix). What would have been the motivation behind the agreements? Why such naked favouritism was shown to private promoters at the cost of public money and trust? Why deliberate attempts were made to exterminate the highly efficient public sector power plants in the state? What made the government to go for privatization when there was a possibility of investing half the amount paid to the private promoters and having most efficient and people friendly power projects in public sector? Wasn't it a violation of all written rules and unwritten ethics of public life? Weren't the combined opposition and the press justified in attributing motives and corruption to the people occupying the positions in the government? Wasn't it irrational and anti-people to sign the PPAs which will drain the public money out? These questions naturally bother the concerned. It is not possible to justify the agreements. One has to conclude that it was a deliberate attempt to cater to the thirst of the private sector at the cost of public sector and public money. The confidence that was bestowed by the people in their representatives was misused to pamper few promoters. We may perhaps conclude by borrowing a statement from *Peoples Democracy* (Vol. 26, no. 2): "If the Financial Institutions are giving the money on the basis of AP Transco's guarantees, why should the IPPs own the projects? Textbook capitalism tells us capitalists get profits as they take risks. Apparently, this is not true of capitalism in India and certainly not in the Power sector. Gone also is the argument that IPPs bring in additionality of resources" (*PD*, Vol. 26, No. 2). Also gone the much-trumpeted opportunities like chance of competition, efficiency, economy and consumer facility.

APPENDIX

Extracts from the Report of the Comptroller and Auditor General of India on GVK I:

- Due to delay in completion of the project and the consequent exchange rate variations, the project cost may go up by Rs. 113.62 crore. This increase entails an additional burden in the shape of higher tariff on the Board by Rs. 17.76 crore per annum.
- The PPA provide for recovery of a maximum of Rs. 30 crore by way of liquidated damages (LD) for the period of delay in

commissioning of the individual units. However, on the basis of time allowed for commissioning for the second and subsequent units, the Board became entitled for levy of LD of Rs. 23.20 lakh. But this was not recovered so far.

- Unlike in the case of payment of taxes on income to the Developer, the Board agreed for payment of return on equity (RoE) on monthly basis instead of on annual basis. Payment of RoE monthly at 16 per cent per annum (Rs. 39.17 crore) thus would work out to 17.17 per cent per annum (Rs. 42.03 crore).
- Depreciation charges were computed for payment of fixed charges on the entire project cost without excluding the cost of land. Since land does not attract depreciation provision, failure to exclude it for computation of depreciation results in an over payment of Rs. 78.40 lakh to the developer per annum.
- The PPA stipulated for computation of incentive for achieving higher PLF (above 68.49%) on the equity instead on RoE. This results in undue benefit of Rs. 1.07 crore per annum to the developer for every one per cent increase in PLF above 68.5 per cent. At 90 per cent PLF the undue benefit would be Rs. 66.81 crore.
- In deviation of PPA conditions, the Developer reduced the proposed equity in Indian currency by Rs. 61.20 crore with a corresponding increase in the equity in foreign currency. This results in increase in the Boards liability towards foreign exchange variations on the return on foreign equity which would be around Rs. 1.35 crores per annum.
- The foreign currency component of the total debt for project financing was fixed in Indian rupees at November 1993 rates of exchange. As this value in Indian rupees is fixed and does not undergo change and vary with exchange rate variations, the Developer had an undue benefit due to exchange rate variations between November 1993 and actual dates of draw of loans. On the loans drawn till May 1996, such gain amounted to Rs. 23.38 crore and there would be a further gain of Rs. 56.06 crore with reference to the prevailing exchange rates on the loans yet to be drawn. The PPA was silent as to the treatment of such gain to the Developer due to exchange variations.

- The Board so far purchased 432.13 MU of energy from the Developer on payment of Rs. 94.69 crore. As against the projected unit rate of Rs. 2.06 the actual purchase cost per unit worked out to Rs. 2.19 resulting in an extra expenditure of Rs. 5.62 crore on the energy so far purchased.
- The land costing Rs. 10 crore acquired by the Developer was adequate for two stages of the project. But, the entire cost of land was loaded into the project cost of first stage (216 MW). Non-apportionment of the cost of land equally between the two stages of the project, results in undue benefit of Rs. 1.13 crore per annum to the Developer.

CAG's observations on Spectrum Power Plant

- Due to postponment of combined cycle commercial operation date the Board had to bear the extra burden of Rs. 17.05 crore towards higher fuel cost (Rs. 11.71 crore) and additional fixed charges (Rs. 5.34 crore) during the period from 29 September 1997 to 18th April 1998.
- By agreeing for payment of RoE monthly on pro rata basis instead of annually the board extended additional benefit of Rs. 2.63 crore per annum to the Developer.
- As the foreign exchange component of total debt for the project was fixed in Indian rupees at December 1993 rates of exchange, there was an exchange gain of Rs. 38.94 crore to the Developer and further exchange gain of Rs. 1.27 crore on the balance debt yet to be drawn. But the PPA was silent on the treatment of such favourable gains in arriving at the final project cost.
- The minimum PLF to be achieved during the stabilisation period was fixed at 51.37 per cent. This was low when compared to the PLF of 68.49 per cent fixed in respect of another project implemented around the same time. The fixation of PLF on lower side during stabilisation period resulted in forgoing recovery of Rs. 9.50 crore from the Developer by way of disincentive.
- The threshold level of PLF at 68.5 per cent fixed for computation of incentive was not realistic as the O & M contractors of the Developer guaranteed operation of the plant at an annual PLF of 85.6 per cent and agreed to pay penalty for every 1 per cent

fall in PLF below 85.6 per cent. At 85.5 per cent of PLF the incentive payable to the Developer by the Board would be Rs. 19.08 crore per annum while the PLF at this level was assured by the O&M contractors of the Developer without any extra payment.

- As against the projected unit cost of Rs. 2.22, the actual cost per unit of energy purchased was Rs. 2.46. This resulted in an extra financial burden of Rs. 18.51 crore in respect of 771.33 MU of energy purchased during the period from 11 February 1997 to 18 April 1998 (Government of Andhra Pradesh, 2001).

Notes

1. Prior to that, the Nizam State Electricity Board and composite Madras State's Department of Power and Energy used to cater to the power needs of the present Telangana districts, and Andhra and Rayalaseema districts respectively. After the formation of Andhra State in 1953, this responsibility was directly carried by the state for three years. In 1956 the Telangana and Andhra regions were united into a single state and in 1959 the state government decided to establish a separate board to manage the power.
2. Even within a small period of 5 years i.e. from 1991-92 to 1996-97, the APSEB achieved a remarkable success in transmission and distribution. On the transmission side the APSEB augmented its network by 26.4 per cent and thus achieved the highest network expansion among SEBs in the country. (The total length of T&D lines was expanded from 1,55,000 in 1978 (IPE: 1982, 131) to 6,08,000 kms by 1999). The distribution system was expanded at a brisk pace during the same period. The number of substations increased substantially from 1135 in '90-91 to 1844 in '98-99. The number of distribution transformers increased from 88,000 in '90-91 to 1,71,083 in '98-99 (Government of Andhra Pradesh, 2002. Also see, Arun Ghosh, 1997, Srihari, 1997 and Hanumanth Rao 1997 and 2002).
3. The VTPS has been turning out a sterling performance every year. It stood First in the country during 1994-95, 1995-96, 1996-97, 1997-98 and 2001-02 by achieving the highest Plant Load Factor. This station has been the recipient of many

prestigious Awards from various organizations including Meritorious Awards instituted by the Government of India. The station has received Meritorious Productivity Award for nineteen consecutive years. The station also got the Incentive Award for ten consecutive years. The station has bagged eight Gold Medals in row since 1994-95. The Rayalaseema Thermal Power Plant stood first in the country in turns of PLF in 1998-99 and 2000-01. It won Meritorious Productivity Awards for five consecutive years and Incentive Awards for six consecutive years. Kothagudem Thermal Power Station V won Meritorious Productivity Awards for three consecutive years and Incentive Awards also for three consecutive years. The Ramagudam 'B' Thermal Power Station achieved the highest PLF for four times at all India level.

4. The REP was a revolutionary programme aimed at taking the electricity to the villages and rural people, particularly to the rural poor, who cannot afford to enjoy the benefits of power. Even the section 18 of the 1948 Act says that, the board should be charged with the general duty of promoting the coordinated development by taking electricity to those areas which were not given this benefit or were not given this benefit adequately (Government of India, Third Five Year Plan: 405-6). Since the First Five Year Plan the government of India had been giving top priority for rural electrification without much success. The number of electrified villages and towns with a population of below 5,000 was only 3,687 (out of 5,61,107). It was decided to electrify 43,000 villages or small towns by 1966. For this purpose a "Rural Electrification Corporation" was set up during third plan. However, it was during IV Plan that rural electrification was taken up on a large scale (IV Five Year Plan: 270-281). The decision of the Andhra Pradesh State Government to give up the metering system in the early 1980s made the situation much worse and proved to be a short sighted one. It had affected the whole system on two fronts. First, it deprived the state government of any mechanism to know how much power was consumed by the agriculture sector and second, it led to the misuse of the facility by a number of farmers. It is common in many places to supply water to others by charging money from them on 'per hour' basis. With the

connivance of the staff of the Electricity department, the theft of power became a regular feature. The affluence of the staff who are posted in rural areas lured others to teach the urban consumers the methods of pilferage and to protect them for a 'Charge'.

The crisis was accelerated by non-investment of money in the power sector by the Telugu Desam Government under N.T. Rama Rao. If we accept that it takes at least 4 years to commission a project, the Telugu Desam Government contributed (from 1987 to 1993) only 560 MW of Power to total Installation (For details on Installation see, APGENCO, 2003 and APSEB 97: 8 and 98: 8). On one hand there was a spurt in the consumption by the agricultural sector, particularly after 1983, on the other, there was no corresponding investment to meet the demand. In 1981-82, 942 million units of Energy were consumed by the agriculture sector. It jumped to 1393 million units in 1982-83 and to 1540 in 1983-84 and finally to 9336 in 1997-98.

Added to this, the problem of declining volume of cheaper Hydel Electricity and increase in the utilization of costly Thermal Electricity imposed enormous burden on the Board. The following table presents the changing ratio of Hydel and Thermal Power from 1990-1998.

Details of Power Generation in MW

Power Gen.	1990-91	1991-92	1992-93	1993-94	1994-95	1995-96	1996-97	1997-98
Hydel	10017	9516	8758	9633	9687	6662	7970	7245-13
Thermal	8102	8726	9114	9639	10842	15103	16719.76	19019.49

Source: APSEB, 1998: 41.

5. Subsidy is not favour. It is mandatory on the part of all state governments. The gap between revenues and 3 per cent of total assets value must be met by the state governments as subsidy. Still, the AP government repeatedly projected the subsidy as a favour to the APSEB.
6. So far no perfect mechanism is available to identify the different components of power loss, agricultural consumption, technical loss and theft are included under the single category, i.e. power loss. Before the reforms, i.e., before 1996-97, much loss was attributed to agriculture by deliberately inflating the power

consumption by agriculture. After reforms much of the loss was attributed to technical loss and theft (see APTRANSCO, 2000. First five tables and Ajay Pandey, 2001: 128).

7. The entire opposition during the Telugu Desam rule openly accused the government of colluding with promoters and allowing them to raise the book value of the fixed cost. Very recently, two vernacular dailies viz., *Andhra Jyothi* (14.7.04 to 21.7.04) and *Prajasakti* (7.8.04 and 9.8.04) and *Deccan Chronicle* (8.8.04) made similar allegations.
8. The liquidity damages in case of Lanco were 50,000 rupees a day for first 90 days and three lakhs a day after 90 days. In case of Spectrum the damages were 8.7 lakhs a day and Spectrum took nine months extra time to complete the project. Almost every promoter took more time to complete the project and the TRANSCO never collected the damages.

REFERENCES

1. Ajay Pandey, 2003. "Power Sector Reforms: A Long Road Ahead" in *Survey of Indian Industry 2003*. Madras: *The Hindu*.
2. APGENCO, 2003. *A Decade of Performance (1992-2002),* Hyderabad: APGENCO.
3. APSEB, 1997. *Power Development in Andhra Pradesh (Statistics) 1997-98*, Hyderabad: APSEB.
4. APSEB, 1998. *Power Development in Andhra Pradesh (Statistics) 1997-98*, Hyderabad: APSEB.
5. Dayal, H.V. 1980. "Analysis of the Power Sector", in Rajendra K. Pachuri (ed.) *Energy Policy for India*, Delhi: MacMillan.
6. Delhi Science Forum, 2003. *Alternative Economic Survey 2001-2002*, Delhi: Delhi Science Forum.
7. Ghosh Arun, 1997. "Break-up and Privatisation of SEB in Andhra Pradesh: An upcoming Scam", *Economic and Political Weekly*, Vol. 32, No. 29.
8. Government of Andhra Pradesh, 2000. *Report of the Comptroller and Auditor General of India, 1966 to 2000.*
9. Government of Andhra Pradesh, 2001. *Strategy Paper on Power*, Hyderabad.

10. Government of Andhra Pradesh, 2002. *Reforms and Restructuring of Andhra Pradesh Power Sector (India)*, www. andhrapradesh.com/07/16/2002.

11. Government of India, 2001. *Public Enterprises Survey 1999-2000.*

12. Government of India, 2002. *Economic Survey* 200-2001.

13. IBRD, 1999. Andhra *Pradesh Power Sector Restructuring Programme*, New Delhi: IBR.

14. Institute of Public Enterprises, 1982. *Organisational Structure and Financial Policies of the State Electricity Boards (Study sponsored by Planning Commission),* Hyderabad: IPE.

15. Murthy, Ramachandra, 2001. *Vidyut Valayam* (in Teugu, tr. The Circle of Power, and analysis of Power Reforms), Lifeline Communications, Hyderabad.

16. Nair, P.N.V. 2002. A.P. Reform Pays, www.project monitor.com

17. Nye, J.S. 2002. "Corruption and Political Development: A Cost-Benefit Analysis" in Robert Williams ed. *Explaining Corruption*, Vol. I, Edward Elgar Publishing Limited, Northampton.

18. Peoples Monitoring Group on Electricity Regulation, 2001. *Petition before the Andhra Pradesh Electricity Regulatory Commission*, Hyderabad.

19. Raghu, K. 2001. *Petition before Andhra Pradesh Electricity Regulatory Commission on Power Purchase Agreement between A.P. TRANSCO and BPL Power Projects (AP) Ltd.* Hyderabad.

20. Raghu, K. and Satynarayana, 2001. *Andhra Pradesh State Electricity Board Engineers's Association petition on 'Mini Power Plants'*, Hyderabad.

21. Rao, Hanumantha, V. 1998. *Veluthurunundi Cheekatiloki: Vidyuth Rangamupi Pariseelana* (in Telugu), Guntur: Prajapandha Publications.

22. Rao, Hanumantha, 2002. *Economy of Andhra Pradesh 1996-2001: An Alternative Survey* (in Telugu), Hyderabad: Prajasakti Book House.

23. Rao, Koteswara, 2004, "Power Sector Reforms in Andhra Pradesh" in Prof. C. Narasimharao ed. *A Decade of Economic Reforms in India*, Serials, Delhi.

24. Srihari, V. 1997, "Is Restructuring of APSEB Inevitable?", *Economic and Political Weekly*, Vol. 32, No. 39.

25. Srinivasan, V.K., 2003, "Achilles Heel of Economy" in *Survey of Indian Industry 2003*, Madras: The Hindu.

26. TRANSCO, 2000. *Andhra Pradesh Power Sector Reforms, "Powering the New Millennium*, Hyderabad.

27. TRANSCO, 2001. *Power Sector Status & Tariff in Andhra Pradesh*, www.ercap.org.com. www.ercap. org.com.

28. World Bank, 1997, *Andhra Pradesh: Agenda for Economic Reforms.*

29. World Bank, 1999. *Project Appraisal Document on Andhra Pradesh Power Sector Restructuring Programme, Report No. 18849.*

REFERENCES

Arora D., "Conceptualizing the Context and Contextualising the Concept: Corruption Recognised", *Indian Journal of Public Administration*, Vol. 39, No. 1: 1993.

Avasthi Maheswari, "*Public Administration*", Lakshmi Narain Agarwal, Agra, 1993.

Caiden G.E., "Toward a General Theory of Official Corruption", *Asian Journal of Public Administration*", Vol. 10, No. 1: 1988.

Caiden G.E., "What Really is Public Administration?", *Indian Journal of Public Administration*, Vol. 37, No. 1, 1991.

Chaudhuri, Nirad C, "Corruption in Indian Politics", in *Public Administration* (Kanpur), Vol. 6, No. 8, August 1968.

Davies C.J., "Controlling Administrative Corruption", *Planning and Administration Journal*, Vol. 14, No. 2: 1987.

Guhan S., and Paul (eds), "*Corruption in India-Agenda for Action*", Vision Books, New Delhi, 1997.

Narayanan K.R., "Next an India for All, Tolerant and Uncorrupt", editorial, *International Herald Tribune*, 13th August, 1997.

Padhay K.S., "*Corruption in Politics: A Case Study*", B.R. Publishing Corporation, Delhi, 1986.

Report of the Railway Corruption Enquiry Committee, Ministry of Railways, Government of India, 1961.

Report of the Santhanam Committee on Prevention of Corruption, 1964.

Shashi B. Sahai, "*Politics of Corruption: The Goddess that Failed*" Gyan Publishing House, New Delhi.

Surech Kohli (ed)., "*Corruption in India: The Growing Evil*", Chetna Publications, New Delhi, 1975.

"The Destructive Costs of Greasing Palms", *Business Week*, 6 December, 2000, pp. 134-135, 1993.

Vishnoo Bhagwan and Vidya Bhushan, "*Public Administration*", S. Chand & Company Ltd., New Delhi, 1998.

White L.D., "*Introduction to the Study of Public Administration*", MacMillan, New York.

31

DOES "SPEED MONEY" REALLY SPEED UP PUBLIC ADMINISTRATION IN INDIA?

A. Ravishankar
Department of Political Science,
Presidency College, Chennai-600 005.

INTRODUCTION

The problem of corruption has been one of the most enduring dilemmas confronting Governments throughout history. Although differences may exist in the nature and scope of corrupt behaviour, and the extent to which anticorruption measures are enforced, the phenomenon can be found at all times and within virtually every political system.

Historically, concern about corruption has tended to run in cycles, in which revelations of official abuses prompted anti-corruption campaigns and administrative counter-measures that subsequently faded from view until the next round of scandals provided further impetus for reform. The desire to reduce or eliminate corruption was at the core of many enduring innovations for good governance. The major public administration reforms of the late nineteenth and early twentieth centuries—such as introduction of a meritorious civil service system, and professional management of government ministries and departments, or the creation of more formalized budget, procurement, and audit processes and agencies had their roots in the desire to avoid earlier abuses of graft and political patronage.

According to L.D. White, "a wholesome public service is characterized by a high prestige, a positive morale and integrity. These are the three generalized tests that certify to the success of management. Prestige means the attribute of social appreciation which may attach to a person, a group or an institution. High morale is a state of mind in which men and women voluntarily seek to develop and apply their full powers to the tasks on which they are engaged by reason of their intellectual or moral satisfaction which they derive from their own self-realisation, their achievements in their chosen fields, and their pride in the service". Each of these attributes reinforce and supplement, the other. Integrity helps to build prestige and high prestige is an aid to high morale.

With mounting corruption in our country, each of these three attributes of civil service has suffered severe erosion. In a democratic nation, civil service is a secondary player under the command of political executive. Corruption is perhaps the most basic issue influencing the rise and fall of societies through the history of man, reflecting the health or sickness of civilization at any given time.

The entire infrastructure of the modern Indian society is built on the edifice of corruption. Unlike other evils which emerge from the bottom of the society, corruption in India starts from the top. Thus proving the age-old Sanskrit adage that the tree has roots at the top and branches at the bottom. Corruption in India has become a convention, a tradition, a psychological need and necessity. It stems from the basic roots of life. It is regular practice, a business transaction.

As we trace the social roots of corruption in our country, we come to understand that the eternal message of tolerance, the sense of forgiveness probably had led to the tolerance of a sin like corruption. In India there seems to be a lack of awareness about the damages of corruption or lack of probity in public life in the well beings of people.

Since independence our political system is based on certain God-like virtues which are not present in those who work for it. All the ideals of socialism and collective wealth which seem to inspire our lawmakers are subverted by the misuse of the enormous power and patronage placed in the hands of ministers and bureaucrats whose appetite and acquisitiveness have been sharpened by their own recent hunger and poverty. This in turn accounts perhaps for the proliferation of laws whose objective appears to be neither a good administration nor justice. The number of laws, rules and procedures governing all professions and affecting the daily living of individuals in our country today is legion. People start breaking those laws which are seen as troublesome rather than pre-requisites for stability and justice in society. The general contempt for law thus developed encompasses much that is also good and necessary in it. It is this public cynicism about the justice or reasonableness of law that contains the first seed of the corruption that overtakes any society.

There are three main reasons for the high incidence of corruption in India. First, it started during the days of British Imperialism when 'cheating' the government was popularly regarded as a 'patriotic' act of defiance, whether you were cheating the railways by traveling without ticket and by removing the bulbs and other fittings from train compartments, or protecting any offender from the police or evasion of income tax. All this was supposed to deprive the British rulers of our money.

Unfortunately, the old habits die hard, and have not changed with the transfer of power in 1947. The people, in a way, are still alienated from the government. For the common people the government is still the 'enemy' whom it is considered legitimate to cheat and defraud.

The second reason is the signs of affluence and luxurious life of the well to do people which lures the officials to indulge in corrupt practices. Apart from this inflation, higher cost of living, rising prices of essential commodities have made it impossible for the officials to resist their temptation of earnings by immoral means.

The final reason is our system of democracy which is based on an expensive electioneering process. The limitation on individual election expenses is largely observed in its breach. The money for election expenses used to come from the big industrialists who could change it to 'company expenses' in the interests of 'public relations'. All this creates a climate of corruption, engulfing the nation as a whole. When a businessman has to oil the palm of officials to get anything done, he becomes unscrupulous with the consumer.

CORRUPTION DEFINED

The term corruption is used as a shorthand reference for a large range of illicit or illegal activities. Although there is no universal or comprehensive definition as to what constitutes corrupt behaviour, the most prominent definitions share a common emphasis upon the abuse of public power or position for personal advantage. "Corruption involves behaviour on the part of officials in the governmental system, whether politicians or civil servants, in which they improperly and unlawfully enrich themselves, or those close to them, by the misuse of the public power entrusted to them.

Some types of corruption are internal, in that they interfere with the ability of government agency to recruit or manage its staff, make efficient use of its resources or conduct impartial in-house investigations. Other corruptions are external in that they involve efforts to manipulate or extort money from clients or suppliers, or to benefit from inside information.

Corruption, among officials and ministers has two sides—the overt and the covert. An official or minister may be receiving bribes or donations for his party funds by doing favours to the 'donors' or 'bribe givers'—issuing licences or permits for which the traders and the industrialists are prepared to do anything. The covert or subtle form of corruption in which the minister may not touch the money, but may be aware that it is being paid into party fund by industrialists, importers and exporters.

It is often useful to differentiate between grand corruption, which typically involves ministers and senior officials, major decisions or contracts, and the exchange of large sums of money and petty corruption, which involves low-level officials, the provision of routine services and goods, and small sums of money. It is also useful to differentiate between systemic corruption, which permeates an entire government or ministry and individual corruption, which is more isolated and sporadic. Finally, it is useful to distinguish between syndicated corruption, in which elaborate systems are devised for receiving and disseminating bribes, and non-syndicated corruption in which individual officials may seek or complete for bribes in an ad hoc and uncoordinated fashion.

LIST OF CORRUPT BEHAVIOURS

- The design or selection of uneconomical projects because of opportunities for financial kickbacks and political patronage.
- Procurement fraud, including collusion, overcharging, or the selection of contractors, suppliers, and consultants on criteria other than the lowest evaluated substantially responsive bidder.
- Illicit payments of "speed money" to government officials to facilitate the timely delivery of goods and services to which the public is rightfully entitled, such as permits and licenses.

- Illicit payments to government officials to facilitate access to goods, services, and/or information to which the public is not entitled, or to deny the public access to goods and services to which it is legally entitled.
- Illicit payment to prevent the application of rules and regulations in a fair and consistent manner, particularly in areas concerning public safety, law enforcement, or revenue collection.
- Payments to government officials to foster or sustain monopolistic or oligopolistic access to markets in the absence of a compelling economic rationale for such restrictions.
- The misappropriation of confidential information for personal gain, such as using knowledge about public transportation routings to invest in real estate that is likely to appreciate.
- The deliberate disclosure of false or misleading information on the financial status of corporations that would prevent potential investors from accurately valuing their worth, such as the failure to disclose large contingent liabilities or the undervaluing of assets in enterprises slated for privatization.
- The theft or embezzlement of public property and monies.
- The sale of official posts, positions, or promotions; nepotism; or other actions that undermine the creation of a professional and meritorious civil service.
- Extortion and the abuse of public office, such as using the threat of a tax audit or legal sanctions to extract personal favours.
- Obstruction of justice and interference in the duties of agencies tasked with detecting, investigating, and prosecuting illicit behaviour.

SPEED MONEY

Speed money can be defined as one which "helps in getting work done quickly by speeding up the wheels of government administration". An honest and over centralized bureaucracy is worse than a dishonest and over centralized one because corruption enables the affected to find their way out of bureaucratic oppression. However, speed money enables the bureaucracy to seek rent and leads to diversion of productive wealth into unproductive channels such as gold and real estate. It deprives the common man from the fruits of development. It is possible to have economic growth along with increase in unemployment, rise in prices, destruction of environment and dependence of foreign countries. Therefore, speed money cannot be justified merely because it gives relief from bad governance.

THE COST OF SPEED MONEY

Speed money has not always been perceived as having a negative impact upon development. Many argue that speed money improves social welfare, both because it is a way to avoid cumbersome regulations and because it is a system of building in rewards for badly paid bureaucrats. Arguments were advanced that it could have beneficial effects. When wages are low enough to live on, some maintained that it is natural for civil servants to augment their salaries by speed money. It is alleged that speed money could advance economic efficiency by helping restore artificial and administratively determined prices. Others maintained that speed money plays a useful redistribute role, transferring resources from wealthy individuals and corporations to those of more modest means, or that it could serve as a tool of national integration by allowing ruling elites to entice or co-opt fractious political, ethnic or religious groups. Finally, some scholars have argued that speed money is a natural stage of development.

But the problem of speed money have several common features. First, they often refer to the benefits stemming from specific illicit acts and do not consider the systemic impact of corruption. Although a given transaction may have positive results, it may also generate negative externalities that degrade the performance of the system as a whole and compromise the nations long term dynamic efficiency.

Second, many of the alleged benefits from speed money, such as streamlining government transactions or enhancing civil service pay, only appear as such against the background of the governmental organization that is failing to perform effectively.

Third, speed money encourages people to avoid both good regulations and bad. There is no guarantee that an importer who bribes a customs official to expedite the clearance of badly needed medication one week will not bribe the official to expedite the clearance of illegal narcotics the next.

The task of evaluating the practical impact of corruption upon our country's development is a complicated one. Although there are instances when illicit acts can improve the economic rates of return, the bulk of the evidence indicates that corrupt actions typically generate for more costs than benefits. Speed money ruined the efficiency of government, crippled the merit system and generated an atmosphere of distruct which pervades all levels of administration.

Speed money has strongly affected development efforts of our country negatively, belying the so-called 'revisionist hypothesis' prevalent in the West which considers speed money as either a necessary step in the development process or means of speeding up public administration. But speed money in reality leads to the favouring of inefficient producers, the unfair and inequitable distribution of scarce public resources, and the leakage of revenue from government coffers to private hands.

Less directly, but no less perniciously, speed money leads to loss of confidence in government. Upon closer inspection, many of speed money's alleged distributive, efficiency and political benefits turn out to be illusory. Rather than enhancing a more equitable distribution of income, speed money distorts the allocation of social resources away from those who are legally entitled to them and toward the rich, the powerful, and the politically well connected. Rather than compensating civil servants for poor pay, speed money undermines the merit system and compromises service professionalism and esprit de corps. Some times, it can even foster additional inefficiencies within governmental organisation. Instead of cementing political loyalties, speed money more often breeds public cynicism and resentment towards the political process and those associated with it.

ANTI-SPEED MONEY ISSUES

The anti-speed money issues are intended to reduce the burden that is widespread upon the development of our nation. These issues are centered upon the following objectives.

- Establishing a transparent public administration.
- Improving the quality of governance by supporting anti-speed money efforts.
- Making ministers and bureaucrats to have ethical standards.

Public administration reform takes place in response to official malfeasance. Such reform may help the government to effect changes that will make speed money behaviour more difficult to engage in and more easily detected once it occurs. There are several priority areas where efforts to upgrade the quality of our public administration will pay dividends in the struggle against speed money.

Efforts to strengthen information systems, relating financial management, should enhance transparency and accountability which strengthen the capacity of government to monitor their expenditures. Measures to strengthen internal audit functions and to ensure adequate control over disbursements can play the dual role of helping monitor and improve performance while making theft and embezzlement more easily detected. Procurement reform can reduce costs while simultaneously making it more difficult to perpetrate fraud and abuse.

Another area where significant progress can be made is civil service reform. Poor salaries, low morale, lack of commitment, uncertain prospects for career development and insufficient linkage of merit to promotion can foster pervasive corruption among public officials. There are number of initiatives to redress these problems. Efforts to decompress pay scales and improve employment conditions throughout the civil service will lower the incentive for illicit behaviour. Initiatives to reduce the number of exemptions and special allowances will make remuneration more transparent. Measures to improve procedures for recruitment and promotion should help avoid abuses of patronage, nepotism and favouritism and to help to foster the creation of an independent meritorious civil service. Efforts to draft and enforce a code of ethics will clarify what is expected to civil servants and ensure adherence to appropriate norms of behaviour.

One can improve the effectiveness of the government while simultaneously reducing opportunities for speed money by narrowing its scope for intervention. Within ministries and departments one of the best approaches is the re-engineering to business process. As procedures are simplified and streamlined, the need for speed money payments to expedite services disappears. At a broader level, deregulation, commercialisation and privatisation can achieve similar objectives. As the sphere of state activity decreases, then as a general rule the opportunity for soliciting bribes will also go down.

Several good governance initiatives relating to the legislative and judicial branches can also help in the fight against speed money. One important means to enhance accountability is to strengthen the Parliament's oversight function and improve the capacity of parliamentary institutions, such as supreme audit agencies, to function effectively. Measures for legal and judicial reform, such as efforts to reduce judicial backlogs through alternate dispute resolution techniques or to improve courtroom management to ensure cases can be tried in a timely fashion, or to enhance the independence and professionalism of the judiciary, will all have positive externalities in the struggle against speed money. These initiatives are non-controversial and widely recognized to be the building blocks of solid public administration.

IMPROVING THE QUALITY OF GOVERNANCE BY SUPPORTING ANTI-SPEED MONEY EFFORTS

In pursuing explicit anti-speed money programmes, efforts must be taken to develop a national anti-speed money strategy; improve the ability of the courts to try corruption cases; respond to request from legislators and bureaucrats for legal opinion in drafting anti-speed money statutes or professional codes of conduct, strengthen the legal mechanisms for review of administrative action, e.g. the creation of an Ombudsman or provision for judicial review; or improve the capacity of anti-speed money agencies to detect or prosecute illicit behaviour.

ETHICAL STANDARDS FOR MINISTERS AND BUREAUCRATS

This calls for more robust internal measures to enhance the integrity of ministers and bureaucrats. These measures will take place along the following dimensions.

- Maintaining the integrity of their departments.
- Observing highest standard of ethics in dealing with contracts.
- Updating code of conduct for ministers and bureaucrats.
- Creating independent internal reporting mechanisms like inspection committee.
- Improving the quality of oversight.
- Advancing staff awareness.

CONCLUSION

The prevalence of speed money in India's public life has become a matter of grave concern which threatens the political, administrative and economic environment of our country. Though public awareness of this problem has increased over the years, significant progress has not yet been made in terms of developing and designing remedies that can adequately deal with its magnitude and severity. The corruption in India can only be controlled by reforming the political process, restructuring and reorienting the public administration, empowering the people and creating sustained public pressure on speed money.

Part - 4

CORRUPTION: CULTURE, ETHICS, RELIGION AND YOGA

32

CORRUPTION CULTURE AND CORPORATE GOVERNANCE

B. Jayanthi
Tamil Nadu Institute of Labour Studies, Chennai

The South Asian Human Development Report, 1999 has pointed out that if corruption level in India is reduced to those in the Scandinavian countries, investment rates could increase annually by some 12 per cent and GDP growth rate by almost 1.5 per cent each year. The word 'corporate governance' has become a buzzword these days because of two factors. The first is that after the collapse of the Soviet Union and the end of the cold war in 1990, it has become the conventional wisdom all over the world that market dynamics must prevail in economic matters. The concept of government controlling and commanding heights of the economy has been given up. This, in turn, has made the market the most decisive factor in settling economic issues.

This has also coincided with the thrust given to globalisation. Globalisation involves the movement of four economic parameters namely, physical capital in terms of plant and machinery, financial capital in terms of money invested in capital markets or in FDI, technology, and labour moving across national borders. The pace of movement of financial capital has become greater because of the pervasive impact of information technology and the world having become a global village.

CORPORATE GOVERNANCE

Corporate governance is one of today's most prominent business challenges. Corporate governance is relationship between those who own the capital and those who control it. In a wider sense, Corporate Governance has been aptly described by Professor Kenneth Scott of Stanford Law School as including every force that bears on the decision-making of the firm. That would encompass not only the control rights of stock holders, but also the contractual covenants and insolvency power of debt holders, the commitments entered into with employees, customers and suppliers, the regulations issued by governmental-agencies and the statutes enacted by the parliamentary bodies.

When investments take place in emerging markets, the investors want to be sure that not only are the capital markets or enterprises with which they are investing, run competently but they also have good corporate governance. Corporate governance represents the value framework, the ethical framework and the moral framework under which business decisions are taken. In other words, when investments take place across national borders, the investors want to be sure that not only is their capital handled effectively and adds to the creation of wealth, but the business decisions are also taken in a manner which is not illegal or involving moral hazard.

Spectacular business failures and more recently, high profile scandals, financial crises and/or institutional failures in Russia, Asia and the United States have brought corporate governance issues to the fore in developing countries, transitional economies, and emerging markets. Yet, recent financial crises provoked by corruption and mismanagement have made attracting sufficient levels of capital particularly challenging these days. These crises cost investors billions of dollars and sabotaged companies' financial viability. They also contributed to increased shareholder activism and competition for investment. Investors, especially institutional investors, are now making it clear that they are not willing to foot the bill for corruption and mismanagement. Before committing any funds, investors increasingly require evidence that companies are run according to sound business practices that minimize the possibilities for corruption and mismanagement.

NEXUS BETWEEN PUBLIC GOVERNANCE AND CORPORATE GOVERNANCE

Since independence from Britain in 1947, India has had a comparatively greater degree of state regulation of industrial activity than the Western norm. This has involved a combination of direct state ownership of 'key' or 'strategic' industries, and legal powers to control and regulate those areas ceded to private entrepreneurship. This tightly regulated system inevitably gave rise to a phenomenon known as the 'licence-permit raj' (literally, licence-permit regime), involving politicians empowered to make decisions, bureaucrats who ran the system on a daily basis and knew its workings far better than politicians, and representatives of domestic capital in a triadic relationship.

The nexus between the Indian political elite and a handful of 'big business' houses, with the bureaucrats as essential intermediaries, is a longstanding one. For decades, the prospects of Indian big businesses have depended on their degree of cosiness with the decision makers (politicians) and administrators (bureaucrats).

The history of corruption in post-Independence India starts with the Jeep scandal in 1948, when a transaction concerning purchase of jeeps for the army needed for Kashmir operation was entered into by V.K. Krishna Menon, the then High Commissioner for India in London with a foreign firm without observing normal procedure. Contrary to the demand of the opposition for judicial inquiry as suggested by the Inquiry Committee led by Ananthsayanam Ayyangar, the then Government announced on September 30, 1955 that the Jeep scandal case was closed.

In 1950, A.D. Gorwala, an eminent civil servant was asked by Government of India to recommend improvements in the system of governance. In his report submitted in 1951 he made two observations: "One, quite a few of Nehru's ministers were corrupt and this was common knowledge. Two, even a highly responsible civil servant in an official report as early as 1951 maintained that the Government went out to its way to shield its ministers".

The need for corporate governance has been highlighted because of the scams we have been having almost as an annual feature ever since we had liberalisation from 1991. We had the Harshad Mehta Scam, Ketan Parikh Scam, UTI Scam, Vanishing Company Scam, Bhansali Scam and so on.

Corporate governance dependes upon two factors namely, the attitude and the values cherished by the management of the business enterprise and the external environment in which the business operates.

The external environment in which the business operates would include the legislation relating to the functioning of business enterprises, covering the entire spectrum from registration of companies, their structure, and settlement of disputes, laws relating to the capital market and punishment for bad practices like insider trading and so on. Corporate Governance represents the moral framework, the ethical framework and the value framework under which an enterprise takes decisions. The importance of the fact is that corporate decisions should not only be concerned with purely the economic aspects but also the ethical dimension.

Public governance on the other hand is broadly connected with the running of the government of a country and ensuring that the rule of law prevails. There has to be fairness and transparency in the system of justice. If the public governance is not conducted on healthy lines and if there is corruption, then there is no fairness. If the public servants are going to exploit their position for private gain then the quality of public governance suffers. If the quality of public governance suffers, corporate governance then becomes more difficult. It can definitely be said that the management of an enterprise can still be ethical and try to maintain its internal corporate governance. If the environment in which it operates is not clean then it may not be successful or even if successful, it will find it very difficult to operate.

THE INDIAN EXPERIENCES

— Narsimha Rao was the first Prime Minister being prosecuted in corruption charges. Cases like Rs. 2500 crore Airbus A-320 with France involving kickback (1990), Harshad Mehta security scam (1992), Gold Star Steel and Alloys controversy (1992), JMM bribery case, Hawala scam of Rs. 65 crore and Urea scam (1996) also came up during the period of Narsimha Rao Government.

— In July 2001, Prime Minister Atal Behari Vajpayee offered his resignation following a series of corruption scandals that involved top-level politicians and businessmen.

— It took the CBI's investigators in the Bofors' case over a decade to compel the Hinduja brothers—transnational tycoons based in London with high political 'connections' in both India and the UK—to come to India to be interrogated.

- The lack of transparency in our capital markets and the scope for insider trading, which this provides, was exposed in the Ketan Parikh Scam. The presence of brokers in the management of the stock exchanges can be a significant factor, which could promote insider trading. There have been comments that the so-called Ketan Parekh scam is not a scam at all and there is no scam for the JPC to look into.
- Lack of effective punishment systems: Leeson of Barings in Singapore who was involved in disastrous speculation was punished within two years.

  In India, it took seven years for Harshad Mehta to be punished at the first stage. (This necessitates the need for building a prompt punishment system along with plugging of the loopholes).
- The UTI scam represented another dimension of the corruption and the lack of corporate governance in the financial sector. UTI which gave the best of both worlds to the investors and assured return and also market capitalisation, could function only when the government was controlling the economy. Greater liberalisation meant that when the investor had a choice either to have an assured return as in a fixed deposit or take the risk involved in a fast changing capital market.
- The announcement by Xerox Corporation that its officials in India had made improper payments to some people, including Government officials, to the tune of Rs. 2.7 crore to Rs. 3.5 crore between 1999 and 2000, raised the question of precise nature of the impropriety committed by Xerox officials in India? According to one view, "it is still not known whether Xerox bagged contracts by paying money to Government officials or whether they were just paying these amounts to put some lubricant in the rusty spokes of babudom for issues like hurrying up their payments". As everyone knows, soliciting and the payment of bribes is an integral part of the functioning of the Indian economy so much so that it is quite inconceivable to think of a business enterprise which has not set aside funds to look after this head of expenditure on a long-term basis.
- When an allegation was made in the case of BALCO disinvestment which was upheld by the Supreme Court itself,

by the Chief Minister of Chattisgarh that Rs. 100 crores bribe was given, it caught the headlines for some time.

— According to a study by PHD Chamber of Commerce and Industry, investment would increase by 2.9 per cent of GDP and GDP growth by 1.3 per cent if corruption index improves by one standard deviation or around 15 per cent. Implication is that India is loosing at least Rs. 63,800 crore worth of additional investment per annum, roughly three times the foreign direct investment (FDI) we are attracting now and Rs. 28,600 crore of consequent national income per annum. The unaccounted money in India is estimated to be in the range of Rs. 350 to 700 thousand crore more than the combined revenue of the Centre and the State government in the last fiscal. A survey of exporters by Exim Bank found that 64 per cent of interviewed face major problems with customs clearance processes and with port authorities. Exporters spend 1-15 per cent of export revenue to grease the corruption machinery.

— In a frank discussion in Singapore, fund managers and corporate executives revealed to the Indian businessmen that the main reason why they were not prepared to mesh India into their global production plans was that even after they had obtained all the clearances from the Central and State Governments, they remained at the mercy of local bureaucrats and politicians. Anyone of them could stop their operations, and threatened to do so if they were not given an adequate 'inducement'. Every change of government in a state led to a fresh set of demands and a fresh set of negotiations with the new incumbents.

In fact the biggest scam is that we have a system that encourages scams and what is worse, does not punish the scamsters. However, various scams and cases of corruption in the post-liberalisation period highlight the need for better corporate governance.

Sound corporate governance practices have become critical to worldwide efforts to stabilize and strengthen global capital markets and protect investors. They help companies to improve their performance and attract investment. Corporate governance enables corporations to realise their corporate objectives, protect shareholder rights, meet legal requirements and to demonstrate to a wider public how they are conducting their business.

FACTORS FACING CORPORATE GOVERNANCE

Corporate governance depends upon two factors —

The first is the commitment of the management for the principle of integrity and transparency in business operations. The dramatic Enron case has highlighted how companies, which were the darlings of the stock market and held up as models for vigorous and innovative growth can ultimately collapse like a house of cards as they were based on fraud and dishonesty. Enron as an enterprise which built a dazzling track record for nearly 17 years collapsed in a welter of scams. An energy-trading company as widely praised as any online wonder at the height of the Internet euphoria. Analysts predicted that it would come to dominate the wholesale market for electricity, natural gas, coal, energy derivatives and bandwidth, and on three continents. Investors loved it enough to value the company at $28 billion in October 2001, less than two months before it skidded into bakruptcy. It was not that Enron lacked substance, but in the end of hype got the better of it. To meet the outside world's unrealistic expectations, it began to fudge the figures. To disguise its liabilities, it wrapped them up in private partnerships and took them off its balance sheet. And to satisfy the wishful thinkers' insatiable demands, it brought earnings forward by selling shares in other off-balance-sheet partnerships, and counting the proceeds as revenues.

The South East Asian economies which were booming and some of the countries were called 'tiger economies', suddenly faced a set back starting with the melt down of the currency in Thailand followed by Indonesia, Malaysia and South Korea. The main cause for this was identified as crony capitalism and lack of corporate governance in the financial sector. The collapse of the South East Asian tiger economies like Thailand, South Korea, Malaysia, Indonesia in 1998 brought home the fact that if there is no proper corporate governance in the financial sector, it leads to crony capitalism and corruption. This, in turn, leads to unsound investments which are speculative and finally the investors lose.

The second is the legal and the administrative framework created by the government. If public governance is weak, we cannot have good corporate governance.

Corruption in government can have a direct influence on business success. With its help the whole climate of doing business can be changed in the bribers favour. Without resort to corruption well-nigh insurmountable problems can arise: deliberate foot-dragging instead of friendly treatment (in passing on information or granting approvals, for example); holding back information rather than imparting it in time (for example, in connection with a crucial deadline such as the latest date for submitting a tender in a public bidding competition); or shelving vs. approving applications (e.g. for import or export licenses or sales authorizations). All this can add up to the decisive difference between business success and failure.

The legal and administrative environment in India provides excellent scope for corrupt practices in business. As a result unless a management is committed to be honest and observe the principles of propriety, the atmosphere is too tempting to observe good corporate governance in practice. We should approach the corporate governance issue in India not merely from the point of view of the Companies' Act or the guidelines which can be issued like the Kumaramangalam code or the Bajaj code but look at the entire network of various rules and regulations impinging on business so that there is an integrated wholistic system created for ensuring that transparency and good corporate governance prevail.

The most relevant shortcomings as far as the government is concerned are:

— Lack of a clear distinction between what is to be considered "public" and what "private", leaving the door open to appropriating public resources for private advantage;
— Lack of transparency in the handling of public finances, lack of independent control agencies, and thus hindrance of presentation of concrete proof;
— Absence of dependable legal machinery for preventing arbitrary application of regulations and laws;
— Weak public institutions, no free press;
— Over-regulation, as evidenced by an unwarranted number of regulations, permits requirements and laws;
— Unclear decision-making procedures hinging on very close personal connections plus capricious interventions by those who hold political power and their abuse of it for their own enrichment.

By and large one can say that the most inefficient a government is and the more "powerful" its bureaucracy, the bigger the corruption problem. When the omnipresence of imprecise or contradictory laws and regulations, the obscurity of the criteria and channels governing decisions, the lack of accountability and democratically sanctioned political controls, all in conjunction with an underpaid and corrupt officialdom, leave a firm otherwise beyond reproach no alternative but to either join the circle of corruption or else withdraw completely from the country.

The ethical temperature of any business or capital market depends on three factors:

The first is the 'individual's sense of values'. The second is the '*social values*' accepted by the business and industry. When Harshad Mehta Scam took place, it was claimed that the manner in which the bank receipts were being treated was the prevailing norm. In other words, practices, which are later on found to be highly objectionable, become acceptable because that was the prevailing market practice. Social values will depend upon the standards set up by professional bodies like the Association of Chartered Accountants or Cost Accounts of India and so on. The third and perhaps the most decisive factor is the system. It is here we face the main challenge. Our system encourages lack of corporate governance.

STEPS TO IMPROVE CORPORATE GOVERNANCE

(a) The Sick Industries Companies Act (SICA) has become so convenient for the unscrupulous managements that we find in our country industries become sick, the industrialist do not become sick. BIFR has also been called the Bureau of Industrial Funeral Rites! It is high time we scrap the entire system. This will mean the abolition of SICA and organisations like BIFR thereunder. Mere tinkering with the system by making amendments is not going to improve the situation.

(b) The entire banking system and the Banking Secrecy Act call for a review. Our banking system is such that if you borrow one lakh of rupees, you are afraid of the bank but if you borrow ten crores of rupees, the bank is afraid of you. With the amount of NPA going beyond 58,000 crores, it is high time that we amend the Banking Secrecy Act to reveal those who are willful defaulters. The Narasimham Committee's recommendation about putting this condition at the time of issuing new loans can cover only to some extent the moral hazard. It is high time that practice of disclosing the name of willful defaulters is made more practical and timely. Publishing the names in the case of suits, which have been filed is of no value at all because by that time the matter is all but over.

(c) Laws like the Benami Transactions Prohibition Act and the Prevention of Money Laundering Act should be implemented effectively and vigorously. Agencies like the CVC can be used to ensure that corrupt practices are effectively punished because it is the atmosphere, which encourages proper corporate behaviour. In India today we have a system where the level of public governance is very poor. There is no fear of punishment at all. In such a situation it is only a saint who will be observing strictly the rules of corporate governance.

I do not deny that there are very honourable companies in India, which are following ethical practices but if the general environment is such that there is no fear of punishment, people are bound to be tempted to indulge in corrupt practices and moral hazards, which go totally against corporate governance.

Thus, corporate governance is the net result of the individual sense of values, the values held in society or part of a society like professional bodies or business associations and finally the system of public governance. If those who violate the norms are effectively punished then there is a fear and there will be adherence of the principles of corporate governance.

GOOD CORPORATE GOVERNANCE

— Constitute the rules and practices that govern the relationship between the managers and shareholders of corporations, as well as stakeholders like, employees, pensioners and local communities.

— Ensure transparency, fairness and accountability. It is a prerequisite for the integrity and credibility of market institutions.

— Building confidence and trust, allows the corporation to have access to external finance and to make reliable commitments to creditors, employees and shareholders. It is this contract that underpins economic growth in a market economy. When this trust is undermined, lenders and investors lose their appetite for risk, and shareholders offload their equity, resulting in lost value and reduced availability of capital. This goes for every stage of the investment process, affecting issues from property protection and ownership registration, to disclosure and the distribution of authority and responsibility among company organs.

Indeed, the central corporate governance principles of transparency and accountability are crucial to the integrity and legal credibility of our market system. We already trust corporations to create jobs, generate tax revenues and provide markets with goods and services. Increasingly, we make use of private sector institutions to manage our savings and secure our retirement income. But to the extent that the market's fall can be traced to scandals and breaches of trust, public support wanes and the market becomes unworkable. The state's reputation is also at stake.

This underscores a widespread public—and hence political—interest in reinforcing corporate governance practices. Such concerns become even more important in an international context where the full benefits of free capital flows will only be realised if there is a mutual understanding on the basic elements of good corporate governance.

BASIC ELEMENTS OF CORPORATE GOVERNANCE

- Government should rigorously enforce existing laws, and should encourage business self-regulation.
- Lawmakers and accounting boards should clarify and simplify existing procedures, so concealing the truth would be more difficult.
- Any new laws should be considered carefully, to avoid creating roadblocks to business growth.
- Corporate boards must insist on ethical behaviour and diligent self-regulation.
- Executives must not allow short-term market pressures to lead to unethical behaviour or distorted reports.

A will to work for better governance and concrete political action to this end are imperative for both sustainable development and the wiping out (or at least minimization) of corruption. This means first of all:

Dismantling over-regulation, for the overload of discretionary administrative rules and regulations provides officialdom at every level with the opportunity to exercise its authority not on the basis of objective requirements but rather in the specific interests of those (low-paid) office holders empowered to decide.

Reform of the public service with a view to abolishing ponderous and nebulous ways of doing and deciding things. In their place introduce more precise and intelligible statutory and administrative regulations together with more efficient information flows; then translate them into real-life jurisprudence and practice. Further, effective superintendence and accountability required of everyone holding an official position as well as irregular personnel rotations in especially susceptible positions, though not at the price of impairing competence. Finally, effective, speedy and justly enforced disciplinary and punitive measures against corrupt officials and employees.

Revised hiring and employment conditions in the civil service, for example, more competition for posts, better remuneration, and Ombudsmen, plus reduction of arbitrarily exercised decision-making authority.

Blacklisting businesses that have been found guilty of corruption and refusing to consider them for government contracts for a certain period—until they have mended their ways.

Build-up or improvement of internal audits and controls by higher authority, applicable to both officialdom and the business sector.

Creation of independent commissions and protection of freedom of the press. Even in industrial countries big cases of corruption have finally been brought to light only thanks to free and independent media.

Corporate governance is a means whereby society can be sure that large corporations are well-run institutions to which investors and lenders can confidently commit their funds. It is now increasingly clear that having a transparent and fair system to govern markets, fair treatment of all stakeholders, and a chance for every entrepreneur with a good product to be successful, are as important to democracy as political institutions and are crucial to sound market economies.

Corporate governance creates safeguards against corruption and mismanagement, while promoting fundamental values of a market economy in a democratic society.

Ultimately, there are two elements for better governance. First is the individual values of the people who are in running the enterprise and the second is the external framework of rules, regulations, organisations and systems. Perhaps a continuous effort at sensitising the people about the need for good corporate governance is required because, however, good may be the operational systems and procedures, if the people who are operating systems do not have the right values, we will not succeed.

REFERENCES

1. *Corporate Boards and Governance*, (1998), ed. by N. Balasubramanian, Indian Institute of Management, Bangalore.
2. Banerjee, A.M. and Chandrasekaran, K.A., (1996) *Renewing Governance: Issues and Options*, Tata McGraw Hill Publications.
3. Charkham J.P., (1994), *Keeping Good Companies: A study of corporate governance in five companies*, Oxford University Press.
4. Chakraborty, S.K., *Value and ethics for organisations: Theory and Practices*, (1998), Oxford University Press.
5. Sengupta, N.K., 1983, *Changing Patterns of Corporate Management*, Vikas Publishing House Pvt. Ltd., Delhi.
6. Report of Kumar Mangalam Birla Committee on Corporate Governance, 2000.

33

THE FALL OF MORALITY AND ETHICAL VALUES IN ADMINISTRATIVE CULTURE

Gaurav Sinha

Department of Public Administration,
University of Lucknow, U.P.

Lord Acton's insightful remarks "Power corrupts and absolute power corrupts, absolutely" appears to have universal validity. Corrupt practices along with fall in morality and ethical values have become like a multi-headed hydra, with no Hercules in sight to stay it. As a matter of fact, the level of morality in public life during the various stages of Indian history has been woefully low with corruption surfacing in bureaucratic behaviour in different degrees of intensity. The impact of a corrupt activity liners on for long and in the course of it is likely to become all persuasive and penetrating. The most significant factor promoting a culture of corruption is the discernible erosion of moral and ethical values in public life as a consequence of growing materialism and consumerism in the wake of westernization, industrialization, globalization & liberalization. This paper highlights some of the significant aspects of decline in morality and ethical values in Indian administrative culture.

The concept of philosopher king was developed in Plato's *Republic* in the forth century, B.C. and that too was utopian vision, not as a realized or realizable ideal. Janak, the king of Videha on the other hand, appears to have been a much older historical figure; he is a major character not only in Valmiki's *Ramayana*, but figure personality also in a long dialogue with Yagna Valkya in the *Brihad Aranyak Upnishad*. He represents the ideal of a ruler combining sovereign temporal powers with high spiritual attainments; one who performed the duties of the ruler with philosophic detachment, remaining above the allurements of power or wealth and following always the moral path. Even if the historical identity of Janak was questioned the value of a most ancient tradition of a king ruling with spiritual enlistment and on righteous principles, remains a beacon light. And so also in the story of Rama banishing his queen, the princes of Mithila, because of a base slander by the citizens. It may be on idealized and romanticized view of the extent of obligation of a ruler to honour public opinion, however ill-informed and wrong it may be. But there is an element of practical value in the story. Those in power have to so conduct themselves, that charges of dishonest and unethical conduct may not be levelled against them with any conviction or credibility.

If we look at the present day scenario, there is a yawing and continuously widening gap between the noble ideals and vision of the founding fathers of the Constitution, the standards set by Jawahar Lal Nehru and the state of affairs that have come into being. Inaugurating a conference of officers of CBI in 1981, the Prime Minister Indira Gandhi with the authority of her great office and with all the information available to her, said that increasing corruption at various levels, not only of bureaucracy and of political life, but also in trade and commerce was a matter of major concern and there is a feeling among the people that the persons known to be corrupt escape the clutches of law because of their position and influence while the small fry are caught in the net. Such an impression, the Prime Minister observed, was detrimental to the credibility of the government as a whole.

In an article published on Independence Day in 1992, the editor of a reputed daily newspaper wrote:

"The state is now in peril. As the saying goes, if the fence begins to devour the field, no one can possibly protect the crop. This is happening to the Indian state. Many of these in-change of its machinery have begin to use it to advance their petty interests at the cost of the future of the country. To say that corruption has become a way of life is to understate the magnitude of the problem. There was corruption before, it has now become 'loot'."

By all accounts there has been a frightening growth of corruption in high places during the last few decades. In the early seventies, it is the corrupt who were singled out. Now it is the honest. Some degree of corruption always existed and was considered unavoidable because of the combination of human nature and power being what it is. But it was unacceptable; it was not only deplored but denounced and at least, there was a sincere effect to deal with the corruption and the corrupt. Today, however, a feeling of helplessness has permeated the public mind. There is a growing feeling that the malady too far advanced to the curable; that the whole system has been contaminated and has got beyond redemption.

BUREAUCRATIC DYSFUNCTIONS

The Indian bureaucracy suffers from certain strange paradoxes. A rigid adherence to procedure combines with a ready susceptibility to personal pressure and intervention. While a bureaucrat may give the appearance being preoccupied with correctness, in practice he may be committing endless improprieties indulging into corrupt practices. Similarly his apparent pursuit of uniform application of justice may contain glaring anomalies.

Indian civil service is characterized by excessive self importance, indifferent attitude towards the convenience of individuals and by an obsession of inflexible authority of department decisions, precedents, arrangement or forms, regardless of how badly with what injustice they may work in individual cases. Additionally the civil service has a mania for regulation and formal procedures, a pre-occupation with activities of a particular unit of administration and an inability to consider government as a whole. Administration is treated as a secret. There is no appreciation of citizen's view point and exercise in public relations are aimed more at publicity and propaganda than on establishing rapport with the community. As a result the civil servant fails to recognize the relationship between the governors and the governed.

The bureaucracy in India is so rigidly hierarchical that there is no mutual trust between various units of the government or even within employees of a particular department. Rather 'mutual suspicion' reigns, leading to authoritarianism among superiors, which in turn is destructive to any team spirit within the organization. When confronted with a difficult decision the Indian bureaucrat seldom makes any attempt to tackle the problem with initiative and imagination. Instead he will refer the matter to another department or make a series of unnecessary reference to subordinates to gain time.

The entire machinery of government is today groaning under its own size. While line jobs remain under staffed; staff positions, which are generally action-shy and comfort loving, have increased indiscriminately. Although there is a core of exceptionally hardworking dedicated and contentious officers, they stand today overwhelmingly outnumbered by the complacent immoral and corrupt officials, who are obsessed with status, rank and emoluments and addicted to habits of personal luxury and indolence.

BUREAUCRATIC MORALITY

It has become a national pastime to talk about corruption in high places, to narrate stories about bureaucratic immortality and to condemn others for corrupt practices. Politicians, government officers and businessmen express the same disturbed concern as do the members of general public. But when they are faced with the temptation to indulge in unethical activities themselves, relativism enters into their thinking. Hence one finds two faces of bureaucratic morality in India. It is not unusual or surprising to find ministers and senior government officers taking a very high moral tone about the increased incidence of corruption in government while at the same time, not hesitating to use their influence to assist their relatives or friends by bending or circumventing the established rules.

The situation, however, by no means applies to all the sectors of the government. There are many officials at various levels of administration who are free from the taint of corruption. At the same time no one can overlook the fact that bureaucratic morality mirrors political morality, and that one can not expect to have clean administration, if political leadership of the country is not free from corruption. In the recent years, Indian administration has deteriorated because of moral decay that marks the conduct of political leaders. A new breed to politicians known as 'party fund raisers' have come to acquire the centre stage in politics. Election have become an expensive business and consequently, the emphasis in each party have shifted from debating political issues to raising funds by any means possible. When a party is elected to office, these fund raisers are often rewarded by within the economic development ministries that issue large contracts and important licenses and permits.

In fact, it is the decline in political morality that creates a vicious circle of unethical behaviour and corrupt practices, huge transactions have been made undertable and black economy has flourished. This in turn has resulted in prolonged inflation which has drastically reduced the real income of the salaried class. The net effect is decline in social behaviour and personal morality. The effect has been aggravated by the phenomenal rise in professional incomes and vast income earned by those operating in black economy. It is unrealistic to expect the salaried to accept austere living in an atmosphere in which other comparable sections of the society are in position to amass large fortunes and indulge in obstentious consumption. Thus decline in the moral standards in political life has been the most signification factor of rise in corruption. Once the track are made by the leader of the society, others always actively tend to follow.

Looking at the impunity with which these power and influences can disregard not only the expected standards of conduct, but even the laws of the land; the lower level; public servant may well be remained that "*laws and regulations are like a spider's web, which catches the small insects, but through which the big ones always break through.*" The bottom line is that even; petty corruption cannot be effectively checked unless there is unquestionable integrity at the political and higher civil service levels and there is improvement in the moral tone of society.

BUREAUCRATIC VALUES

All the officials are human beings possessing value judgment and biases. Human values and orientations are regarded as enduring long term goals which regulate behaviour adaptations. Since values of an official form a part of the work environment and orientation, and since the value system of civil services in India, have been undergoing changes due to factors, such as change in educational system, process of urbanization and industrialization, parliamentary democracy, effect of mass media etc; the impact of these changes on administrative culture is bound to be significant.

The most significant factor promoting a culture of corruption is the discernible erosion of moral and ethical values in public life as a consequence of growing materialism and consumerism in the wake of westernization, urbanization, globalization and liberalization. Obviously, the forces of morality, including the Gandhian principles of ethical life, have been too superficial to penetrate the psyche of an Indian so as to influence his conduct in personal and occupational life. Lust for wealth and power has occupational life. In absence of a strong social and cultural deterrents, corruption has accelerated incessantly. What has further worsened the situation is the social respect shown to the rich and powerful, irrespective of their source of wealth and power. Members of one's family and of the wider community seem to encourage immoral orientations and dispensations for the benefits of such attitudes appear to be much greater than the realistic hidden costs.

While the bulk of our people remain abysmally poor and deprived, there has been, particularly among the privileged minority a conspicuous growth of acquisitiveness. There is a feverish pursuit of wealth untrammeled by moral consideration, ethical values or those of responsibility towards the society. Money has increasingly become a major criterion on the persons social status, and many with ill gathered wealth go about as leaders of the society, wielding power and influence. The question arises that how such a situation has come about? Human beings, as they do seek material possessions and need economic incentives and ethical conduct does not usually occupy the fore ground of their minds. There is in fact a view that economic energy with political liberty tends to engender some immorality and selfish advancement of private goods at the expense of public interest. Perhaps that is what Nehru had in mind, when he said in Lok Sabha in 1961 "corruption if I may say to is a result of development process and I am a little afraid that as the process grows, corruption is also going to the village."

CONCLUSION

The foregoing analysis makes it clear that administrative corruption is rooted in administrative as well as non-administrative sources. The need is to catalogue all the possible factors effecting the problem of corruption and then tackle those which fall within the zone of feasibility. Here again there may be short term as well as long term measures. What is required is that both sets of measures should be initiated concurrently in a planned manner.

It has to be kept in mind that no amount of legal or administrative action can be successful in combating corruption, unless social climate evolves where corrupt powers, however successful they may be, suffer social opprobrium. In most developing countries, including India, it is success and not character, that is looked at with awe and approval. The corrupt, if successful, become role models for people aspiring to be rich and famous. When a 'greed based' corruption gains acceptance as a 'need based' corruption, there is nothing to check immorality to reach its nadir.

This leads us to the issue of values. In a heterogeneous society, like India, a consensus on "right" norms and values is difficult to evolve. Consequently, there is a co-existence of all shades of values, creating a situation, what Fred Riggs calls "polynormativism". Corruption thrives in such conflicting situations, since there is no agreement on what corruption is. In culturally homogeneous societies, on the other hand, where there is a consensus on values, corruption if minimal. In a bureaucracy, rigorous training in rules and procedures and indoctrination of a careful code of ethics, which is understood by all levels of officials, can be helpful in orienting the administrative system with a positive value pattern.

Education for administration also require a fresh orientation. The International Association of Schools and Institutes of Administration (IASIA) has recommended that the instructions in Public Administration should include, *interalia*, standard of conduct which prohibit the use of a public office for self interest, promote respect, fairness and justice by public officials, encourage responsiveness and loyalty to professional colleagues and ensure that the public resources are utilized in an effective and efficient manner. Likewise, training of civil servants should also focus on its ethical component. So far the methodology devised for ethical training has not advanced to a satisfactory level.

Perhaps the most disturbing feature of public institutions in India, is a lack of work culture. Little wonder, the average productivity of an Indian worker is much lower than that of an average Chinese or Japansese worker. Atrocious indiscipline perpetuated by laxity in controls and the attitudes of employees union have eaten into vitals of the Indian nation. The trade unions have fought for their rights and have rarely looked at their duties towards the society and the nation. Senior officers take the path of least resistance and rarely exert their authority and influence to punish or reform the wrong doers. Ironically they, also succumb to the temptations of abdication of responsibility. Thus not only has accountability to be rigorously enforced in various segments of social life, including public officials; but a concerted effort must be made to evolve a culture of moral conduct in all dimensions of life.

The Indian judiciary can be one of the fastest in the world, if it so desires. But mostly it is content to remain slow. Overburdened and dragged by tardy system of postponement of cases, the Indian Judiciary is unable to give speedy judgments on matters involving corruption. If right people suffer and wrong people enjoy immunity form punishment the motivation to remain moral is always low. Time bound disposal of cases involving corruption can be attempted by the judiciary through a more systematic administrative system.

With the ushering in an era of liberalization and globalization in the economic system, the quantum of license, permits and quotas is bound to diminish. There absolute elimination will neither be possible nor desirable. In the interest of the people and the economy whatever control would be necessary will have to continue out in a manner that these do not promote inefficiency and corruption. Thus a more rational and balanced approach to controls in the economy will need to be adopted.

In sum, a systematic ecological or what is called "holistic" approach to understanding and combating the menace of corruption is required. For actualizing that orientation, all the segments of the society must have the will as well as the competence to transform the moral order. In India, the common man and not the common politician and the common bureaucrat, has been concerned about rising corruption. In fact, combating corruption has not been a perceptible priority of the Governments in India, at central state or local level. Instead it has been accepted as a corollary of development, an inevitable symptom of growth and even an insurmountable necessary evil. This approach has created complacency in the centres of governance, leading to discernible apathy towards the need for effective action in countering a culture of corruption that is gaining ground. Hence, public awareness should be accompanied by a sense of social responsibility in the ruling elite.

34

CORRUPTION AND ETHICS

Tripti Barthwal and Amit Pandey

Lal Bahadur Shastri Institute of Management & Development Studies, Lucknow

Human beings have innumerable needs. Out of these there are three basic needs viz., food, clothes and shelter. The satisfaction of these needs is necessary to ensure proper survival. But beyond these basic needs every person craves for a luxurious and comfortable life. Some people slog and work hard to satisfy these needs but most of us have an urge to fulfil these desires in the quickest time and the easiest way. To compound the problem when a person attains a particular desired level, he fixes a new higher desired level and starts aiming at it. Since there is no scale of extent of comfort a man can desire and the means to fulfil these desires are limited, the urge to satisfy them leads to corruption.

Kautilya stated in his *Arthashastra* "Man is the shaper of his destiny". When man fixes up his density he would try to achieve it in his normal way provided he has all the qualities in desired proportions. When he does not have the desired qualities he then tries in different way by using his other qualities like "Variableness", "Exploitativeness", and "Corruptiveness" in-built in him to some extent to reach to his destiny. According to *Arthashaṣtra* corruption is in built in human character. So whenever man gets an opportunity, he indulges into corruption.

One thing is noteworthy here that generally nobody indulges in corruption for the satisfaction of basic needs. Corruption always is to lead a lordly life or to show superiority over other persons. It has, therefore, no limit. Want of greater comforts and better lifestyle which cannot be met by a class of people generate greed, dissatisfaction, mental agony and tension. This state of mind gradually culminates into an urge for additional income to cope up with the situation. Corruption becomes a means of additional income. In many cases corruption has become a practice or custom irrespective of the class or level of people. Here known source of income or legal income or level of income becomes immaterial. Thus now corruption has become a universal practice and has been institutionalised making people to think and say that "Corruption will be there to some extent till society or community will exist". It has grown out of bounds, it has no limit and is present in all areas including education and health related services.

Despite offices displaying notices cautioning bribing and many slogans against corruption, several laws and acts, etc. to punish corruption huge sum of money being spent to prevent corruption. It is still rampant in India.

We have huge income-tax department, sales tax department, weights and measures division, customs department, excise department, widespread network of railway ticket checking/ examination section, drug controllers centres, licensing authority, police and security forces both internal and border maintained by state and central governments, central industrial security department so on and so forth.

Besides these, some organisations organise their security arrangements themselves by employing private security agencies. Further we have consumer forum to safeguard the interest of the consumers. In spite of all these what we see, we see corruption, corruption in every place including in very high positions.

Corruption seems to have become an indispensable aspect of today's life. Talk of clearing a building plan sanctioned from Corporation, Municipal or Panchayat, or of admission to school, college or any professional educational institute, or getting a license, or getting proper medical care, corruption is found everywhere. This is only one aspect of corruption. There is another aspect of corruption which relates to the selection of manpower to manage and run the organization. Look at the top management level managing the show. How many of them will pass the competence level. If it would have been, then organization would not have been sick and extinguished. Why do we do? We do it to obtain small gain for self in a little span of time leaving aside the greater interest. But what is the result? The entire country suffers and suffers lot. Finally when the organization dies we throw a good number of people to unemployment. This is a social evil. Today corruption has entered into selection of students in professional educational institute and selection of candidates for employment. The merit has become secondary. The result is incompetency or generation of incompetent human resources. The rein of incompetency brings the disasters in all fields.

Thus corruption can be divided into:

- Money/facility related corruption
- Human resource deployment related corruption.

We often talk more about money/facility related corruption by passing the human resource related corruption. But it is the human who only is corrupt and hence more stress has to be given to human quality to prevent corruption . Just think if an evil man is selected to key position only evil things would be encouraged and would happen which would not only destroy the work, but also people and the organization at last. It is, therefore, more pertinent necessity to pay more attention towards selection of people to high post with regard to their quality it would be relevant if we read what Peter Drucker has written in his book in this regard.

"A man might himself know too little, perform poorly, lack judgement and ability and yet not do damage as a manager, but if the lacks in character and integrity—no matter how knowledgeable, how brilliant, how successful-he destroys. He destroys people, the most valuable resource of the enterprise. He destroys spirit and he destroys performance." It is the human resource which makes miracle and also destroys. Proper selection of human resource stops destruction. It is necessary to be very careful in selection of human resource".

People say corruption is at the lower levels in an organisation i.e., it is down-top. But I would say it is top-down. If the corruption is in the downward level it could be prevented easily with least efforts. But if corruption is at top and middle level it would be very difficult to restrain. It only spreads in multi-direction making corruption universal. Today corruption is universal, it is in every direction and every sphere of life. You cannot think or live without corruption.

Today corruption is top driven with bottom support. In every organization when the top is corrupt, the support of bottom is easily obtained by frightening the bottom with transfers or closing the path of promotion and other opportunity. All of us have such experiences and can narrate a great number of stories in this respect. The top driven corruption is the sole reason for degeneration and crush of organisation.

To understand how corruption takes place at levels, lets' take the example of setting up of an industry. Corruption takes place in the industry from the day of its inception. When a company is set up, it is to be registered. For registration of a company money is to be paid to various agencies. The payment of money may likely culminate into registration of fake and financially weak company. Such fake and weak company leaves business in no time swallowing loan money and creating problem for the lender as well as for the Government. If the money is not paid again there is fear that the registration will be delayed and would need lot of proper work and face other incidental problems. Thus even a good company need to pay this money for registration. The agency which takes care of registration on behalf of the company takes fees but does not issue any receipt. If at all it provides such receipt, the receipt is of lower value. Both the cases the agency avoid paying taxes or lower amount of tax.

After registration is completed, the company has to take a trade licence, tax clearance, and open a bank account. In all these steps it has to pay money appropriately.

The company now goes into setting up of the industry. It has to appoint a consultant to prepare a techno-economic feasibility report (TEFR) highlighting types of products, facilities with process, raw material sourcing, site, financing and economic appraisal with profitability statement. While preparing such TFR a tailor-made report is prepared protecting the full interest of the client. Here again in many cases a compromise need to be made by the consultant keeping in view of the future involvement in the project execution. This compromise may lead to a type of corruption which remains hidden in the project. As for example the capital cost is kept at a lower value than actual requirement to show enhanced profitability for making the project lucrative.

Once the project is prepared, environmental clearance is to be taken from appropriate authority to establish environment friendliness of the concerned project and for which money has to be paid to hasten the clearances. Without this again the project cannot be implemented.

To obtain the land and service facilities from appropriate authority where the project is set up, money is to be paid for quicker action and provisions.

The project now needs the appropriate finance. The company now goes to development bank with TEFR and all clearances. Here the company has to bear a portion of the finance and balance would come from the bank or financial institution. The company may raise fund from the market. The company may also obtain loan from a number of banks and financial institution. While obtaining sanction for loan or raising fund from any source the company need to pay money.

The company's share of capital investment for the project is usually borne by the vendors who supplies the plant and equipment through over invoicing. This over invoicing has become a regular practice in private companies. In this case the vendors raise an invoice on the company for his equipment and services provided for the project for payment showing certain per cent or amount higher than the actual value of their work receivable from the company. Since the invoice shows higher value than actual amount, it is called over invoicing. The difference between higher value and actual value in vendor's invoice is shown as company's contribution towards the project. Thus really the entrepreneur is not supplying any real fund but in paper he is putting his own money.

For setting up of the project, now vendors are selected to supply the various equipment. Some other vendors are selected for construction and project management. While selection of vendors, the selected vendors pay money for enlisting as well as securing the order. The vendors get back these money through supply of equipment and other services.

The vendors includes taxes and duties in their supplies. While payment of taxes and duties or clearance from ports with imports of plant and equipment, the vendors pay money employing clearing agent. The vendors evade taxes and duties and by taking order in the name of a sister company whose turnover is lower.

During inspection and despatch of material money is paid by vendors.

The truckers while carrying the goods to project sites pays money at various points.

The site contractors pay money to local mafias and other agents.

The vendors and contractors pay money while clearing their bills and invoices. This may be in kinds also.

The vendors pay money for getting undue advantages.

Because of under estimates, time over-run or other reasons, there are every possibility of cost over-run. In case of any cost over-run, the company has to make a revised cost estimate. It has to get the clearance of additional fund from the financial agency. It pay money. Selection of incompetent project personnel leads to corruption. This is human resource related corruption.

Once the project has been implemented, it has to go to the commercial production. In operation stage the corruption takes place in many areas. Some of them are as under:

- While taking loan for working capital.
- In selection of contract labours.
- In selection of raw material supplier.
- Payment on supplier's bills/in-voices.
- Payment during inspection and despatch.
- Payment by trucker and carriers.
- Despatch of finished product out of the factory.
- Sales and purchase of shares.
- Payments by employees at various points for obtaining different services for their living.
- Donations by the industry.

The process goes on and on in every industry but the nature and type may be different. In Government sectors the major corruption occurs while selection of vendors and during the placement of orders on them. Another source is during the construction and release of vendors' bills. In private sectors the major corruption occurs while obtaining finance, over invoicing by vendors and during despatch of finished goods. The human resource related corruptions mostly occurs in Government sectors. In case of private sectors becoming sick and non-payment of dues to share-holders are the biggest form of corruption. Over invoicing and despatch of finished goods become the other important sources of corruption in this sector. Analyzing the form of the corruptions, the location where corruption occurs and areas can be assessed very quickly. The persons who are at the helm of affairs in these places, are corrupt or turned to be corrupt slowly.

ETHICS

An issue which is closely associated with corruption is ethics. Ethics may be defined as the guiding principles which help us to differentiate between what is right or wrong and what is good or bad. A well-defined ethics policy along with an outline of related standards of conduct provides the framework for ethical, moral behavior within your company. The benefit of developing such a policy is higher employee morale and commitment which in most cases leads to higher profits. But mere higher profits should not be the motivating factor in defining your ethics policy.

When you are developing your ethics policy, you must decide what it is you want your company to stand for, put it in writing, and enforce it. According to Kenneth Blanchard and Norman Vincent Peale, authors of *The Power of Ethical Management,* you can base your policy on five fundamental principles:

- **Purpose.** A purpose combines both your vision as well as the values you would like to see upheld in your business. It comes from the top and outlines specifically what is considered acceptable as well as unacceptable in terms of conduct in your business.
- **Pride.** Pride builds digits and self-respect. If employees are proud of where they work and what they are doing, they are much more apt to act in an ethical manner.
- **Patience.** Since you must focus on long-term versus short-term results, you must develop a certain degree of patience. Without it, you will become too frustrated and will be more tempted to choose unethical alternatives.
- **Persistence.** Persistence means standing by your word. It means being committed. If you are not committed to the ethics you have outlined, then they become worthless. Stand by your word.
- **Perspective.** In a world where there is never enough time to do everything we need or want to do, itis often difficult to maintain perspective. However, stopping and reflecting on where

your business is headed, why you are headed that way, and how you are going to get there allows you to make the best decisions both in the short-term as well as the long-term.

A company policy is a reflection of the values deemed important to the business. As you develop your ethics policy, focus on what you would like the world to be like, not on what others tell you it is.

According to Blanchard and Peale, there are three questions you should ask yourself whenever you are faced with an ethical dilemma.

- **Is it legal?** In other words, will you be violating any criminal laws, civil laws or company policies by engaging in this activity?
- **Is it balanced?** Is it fair to all parties concerned both in the short-term as well as the long-term? Is this a win-win situation for those directly as well as indirectly involved?
- **Is it right?** Most of us know the difference between right and wrong, but when push comes to shove, how does this decision make you feel about yourself? Are you proud of yourself for making this decision? Would you like others to know you made the decision you did?

Most of the time, when dealing with "gray decisions," just one of these questions is not enough. But by taking the time to reflect on all three, you will often times find that the answer becomes very clear.

HOW TO REDUCE CORRUPTION?

Ethics definitely go a long way in checking corrupt practices by emphasizing on right and acceptable behavior. But, beyond ethics certain other things can also be useful.

Objectivity needs to be brought in prevention of corruption. There should be a whole-hearted desire that corruption should be prevented. Once the desire has been truly established prevention will not be difficult. So far there has been no sign of sincere desire.

Human being must control his desire level and fix it in such a level which can be maintained by him from his income. It is normally not done. This has to be culminated to people through deliberation. The salary structure must be made accordingly. However even it is made the corruption could not be controlled. Thus each department must keep a close vigil on their employees. This can be done and desired result attained only by quality leadership.

Top-down corruption is very harmful. We must first attack the top. All top positions must be selected from people who has strong character and integrity. People against whom there is slightest doubt about their variability, exploitation and corruption should never assume the top positions. They should be deprived of all-powers, side tracked and isolated. When the top is good, good things will happen. I am sure about 60-70 per cent of corruption can be prevented by this way.

We take months, even years to enquire about a man's guilt. This long time allows the man to erase out all evidences from back doors. This has to be stopped. All such cases must be finalised quickly to generate a sense of fear to others. This quickness will not allow to die out the matter. The victim must be isolated.

All systems must be made very simple so that people can understand easily and act accordingly. The language must be simpler. The action required also shall be simpler. All these can be effected when there is transparency in the system.

On identifying the points of corruption, they can be prioritised depending upon the magnitude and amount action accordingly. The action must be direct. We must search the houses and watch the living style of the people manning these points.

The data collected could be compared with the known source of income of the manned personnel. They should be booked very quickly for discrepancies. We have so many enquiring authorities and so many vigilance departments. Mere having them corruption can be prevented. Direct action is required. We should only have one agency in every state for this purpose with enough powers. There are too many people and too many departments probably diluting the subject. This new group can be formed from the existing different departments and we may dissolve existing unit to form this group.

Corruption shall be totally separated from other criminal activities and it should never be a part of another group. Once we have the good people at the top not much of corruption enquiry would be required. The departmental head would be enough. Surprisingly so much of corruption taking place, we do not heard many incidences about booking of employees by departmental heads, when every department spends lot of money for their own vigilance groups. These groups have become only ornaments.

Time has now come to stop corruption. The parallel economy would destroy our economy and will destroy us. The parallel economy would be so big that the real white economy will give away to it. It would be quite dangerous. More writing "Do not pay bribe" will not stop bribing. Sounding should stop, action should start. The engraving "*Satyameva Jayate*" in our national sign will remain only as an engraving. If we honestly try, make the people disciplined, segregate the performer and non-performer we can achieve it. There is a word called "dignity". We have not forgotten this word. We are defining it wrongly now. Every post carry certain dignity. We have probably forgotten this totally. Let us all act together to keep the real meaning of this word intact. If we can make a small start in this direction without waiting for others to take the initiative things are bound to improve.

35

FIGHTING BUREAUCRATIC CORRUPTION THROUGH MORAL EDUCATION

Durga Nandan Mishra, Arabindbandhu Misra and Sanjukta Rani Tripathy

P.G. Dept. of Psychology, G.M. College Sambalpur-768004;
Police Training College, Angul-759122
&
Dept. of Home Science, Govt. Women's College, Sambalpur-768001

Corruption is the wrongdoing by those in special positions of trust. The term is commonly applied to self-benefiting conduct by public officials and other dedicated to public service. The Supreme Court in a landmark judgment (2000) has noted that corruption by public servants has acquired a "monstrous dimension" and its "tentacles have started gripping even the institutions created for the protection of the Republic. Unless those tentacles are intercepted... through strong legislative, executive as well as judicial exercises, the corrupt public servants could even paralyse the functioning of such institutions". Almost every country in this world, big or small, developed or developing is painfully aware of the embarrassing fact that only a miniscule segment of any level of Government or private enterprise is immune to bribes/kickbacks. Simon Bolivar (South America, 1819) in one of his speeches warned that freedom becomes difficult to maintain when people's development gets stunted by the "triple yoke of ignorance, tyranny, and corruption". The Frankenstein of corruption is now poised to strike a serious blow to our democratic credentials. Notwithstanding our constitutional provisions to contain corrupt practices, our position would be like the proverbial monkey (on the greasy pole) taking a long time to assert ourselves as a corruption-free nation.

Max Weber has posited that "ideal bureaucracy" which encompasses formal rules and regulations, job specification, formal selection, authority hierarchy, impersonality (avoiding involvement with personalities to ensure uniform application of rules), and career orientation is a myth but may be conjured up as a basis for theorizing about work and its execution in large organizations. The Indian bureaucracy has got extreme ratings from being a thoroughbred horse who knows its rider well, to being a rusted remnant of the once "steel frame" (Georage Lloyd's description during the Raj). The complex mindset of our bureaucrats believed to be the outgrowth of their insecurity and arrogance (Claude Smadja, the erstwhile MD of the World Economic Forum) even could not be reformed by Pandit Nehru. In tandem with the increasing criminalisation of politics and politicisation of criminals, there was a distinct transformation of the bureaucrats from being inefficient and arrogant to being corrupt; and "trying to be masters rather than facilitators of reform (Shri A.B. Vajpayee's address at FICCI, 2001).

Walter Lippman, the American newspaper columnist, editor, and author rues the growing incidence of corrupt practices amongst bureaucrats:

> "... people expect their officials to work at a level less self-seeking than that of ordinary life ... democratic people had begun to see much greater possibilities in the government than ever before. They look to it as a protector from economic tyranny and as the dispenser of the prime institutions of democratic life. But when they went to the government, what they found was a petty and partisan, slavish and blind, clumsy and rusty instrument for their expectations. ... When they had no vision of what a democratic state might do, it did not make so much difference if officials took a rake-off. The cost of corruption was only a little money... But when men's vision of government enlarged, then the cost of corruption and inefficiency rose... There has always been corruption ..., but it did not worry people very much, so long as the sphere of government was narrowly limited. Corruption became a real problem when reform through state action began to take hold of men's thought." (Bibliobase, 1998)

Nearly a centruy later similar sentiments are expressed in an editorial: "... the present circumstances are such that people have reconciled to the reality that there is no scope for consternation as not to offer bribes in lieu of their desired work accomplished easily and without hassles (The Dharitri, October 2004).

Any social aberration/malaise such as corruption in public places has several causes behind it. Elaborating them is beyond the scope of the present paper. But it is true, corruption has become widespread as the line differentiating right from wrong has become blurred. The individual's personality traits, his living style, and his background influence his corrupt practices. In a recently concluded raid in the state of Maharastra, property and cash worth rupees five crores was seized from an official. To the utter surprise of the raiders, they found in his diary, the delinquent expressing his desire to donate ten per cent of his ill-gotten wealth to a South Indian temple. Corruption is addictive. Our perception of things is more important than any other factor. Those who believe, their lives are controlled by outside forces other than themselves (externalists) are less satisfied with their jobs, more alienated from the work setting, and are less involved than are internalists (Spector, 1982). Bureaucrats of the former type, to save their skin, generally pass on the buck to others (viz., the 'neta logs'). There is overall decadence of morality; and the abuse of ethical practices continues unabated. When corruption is tackled resolutely in countries like Singapore where it was so deep-rooted in the recent past, it passes comprehension why another Asian gaint i.e., our country with such a brilliant track record is 'pussy footing' on the introduction of innovative measures to arrest this scourge.

Of late, the government is considering a proposal (P C Hota Committee, 2004) to introduce an entrance examination for all India and Central services for higher secondary pass-outs on the pattern of NDA, IITs, and medical colleges. It is heralded as a revolutionary step but with many detractors. This is indeed part of the measures toward administrative reforms and underscores the need to plug the palpable 'ethical deficit' in our bureaucracy. All these indicate that we are seized of the inherent shortcomings in the cadres. In the meantime, the Administrative Staff College of India has been asked to draft a code of ethics and a code of best governance practices. As a part of reforms, steps are also underway to firm up the administrative machinary and the delivery mechanism at the district level. These steps suggest that we are now seized of the matter. It is needless to say, there has been general decline in ethical standards in the workplace (in US) since the late 1970s (Robbins, 2001) and it is mostly due to the conduct of the bosses (Posner & Schmidt, 1992). In the Indian diaspora, the situation is not heartening either.

Catch them 'young' is the new buzzword which promises to rejuvenate the bureaucratic set-up. A relatively corruption free environment such as our defence forces continue to grow stronger over the years owing largely to the members' commitment for high quality—right from the stage of selection (i.e., Services Selection Boards) and training of young aspirants preparing for a challenging career ahead. What we basically search for in administrator along with other qualities is 'high ethical standards' which are no doubt based on certain values. Values are primary convictions that a specific mode of conduct or end-state of existence is personally or socially preferable and contain judgmental element as to what is right or wrong (Rokeach, 1973). Values are relatively stable and enduring Rokeach & Ball-Rokeach, 1989); and they influence attitudes and behaviour (Meglino & Ravlin, 1998). By ranking an individual's values in respect of their intensities, we may reflect on his/her values system (Robbins, 2001).

Presently, by the time prospective candidates are recruited, their value systems are already well entrenched and social scientists express apprehensions about their receptivity to value-based in-service training (Weaver, Trevino, & Cochran, 1999). It may be mentioned that the constructs of leadership (which the bureaucrats have in large doses) and ethics overlap. And charisma, a leadership trait, has an ethical component. Ethical and unethical leaders are likely to use their charisma entirely for different purposes. Whereas the former may use it in socially constructive way to serve others, the latter may eventually use it to enhance power/ control over their followers and pursue self-servicing goals (Howell & Avolio, 1992). Moreover, transformational leaders while changing the attitudes and behaviour of their followers also enrich their moral virtues (Burns, 1978). To what extent, the present day bureaucrats align with which forms of above behaviour is anybody's guess. It was not without reason that our ex-Prime Minister Mr. Gandhi once commented that out of every rupee spent for rural development hardly fifteen paise reach the beneficiaries.

Hence, there is a crying need to lower the age of entry of aspirants into the corridors of power. It is conjectured, the future crop of young bureaucrats would have a strong sense of ethics and social commitment/responsibility and these values would pervade on all their dealings.

However, strong our clamour for e-governance may be (which would eventually dispense with a large number of officials) but bureaucrats are here to stay and possibly in a new avtaar. What we need to do is to change the mind-set of these officials and inculcate in them high sense of morality. While not denying the importance of childhood ethical training, some psychologists speak in favour of helping officials to recognize and handle moral dilemmas (situations in which they are required to define right & wrong conduct) through various means.

To improve ethical quotient of employees, organizational endeavours have become multidimensional. In addition to exposing officials to various seminars and workshops, written codes of ethics should be available to them to resolve conflicts. Victor and Cullen (1988) were of the opinion that corrupt practices are eliminated in a positive work ambience. Its indicators are unambiguous job descriptions and opportunities for evaluating and rewarding both the means and the ends. Presence of positive role models is its other forte. Such a work culture emits distinct impressions that it encourages persons (whistle blowers) to uncover dubious practices. Basing on these issues we may restructure our strategies to build up ethical values in our bureaucrats to stem the rut masquerading as corruption.

Frankly speaking our inability to decide which to eliminate first: inefficiency or corruption has made our dealings on the whole issue messy. In order not to jeopardize our future, it is high time that we weed out the corrupts from our bureaucracy. On the other hand, the inefficient may be asked to bloom elsewhere through redeployment.

In a changed scenario, the 'whistle blower' would lose nothing except his/her anonymity. A public servant worth his salt cannot afford to be unconcerned to the 'learned hopefulness' of his countrymen. In a democratic state like ours, citizens rarely abandon any hope of challenging corruption and guard against any 'negativism' while working for a still better future. The ultimate litmus of personal morality is to voluntarily return unto the society more than what one has received and the bureaucrats are no exception.

REFERENCES

1. Burns, J. M. *Leadership*. Harper and Row, New York, 1978.
2. Howell, J.M. and Avolio, B.J. *The Ethics of Charismatic Leadership: Submission or Liberation?* Academy of Management Executive, pp. 43-45, May 1992.
3. Lippman, W. "*Drift and Mastery*", in Michael A. Bellesiles (Ed.), *Bibliobase*, Houghton Mifflin Company (US), 1998.
4. Meglino, B.M. and Ravlin, E.C. Individual Values in Organisations: Concepts, Controversies, and Research, *Journal of Management*, Vol-24, no. 3, pp. 351-89, 1998.
5. Posner, B.Z. and Schmidt, W.H. Values and American Manager: An Update Updated, *California Management Review*, p. 86, Spring 1992.
6. Robbins, S.P. *Organizational Behavior* (9th Ed.).Prentice-Hall of India, New Delhi, 2001.
7. Rokeach, M. *The Nature of Human Values*. Free Press, New York, 1973.
8. Rokeach, M and Ball-Rokeach, S.J. Stability and Change in American Value Priorities, 1968-1981. *American Psychologist*, pp. 775-84, May 1989.
9. Spector, P.E. Behaviour in Organizations as a Function of Employee's Locus of Control, *Psychological Bulletin*, May 1982.
10. Victor, B. and Cullen, J.B. The Organizational Bases of Ethical work climates. *Administrative Science Quarterly*, pp. 101-25, March 1988.
11. Weaver, G.R., Trevino, L.K., and Cochran, P.L Corporate Ethics Practices in the Mid-1990's: An Empirical Study of the Fortune 1000, *Journal of Business Ethics*, pp. 283-94, February 1999.

36

CORRUPTION: A PSYCHOLOGICAL VIEW & IT'S SOLUTION THROUGH YOGA

Kamakhya Kumar

Deptt. of Yoga

Dev Sanskriti University, Haridwar, Uttaranchal

INTRODUCTION

Man is a social creature. Maximum part of personality is associated with his behavior towards the others in the society and how is his social interaction. On the basis of his thought when someone's social interaction. Becomes rigid and his need becomes not suitable for the society maladjustment develops in the behavior of a person.

Kiesler (a great psychologists) 1982 said "Abnormal behavior consists of a rigid, constricted and extreme pattern of interpersonal behaviors by which the abnormal person, without any clear awareness, engages other who are important in his or her life.

Corruption also is a illegal or immoral behavior, especially from someone with power. Hence the word illegal means "a way from the legal" it implies deviation from some clearly defined norms. In the case of physical illness the norms is the structural and functional integrity of the body. As well corruption is the illness related with morality and behaviourism the psycho-physiological aspect of yoga is of profound importance. This ancient science never regards man as a more biological entity. The ancient thinkers paid great attention to the functioning of the mind and the inner mechanism. Today psychology has also accepted this basic aspect in its scope of investigation and in increasingly recognizing the correlation between the body and the mind.

If this becomes patent that for the progress of man in any field of activity it is necessary that he should possess not only a healthy body but also a healthy mind. Yoga has always aimed at the emergence of a healthy and integrated personality in man as the indispensable condition for his ability to take a higher flights in Yoga.

REVIEW OF LITERATURE

During the early 1960s a number of investigators notes the growing prevalence of individuals who committed corruption (criminal acts) primarily for ego-sates factions and "kicks." A thrills derived from performing come taboo act—usually a senseless act of violence—which serves to intensify the present moment, clearly differentiating it from the routine of daily life. Whereas most "old" types of criminal carefully calculate their acts usually with an eye on material gain with minimum risk, this new criminal type commits violent acts on impulse, simply because it "makes me feel good." As an young told Yablonsky (1962) after a gang killing.

"If I would of got the pistol, I would have stabbed him, that would of gave me more of a build up people would have respected me for what I have done and think liplike that. They would say there goes a cold killer."

Typically, the illegal acts of such criminals are spontaneous and un-premeditated, in most cases there is no evidence that he has even had piror contact with his victim. Even when he does participate in planned criminal acts, he instill interested primarily in kicks. Unlike most other criminals he seeks no gain other than the pleasure to no derived from the criminal act itself.

Typically the professional criminal specialized in a particular type of crime, such as forgery or burglary, and develops a particular style of operation. This goal is to make money in the quickest and safest way possible. In general, he attempts to avoid violence, since it would greatly increase the risk of detection and imprisonment; these crimes are usually well planned and may even be rehearsed.

By and large, professional criminals do not appear to show significant personality deviation aside from their adherence to the values and codes of their own group. But Stojanovich (1969) has sounded a note of cartoon. While many professional criminals he studied did manifest so-called dissocial characteristics.

The term dissocial personality is used to refer to individuals who are not psychopathic personalities but who fallout a predatory criminal lifestyle people such as hired kickers, burglars and forgers, such individuals are economically motivated, usually nonviolent, often highly skilled. Typically they come from subculture in which they were exposed early to deviant codes of behavior and corrupt models.

A number of early investigator attributed criminal behaviour to heredity. Prominent among these investigators were Lombroso and his followers, who become known as the "Italian School of Criminology (Lombroso-Ferrero-1911). According to Lombroso, "the criminal was a born type" with stigmatizing features—such as a low forehead an unusually shaped head and jaw eyebrows going together above the bride of the nose, and protracting ears—that clearly distinguished him from normal people. This stigmata were considered to be a throw back to "Savage man" and were believed to predispose the individual to criminal behaviour.

Focusing ever the review of literature the illegal or immoral behavior as we defined as corruption is due to the following causes.

1. Unsatisfaction
2. Ignorance
3. Ego-satisfaction
4. Fear
5. Frustration
6. Delusion
7. Depressive reaction etc.

Here comes the practice of yoga to deal with this psychological problems deeply related with the behaviour.

While abnormal behaviour stems from super natural causes. Behaviors or thoughts are maladoptive and that causes the persons who experience them considerable distress as well as depressive reaction.

ROLE OF YOGA

Layman has very vague and often strange ideas on yoga. But even those who have some knowledge of this ancient science and have come into practical *contact* with it often find it difficult to appreciate some of its more obvious truths. Indeed a few of the ideas propounded in this context, may appear to be new and will very likely uproot many pet theories on yoga.

The power of the human intellect and energy is just like a candle's light that removes the drakness. If someone puts his energy to the study and practice of fine arts he will be known as an artist. If some one directs it towards music he will be known as musician. If some one puts it towards scientific research he will be known as a scientist. If someone puts into illegal acts he will be a criminal. The same energy, when employed for the exploration of the unseen powers and laws of nature is known as Yoga.

Yoga is a school of thought, which teaches the technique by which to transcend the limitation of the body and the mind. One, who employs or utilizes his energy for the study and practice of Yoga, broadens and improves his vision by redirecting the downward trend of his energy. Yoga nidra is one of the most scientific methods of relaxation yet devised. It acts at the deepest levels of our being reducing goes tensions which cause most of our disorders and imbalances of the mind. In dealing with the illegal and immoral behavior of a person the practice of yoga nidra will be an ideal practice. Because of all the metal imbalances, which have been discussed earlier, can be solved through the level of consciousness only.

During the practice of yoga nidra Body and mind relaxes and the consciousness remain awake. Here through the level of consciousness the behaviour can be changed.

DISCUSSION AND CONCLUSION

All the root causes of corruption as well as crime is related with the behaviour of a human being. Running away from the difficulties of life is not the way to deliverance. Those who sincerely practice yoga remain undisturbed like an ocean, which receives the turbulent waters of rushing rivers.

The esoteric aspect of yoga deals with the energy of *atman* (the consciousness). The Yogic practices may give a proper solution of the problem of corruption.

REFERENCES

1. Acharya, Sri Ram Sharma; *Extrasensory Potentials of Mind*; Shri Vedmata Gayatri Trust; 2001.

2. Baron, A Robert; *Psychology*; Prentice Hall of India 2000.
3. Coleman, C James; *Abnormal Psychology*; 1988.
4. Paramhamsa, Niranjananada; *Yoga Darshan*; Bihar School of Yoga; 1998.
5. Saraswati, Swami Satyananda; *Dynamics of Yoga*; Yoga Publication Trust; 2002.

37

CORRUPTION IN THE NAME OF GOD

Ramesh Madan
Assistant Director, ICSSR, New Delhi

Indian society, especially in the recent decades, has undergone drastic changes in moral, religious and political arenas. Some of these changes are new due to the social and political circumstances, and some are an extension of sub-continental culture. Corruption as a social and political phenomenon is rampant in our society. Of late, corruption has taken to the dimension of a form of economy. This economic dimension of corruption has even entered religious sphere. This has attained many overtones and multitudinous manifestations such as casteism and communalism, land mafias, collection drives and corruption among the priestly classes and management of religious citadels and institutions under their control. This paper is an attempt to analyse some of these developments.

Traditionally, people resorted to religion, prayers and God to get peace of mind and for soothing one's soul. The enlightenment of the Buddha was in response to the questions on birth and death that troubled him and the quest for the truth. Today, some people resort to God for some other reasons. Nowadays, the concept of God has become so commercial that reason people even think about God or religion is if they want material wealth, may be a few cars, a big bungalow and luxurious life.

The craze for making a fast buck has led many a mind astray. Pour-money and-get-your-job-done policy is written over all faces in every office these days and more the money faster is the rate of work done. Above all there is also the muscle power to worry about for if one fills a tender for any purpose one is sure to face competition from one or more of our ex-gun totting friends. But the saddest of all is the part when you have to part from a few notes even to enter the abode of the gods and goddesses. The special rates in Kamakhya temple are a ready instance of this practice. In Kalighat (Kolkata), the Pandas have taken upon themselves the right to curse the devotees if they refuse to hand them a couple of hundreds. Our entire system beginning from democracy to devotion reeks of corruption. And the day is not far when *moksha* could be purchased for a pittance.

RITUALISTIC HINDUISM AND MATERIAL WEALTH

Why is Indian society so corrupt morally? Why can people no longer tell the difference between right and wrong? In a country where the majority religion so emphatically states that materialistic pursuits are not important, why has the exact opposite happened? In fact, Hinduism gives the absolute and total freedom to create wealth, power etc. What it warns against is the state of being slave to your senses and thus to the five vices. Instead, it advises humanity to gain complete mastery over them. Our ancient greeting of '*vijayee bhav*' '*tejasvee bhav*,' etc are prime evidence that current understanding has gone astray. Religion is used as an excuse for doing nothing or rejected for irresponsible self-gratification.

How is living without materialism possible in a relative world? Is it because the morals, values and ethics taught in the scriptures (of Hinduism) no longer make sense to most people? Has Hinduism become so esoteric than the common person cannot understand anything but the most ritualistic parts? It is basic misunderstanding of Hinduism. But then, non-ritualistic Hinduism was never really a religion for the masses. Hinduism urges one to be one's own guide for which self-inquiry is a pre-requisite and which in turn relies on the intellect. Interestingly, now those who make use of Hindu faith for political and financial purposes are not the innocent masses.

CORRUPTION: INTEREST IN MONEY MATTERS, AND NOT IN SPIRITUAL MATTERS

Charity and trust in the name of god and goddesses are built up and often misused. Vested interests report to spirituality to amass wealth. Some people put idols in places meant to grab and start worshipping and rituals, and then fence the needed area.

Collection is also done from innocent adherents and faithful and privatised. This practice is very strong among the Hindus. But, no group is exception, including Sikhs and Muslims. Property disputes are reported from Christians too. A group of concerned church leaders and activists in southern India has launched a campaign to combat 'the deep-rooted cancer of corruption' within churches.

The campaign has been established following the murder of a bishop, the imprisonment of another, and a rise in concern among church members that corruption is rife in church hierarchies, particularly in denominations, which receive funding from abroad. A seven-member task group of officials from church-related organizations 'to fight corruption and violence within the church' has been set up following a meeting by more than 20 church leaders at the Inter-Church Service Association in Chennai.

Moses P. Manohar is the coordinator of the anti-corruption campaign. K. Rajaratnam, a prominent Lutheran leader and former president of the National Council of Churches in India chaired the meeting and told: 'Corruption is rampant among church leaders. The mission of the church is not on the agenda of many church leaders. Their real agenda is power and money.' Rajaratnam is also the executive secretary of the United Evangelical Lutheran Church of India (UELCI), a forum of 11 Indian Lutheran churches. After the meeting, the church leaders issued a statement saying the campaign had been prompted by the recent 'killing of a head of a church on property-related issues and the award of two months' imprisonment by the judiciary to another bishop.'

Bishop G. Emmanuel, president of the Andhra Evangelical Lutheran Church (AELC), was stabbed to death in the AELC complex, allegedly because of a dispute over the lease of AELC property. Bishop M. I. Kesari, of the Church of South India (CSI) diocese of Kanyakumari was sentenced to two months' imprisonment for corruption and contempt of court. Bishop Kesari was jailed for defying a court order not to declare the outcome of a church election allegedly rigged by the bishop's faction. The bishop has appealed against the sentence, and the prison sentence has been put on hold. The church leaders' statement declared that a movement must be initiated to bring rethinking and revival in the church. The movement is not just aimed at a few individuals, but is meant for creating a new ethos where people should be ashamed of becoming suddenly rich and the people in general must be prepared not to be tolerant of corruption.

Such efforts against corruption should have come from every sections of the society. Unfortunately, this is not so.

EDUCATIONAL INSTITUTIONS UNDER RELIGIOUS CONTROL

Despite favouritism, some of the religious institutions do charity work in social and educational arenas. But recently, some of them enter into areas of privatisation and cater to the interests of the wealthy and mints money instead of supporting the needy. The capitation fee industry in professional courses, which are supposed to educate students into service-oriented people, is encouraging a corrupt system.

CASTEISM AND COMMUNALISM

Communal and caste tensions are also instigated in the name of gods. The Hindutva aggression against Muslims and the Muslim fundamentalism during the 1990s was neither a reawakening of ancient hatreds nor a consequence of religious fundamentalism. Rather it occurred because of the interaction between the various socio-economic developments in India during the 1980s and 1990s and the strategies and tactics of India's politicians.

Rapid urbanization has uprooted individuals from their previous occupations and communities and placed many in competition for new livelihoods. Newcomers who succeed frequently arouse resentment, and many riots have targeted successful Muslim merchants, business owners, and Muslim returnees from the Persian Gulf states, where they often earn incomes many times higher than they would have earned in India. High-caste Hindus, fearing the loss of their social prestige, have provided an important social base for Hindu militancy. Hard-pressed members of these high-caste groups have been an especially receptive constituency for appeals to curtail the 'special privileges of pampered minorities.'

In addition, the economy was unable to provide job for all who entered the labour market, and the 1980s and early 1990s saw an increase in the ranks of the unemployed. Some of the unemployed have become involved in gangs whose strong-arm tactics are used by politicians wishing to intimidate or incite communal tensions. Other unemployed youths join militant religious organizations like the Bajrang

Dal and Shiv Sena. The Militant groups provide security for temples and members of their religion but are also sources of communal violence.

Changes in the nature of India's political process also have contributed to the rise of religious tensions. India's politicians showed increasing willingness to exploit religious and ethnic tensions for short-term political gain, regardless of their long-term social consequences. Political scientist, Rajni Kothari, charges that there has been a general decline in the morality of Indian politicians, as they play a 'numbers game,' in which they appeal to chauvinistic caste and religious sentiments to win elections, despite the longer-term social tensions that their compaigns create. The support of the Congress for Article 370 of the Constitution, which provides a special status for the Muslim majority state of Jammu and Kashmir, and the measures taken to provide India's Muslim community with distinctive rights have contributed to the popular resonance of the BJP's charges that the Congress (I) stands for minority appeasement and 'pseudo-secularism'. The violence of religious militants in Punjab and Jammu and Kashmir has also contributed to sentiments among the Hindu majority that religious minorities employ agreessive tactics to win special concessions from the government.

The Shah Bano controversy in 1985 put state-religion relations in the forefront of the political agenda. Shah Bano was a 73 years old Muslim woman from Madhya Pradesh who filed for alimony after being divorced according to Muslim law by her husband after 43 years of marriage. The Supreme Court ruled in Shah Bano's favour, creating outrage among Muslims who felt that the sharia (Islamic law), which does not provide for alimony, had been slighted. In apparent capitulation to this important political constituency, Rajiv Gandhi pushed the Muslim Women (Protection of Rights on Divorce) Bill, which removed Muslim divorce cases from India's civil law and recognized the jurisdiction of sharia. The legislation, in turn, engaged large sections of Hindus, whose personal conduct is judged under India's secular civil code.

Shortly thereafter, in a ploy that Rajiv Gandhi may have misguidedly conceived to placate Hindu militants, the courts ruled that the doors of the Babri Masjid should be opened to Hindu worshipers. The VHP was joined by the BJP in a campaign to reclaim the disputed birthplace of Ram. In 1989, the VHP launched a campaign encouraging Hindu devotees from across India each to bring a brick from their villages to Ayodhya. Outbreaks of violence between Hindus and Muslims spread as the compaign progressed, and the BJP successfully prevailed upon the VHP to withdraw the campaign before the 1989 elections. Tensions heated up again in the summer of 1990 when BJP leader Advani embarked on a 10,000 kilometer tour of the country in a Toyota van decorated to resemble the mythological chariot of Ram. Advani's arrest did not prevent clashes at Ayodhya between paramilitary forces and Hindutva activists. The clashes sparked a wave of communal violence and left more than 300 dead.

The Ramjanmabhumi Temple mobilization appeared to pay substantial dividends in terms of the BJP's remarkable growth of support in North India in the 1991 elections, and the VHP and BJP kept the issue alive despite the fact that their actions put tremendous pressure on the newly elected BJP state government in Uttar Pradesh. Its July 1992 *Kar Seva* to build the temple ended peacefully only through last minute negotiations with Prime Minister Narasimha Rao. BJP leader L.K. Advani had promised Rao that the December 6, 1992, *Kar Seva* would also be peaceful. Despite Advani's promise, thousands of Hindu activists broke through a police cordon and destroyed the Babri Masjid. This event and the subsequent riots throughout the country left tensions between Hindus and Muslims at a high pitch.

During the following week after the demolition of Babri Masjid, riots spread throughout the countryside, killing some 1,700 people. Riots broke out again in Bombay from January 9 through January 11, killing 500 more people. In March 1993, the Bombay Stock Exchange and other prominent places in the city were shaken, and some 200 people were killed by bombs placed by members of India's criminal underworld at the behest of Muslim fundamentalist elements. The manipulation of India's religious tensions by militants, criminals, and politicians highlighted the extent to which religious sentiments in India had become an object of exploitations and corruption.

It should be understood that all this happened in the name of God. As Hindu-Muslim tensions exist, Christians were also made target. Throughout India, Hindu extremists assaulted priests and nuns and ransacked Christian churches and schools. Christian leaders fear the worst is yet to come amid the country's growing atmosphere of intolerance and communalism. Hindu organizations such as the

Rashtriya Swayamsevak Sangh (RSS) and the Vishwa Hindu Parishad (VHP) received support from the then ruling Hindu nationalist Bharatiya Janata Party (BJP).

About 400 VHP activists desecrated and forcibly took over a church belonging to the Evangelical Church of India in Surat district in Gujarat. The church's cross was removed from the altar and replaced by Hindu idols. In addition, a saffron flag, symbolizing that the church was now a place of Hindu worship, was hoisted. A five member fact-finding team headed by John Dayal, the secretary-general of the All India Christian Council, alleged that Hindu fundamentalist organizations were trying to convert the church into a temple. The matter, now a national controversy, is pending in court. In the incident, about 80 Christian families, some 200 tribal Christians in all, were driven out of the village, taking refuge in a nearby forest. VHP activists have warned that the Christians will only be allowed back if they embrace Hinduism. Christians in the area blame the district police of aiding the VHP.

In Gwalior, several men forced their way into the home of a 64 years old priest, C. Alphonse. They beat him with sticks and iron rods, leaving him with a head injury and fractured arms, legs, and teeth in the attack at midnight. Meanwhile, members of the radical Bajrang Dal group and the VHP assaulted a Pastor, Amulya Pegu, in Majuli, Assam, apparently to curtail the growing Christian influence in the area. In Uttar Pradesh, armed men held captive nuns of St. Mary's Convent in Haridwar district while looting cash and other valueables. In Kolar district of Karnataka, a mob of about 100 threw stones at Christians and a church, alleging that conversionist pamphlets and books were being distributed. In Bokaro village, near Ranchi, more than a dozen armed men assaulted the St. Anna High School's principal and three nuns. After raping the cook, they fled with cash and other valuables. School officials accuse local authorities of failure to take action against the culprits. In northeast Manipur, gunmen abducted and murdered a 32 years old priest, Shajan Jacob Chittinapilly. He was taken to a field and shot in the forehead, at direct range.

Minorities are forced to broaden their campaign against violence, in which the Christians seek the support of other communities such as Buddhists and moderate Muslims. The solidarity of secular Hindus and civil society is expected to exert moral and political pressure on the government. The violence is linked to Christian efforts to serve the downtrodden in India, such as the Dalits. The situation is going to worsen; the more they work for the poor and Dalits, and the more they are going to demand their rights, the more the violence will escalate. The missionaries pay price to fight for equality and justice. In September 2004, the followers of Mother Teresa were attacked in Kerala, and the search is on to find the culprits.

Caste hierarchy and casteism dominates in deeds in the name of God. In India, this phenomenon is not exclusive to Hinduism. An extensive study on the social background of India's non-Catholic clergy over two decades has spelt out for the first time what the authors describe as 'some of the most difficult and presssing problems of churches in India.' Sociologists, T.K. Oommen and Hunter P. Mabry, authored the recently published book, *The Christian Clergy in India, Volume 1: Social Structures and Social Roles*.[1] This study of non-Catholic clergy, both Protestant and Orthodox, exposes the deep imbalances within the nation's Christian community.

According to the study, Christianity in India (which represents 2.3 per cent of India's one billion citizens) is primarily a 'church of the oppressed' with Dalits accounting for 40 per cent of church members, under-developed communities 30 per cent, and tribal people 20 per cent. Only 10 per cent of Christians are from India's powerful upper castes. But the upper castes hold most positions of power in the churches, while the Dalits and under-developed communities are grossly 'under-represented' among clergy.

Describing the influence of upper-caste clergy, Professor Oommen in an interview said that from the earliest conversions in India, 'the clergy always came from the upper castes. With the majority of the people being lower castes, they always had a feeling of frustration and discontent about it.' Although the percentage of Dalit clergy is rising in denominations such as the Church of South India and Church of North India (both of which have many Dalit members) lower-caste Christians are still not adequately represented among the clergy, particularly in church hierarchies. 'There is a clear imbalance in the representation of these (Dalits, underdeveloped, and tribal groups) categories in the theological and church establishments—with upper-castes overrepresented,' the authors conclude in a chapter on social status. A table in the book shows that Dalits and lower castes constitute 70 per cent of non-Catholic Christians, but account for only 25 per cent of the heads of their churches. But the upper castes who account for one-tenth of non-Catholic Christians, provide 42 per cent of church heads, 31 per cent of theological teachers and 36 per cent of 'theologically trained women.'

Caste system exists among Muslims also. Lakshadweep Muslims are put in the list of Scheduled Tribes. In North India, Kshatriya and Brahmin converts and Pathans among Muslims do not have marriage relations with backward and dalit Muslims in the normal circumstances.

CAN WE BE OPTIMISTIC?

Every society in the world has gone through such cycles of difficulties and India is no exception. World history has numerous examples for vicissitudes of moral, ethical and social values. Every country in this world had suffered and revived sometime or other in the past. Countries such as India, Egypt, Persia, China and most of Africa and Latin America have experienced such cycles. In the modern times, news about dishonesty, immorality and corruption get more publicity and attention than ever before. This is a question how things are highlighted.

Most of the time, we see the urban India and make inappropriate inference. As Mahatma Gandhi once said that, the real India is in Indian villages and he is correct. India is changing fast in cities but such changes are much slower in the rural areas. India was successful in the modernization of Industries, transportation, communication and infrastructure facilities. Gandhi was concerned that such changes could cause India to lose its identity and its cultural heritage. Gandhi had a fear that modernization will provide more comforts and may instigate corruption. It appears that when the public wants more comforts and pleasures, they disregard honesty and morality. Consequently, those people do not distinguish between right and wrong. However, this is question of perception.

India had gone through several religious and moral revivals in the past. Saints, kings and political leaders have emerged at appropriate times as role models to educate, correct and motivate the people who lost faith in moral and ethical values. Notable among those are Vyasa, Buddha, Mahavir, Guru Nanak, Kabirdas, Ravidas, and Alwars (Vaishnava saints) and Saiva Saints of the South. In later times, we had Ramakrishna Paramahansa and Swami Vivekananda. Political leaders like Mahatma Gandhi have established and practised high ethical standards and moral values. Just like the saviours in the past, can we expect that a great leader will appear at appropriate time to change the course of current conditions in India? The awakening has happened so many times in the past. Should we wait or act now? Better act.

REFERENCES

1. Published by Christian Institute for the Study of Religion and Society (CISRS), Bangalore and New Delhi.